AF686413

MODERN MANAGEMENT OF RENOVASCULAR HYPERTENSION AND RENAL SALVAGE

MODERN MANAGEMENT OF RENOVASCULAR HYPERTENSION AND RENAL SALVAGE

KEITH D. CALLIGARO, M.D.
Chief, Section of Vascular Surgery
Pennsylvania Hospital
Associate Professor of Surgery
Thomas Jefferson University Medical College
Philadelphia, PA

MATTHEW J. DOUGHERTY, M.D.
Assistant Professor of Surgery
Thomas Jefferson University Medical College
Attending Vascular Surgeon
Pennsylvania Hospital
Philadelphia, PA

RICHARD H. DEAN, M.D.
Director, Division of Surgical Sciences
Professor of Surgery
The Bowman Gray School of Medicine
Wake Forest University
Chief of Surgery
North Carolina Baptist Hospital
Winston-Salem, NC

SANS TACHE

Williams & Wilkins
A WAVERLY COMPANY

BALTIMORE • PHILADELPHIA • LONDON • PARIS • BANGKOK
BUENOS AIRES • HONG KONG • MUNICH • SYDNEY • TOKYO • WROCLAW

1996

Editor: Carroll C. Cann
Managing Editor: Susan Hunsberger
Production Coordinator: Marette D. Magargle-Smith
Book Project Editor: Arlene C. Sheir-Allen
Designer: Nancy Abbott
Typesetter: Maryland Composition
Printer: Maple Press
Binder: Maple Press

ISBN 0-683-01357-2

9 780683 013573 90000

Copyright © 1996 Williams & Wilkins

Rose Tree Corporate Center
1400 North Providence Road
Building II, Suite 5025
Media, Pennsylvania 19063-2043 USA

All rights reserved. This book is protected by copyright. No part of this book may be reproduced in any form or by any means, including photocopying or utilized by any information storage and retrieval system without written permission from the copyright owner.

Accurate indications, adverse reactions, and dosage schedules for drugs are provided in this book, but it is possible that they may change. The reader is urged to review the package information data of the manufacturers of the medications mentioned.

Printed in the United States of America

Library of Congress Cataloging in Publication Data

Modern management of renovascular hypertension and renal salvage /
[edited by] Keith Calligaro, Richard H. Dean, Matthew J. Dougherty.
p. cm.
Includes bibliographical references and index.
ISBN 0-683-01357-2
1. Renovascular hypertension—Surgery. 2. Renal artery
obstruction—Surgery. 3. Renal artery aneurysms—Surgery.
I. Calligaro, Keith D., 1956– . II. Dean, Richard H.
III. Dougherty, Matthew J.
[DNLM: 1. Hypertension, Renovascular—surgery. 2. Renal Artery
Obstruction—surgery. 3. Vascular Surgery—methods. WG 340 M691
1996]
RD575.M63 1996
616.1′32—dc20
DNLM/DLC
for Library of Congress 95-38950
CIP

The Publishers have made every effort to trace the copyright holders for borrowed material. If they have inadvertently overlooked any, they will be pleased to make the necessary arrangements at the first opportunity.

96 97 98 99
1 2 3 4 5 6 7 8 9 10

Reprints of chapters may be purchased from Williams & Wilkins in quantities of 100 or more. Call Isabella Wise in the Special Sales Department, (800) 358-3583.

Dedication

Dedicated to our wives, Ina Lee, Mary Sue, and Stephanie, for their patience and understanding.

Keith D. Calligaro
Matthew J. Dougherty
Richard H. Dean

Preface

Renovascular disease remains one of the most controversial and challenging subjects in vascular surgery. Initial recommendations concerning treatment of renovascular hypertension and renal salvage were made in the 1960s. Thirty years later, diagnosis and management of renovascular disease remain complicated. Although indications for treatment of aortic aneurysms, limb-threatening ischemia, and carotid artery stenosis are generally well-defined, endovascular and surgical intervention for renal artery stenosis continue to evolve.

Management of renovascular disease in the 1990s requires a well-designed and creative management strategy. The purpose of this book is to provide a comprehensive review of current knowledge concerning the pathophysiology and diagnosis of renovascular disease. Additionally, indications and techniques for renal revascularization for renovascular hypertension, renal salvage, and other conditions are extensively reviewed. The most respected national and international authorities in the field have contributed their experience and recommendations concerning this subject. The Editors wish to sincerely thank these authors for their efforts. We would also like to sincerely thank Susan Hunsberger of Williams & Wilkins for her tireless efforts and interest in this project. Our hope is that this book will serve not only as a useful reference but also as a practical guide for the vascular surgeon, nephrologist, and interventional radiologist faced with treating all aspects of renovascular disease.

Keith D. Calligaro
Matthew J. Dougherty
Richard H. Dean

Contributors

Clyde Barker, M.D., Chairman, Department of Surgery, Hospital of the University of Pennsylvania, Philadelphia, PA

Richard A. Baum, M.D., Departments of Surgery and Radiology, University of Pennsylvania School of Medicine, Philadelphia, PA

Henry D. Berkowitz, M.D., Chief, Division of Vascular Surgery, Presbyterian Medical Center of Philadelphia, Philadelphia, PA

Kenneth L. Brayman, M.D., University of Pennsylvania Medical Center, Department of Surgery, Philadelphia, PA

David C. Brewster, M.D., Associate Clinical Professor of Surgery, Harvard Medical School, Massachusetts General Hospital, Boston, MA

Keith D. Calligaro, M.D., Chief, Section of Vascular Surgery, Pennsylvania Hospital, Associate Professor of Surgery, Thomas Jefferson University Medical College, Philadelphia, PA

Richard P. Cambria, M.D., Associate Professor of Surgery, Harvard Medical School, Associate Visiting Surgeon, Massachusetts General Hospital, Boston, MA

Jeffrey P. Carpenter, M.D., Assistant Professor of Surgery, University of Pennsylvania Medical Center, Director of Vascular Laboratory, Department of Surgery, Hospital of the University of Pennsylvania, Philadelphia, PA

Richard H. Dean, M.D., Director, Division of Surgical Sciences, Professor of Surgery, The Bowman Gray School of Medicine, Wake Forest University, Chief of Surgery, North Carolina Baptist Hospital, Winston-Salem, NC

Matthew J. Dougherty, M.D., Assistant Professor of Surgery, Thomas Jefferson University Medical College, Attending Vascular Surgeon, Pennsylvania Hospital, Philadelphia, PA

Robert E. Gerhardt, M.D., Pennsylvania Hospital, Philadelphia, PA

John W. Hallett, Jr., M.D., Section of Vascular Surgery, Mayo Clinic/Mayo Medical School, Rochester, MN

Abigail K. Hanna, M.D., Departments of Surgery and Radiology, University of Pennsylvania School of Medicine, Philadelphia, PA

Kimberley J. Hansen, M.D., Division of Surgical Sciences, The Bowman Gray School of Medicine, Wake Forest University, Winston-Salem, NC

George Holland, M.D., Departments of Surgery and Radiology, University of Pennsylvania School of Medicine, Philadelphia, PA

Brian Johnson, M.D., Department of Surgery, University of Washington School of Medicine, Seattle, WA

Laurie M. Kuestner, M.D., Vascular Fellow, Division of Vascular Surgery, University of San Francisco Medical Center, San Francisco, CA

Louis Martin, M.D., Professor of Radiology, Division of Interventional-Vascular Imaging, Emory University School of Medicine, Emory University Hospital, Atlanta, GA

George H. Meier, M.D., Associate Professor of Vascular Surgery, Yale University School of Medicine, New Haven, CT

Louis M. Messina, M.D., Section of Vascular Surgery, Department of Surgery, University of Michigan Medical School, Ann Arbor, MI

Ashby C. Moncure, M.D., Associate Clinical Professor of Surgery, Harvard Medical School, Massachusetts General Hospital, Boston, MA

Andrew C. Novick, M.D., Chairman, Department of Urology, The Cleveland Clinic Foundation, Cleveland, Ohio

Kenneth Ouriel, M.D., Associate Professor of Surgery, Section of Vascular Surgery, Department of Surgery, University of Rochester Medical Center, Rochester, NY

Linda M. Reilly, M.D., Division of Vascular Surgery, University of San Francisco Medical Center, San Francisco, CA

Thomas Sos, M.D., Department of Radiology, The New York Hospital–Cornell University Medical Center, New York, NY

James C. Stanley, M.D., Professor of Surgery, Head, Section of Vascular Surgery, The University of Michigan Medical Center, Ann Arbor, MI

Ronald J. Stoney, M.D., Professor, Division of Vascular Surgery, University of San Francisco Medical Center, San Francisco, CA

D. Eugene Strandness, Jr., M.D., Professor and Chief, Division of Vascular Surgery, Department of Surgery, University of Washington School of Medicine, Seattle, WA

David W. Trost, M.D., Division of Cardiovascular and Interventional Radiology, The New York Hospital–Cornell University Medical Center, New York, NY

Contents

Part I

Pathophysiology and Diagnosis of Renal Artery Disease

1

Pathophysiology of Renovascular Hypertension

Robert E. Gerhardt

Although there have been many advances in the therapy of renovascular hypertension over the years, the basic pathophysiology of renovascular hypertension has been understood for approximately 15–20 years with only minor refinements in understanding in recent years. Although impossible in any one chapter, I will review and summarize the current knowledge of the pathophysiology of renovascular hypertension.

EXPERIMENTAL HYPERTENSION

The understanding of renovascular hypertension begins with the work of Tigerstedt and Bergman in 1898.[1] These researchers demonstrated that a watery extract of rabbit kidney could increase blood pressure and named the active pressor "renin." In addition, they demonstrated that renal vein blood increased the blood pressure in nephrectomized animals and noted a greater response to "renin" in nephrectomized animals.[2]

Beginning in 1933 and continuing through the late 1940s, Harry Goldblatt and his associates performed and reported a number of animal studies that provided the framework, still valid, for understanding much of the pathophysiology of renovascular hypertension.[3–6] Although his initial studies served to document that the kidney was the major source of hypertension during renal arterial constriction,[3] his subsequent classical experiments were much more revealing. Goldblatt developed a methodology by which he could chronically restrict, by means of an adjustable implantable silver clamp, the blood flow to one or both renal arteries.[3] In reality, he used three models of renovascular hypertension: (1) unilateral nephrectomy with a clamp placed on the remaining renal artery (one-clip, one-kidney model); (2) a clamp on a single renal artery with both kidneys in place (one-clip, two-kidney model); and (3) a clamp on both renal arteries (two-clip, two-kidney model). In addition, Goldblatt produced many variations on this basic theme, including clamps on splenic, femoral, and visceral arteries to demonstrate that blood pressure elevation was, in fact, caused by the kidneys alone.[4]

With his large number of studies, Goldblatt showed that tightening the clamp in a one-clip, one-kidney model resulted in sustained hypertension. Similarly, tightening bilateral clamps (two-clip, two-kidney model) in either a simultaneous or sequential pattern produced sustained severe hypertension. Tightening a single clamp in an animal with two kidneys (one-clip, two-kidney model) resulted in acute hypertension, but the hypertension was frequently not sustained.[5] Goldblatt also reported that removal of the clamps on the renal arteries reversed the hypertension in most studies; in very chronic studies, this may not always occur.

By 1947, although the effector substances produced by the ischemic kidney were not chemically well characterized, it was understood that renin was an enzyme produced by the kidney in response to decreased blood flow to the kidney and that this acted on renin substrate (which was produced elsewhere) to produce a third substance (then called angiotonin), which was an active vasoconstrictor.[6] Angiotonin (angiotensin) also increased salt and water retention—both mechanisms resulting in increased blood pressure. This "angiotonin" was subsequently degraded by an enzyme in the blood. Thus, by the late 1940s, the fundamental pathogenesis of renovascular hypertension was reasonably well understood.

Subsequent studies by Laragh and his colleagues demonstrated that hypertension in the Goldblatt one-clip, one-kidney model had a different etiology from the one-clip, two-kidney model.[7] These studies used angiotensin II inhibitors (i.e., angiotensin-converting enzyme inhibitors, ACE I) administered to Goldblatt model animals. The drug had little effect on one-clip, one-kidney animals but markedly decreased the blood pressure in one-clip, two-kidney models **(Fig. 1–1)**. Laragh's group interpreted this as demonstrating that the renin levels were high in the one-clip, two-kidney models but normal in the one-clip, one-kidney model.

However, while administration of angiotensin II inhibitor to one-clip, one-kidney sodium repleted animals had no effect, the same dose of inhibitor given after sodium depletion in the same model produced a marked decrease in blood pressure[8] **(Fig. 1–2)**. From this and other studies, it was thought that the experimental models of hypertension could then be broken down into **acute phase** and **chronic phase** in both models. In both experimental situations, the tightening of one clamp resulted in hypertension secondary to an initial release of renin. In the chronic phase other

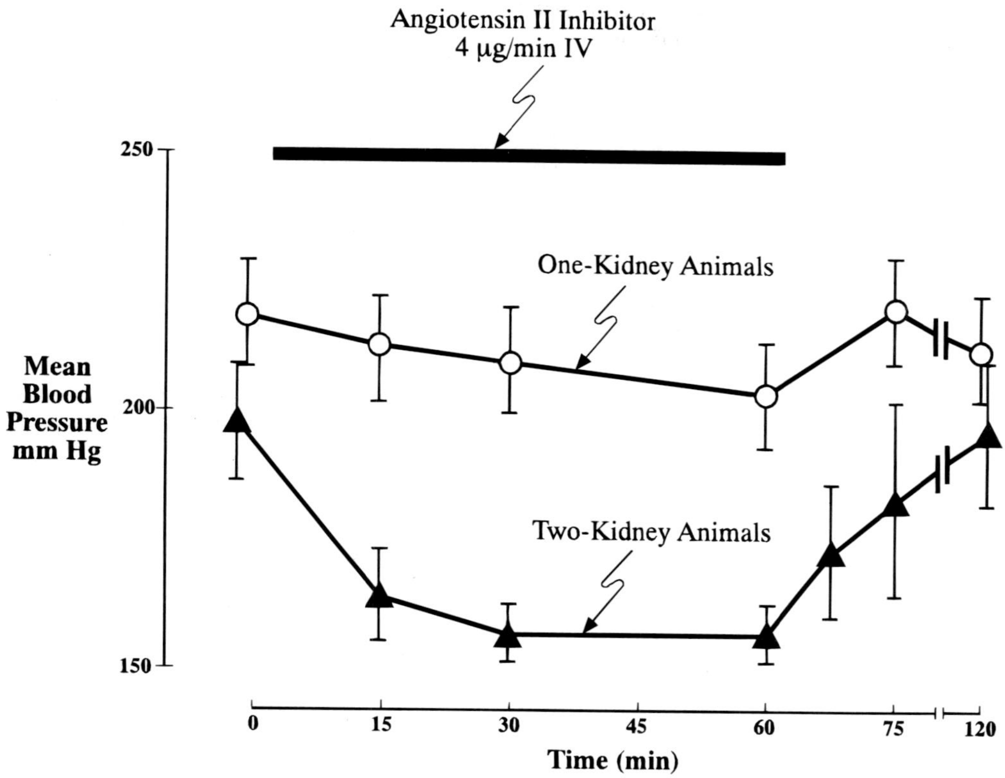

Figure 1–1. Effect of angiotensin II inhibition (angiotensin-converting enzyme inhibitor) on one-clip, one-kidney and one-clip, two-kidney experimental hypertension. one-kidney animals = one-clip, one-kidney model; two-kidney animals = one-clip, two-kidney model. Reprinted with permission from Brunner HR, Kirshman JD, Sealey JE, Laragh JH. Hypertension of renal origin: evidence for two different mechanisms. Science, 1971;174:1345.

factors come into play.[9] In the one-clip, two-kidney model, any excess sodium or water retained by angiotensin is excreted by the normal unclamped kidney and the hypertension is sustained by excess renin-angiotensin production alone (thus the marked decrease of hypertension when angiotensin inhibitors are administered). In the one-clip, one-kidney model, excess salt and water retained by initial renin production cannot be excreted adequately and results in a volume component to the hypertension. The renin component is masked by the increased volume unless the animal becomes volume depleted at which time the hypertension is maintained by renin increase.

In the two-clip, two-kidney model, which may be the most im-

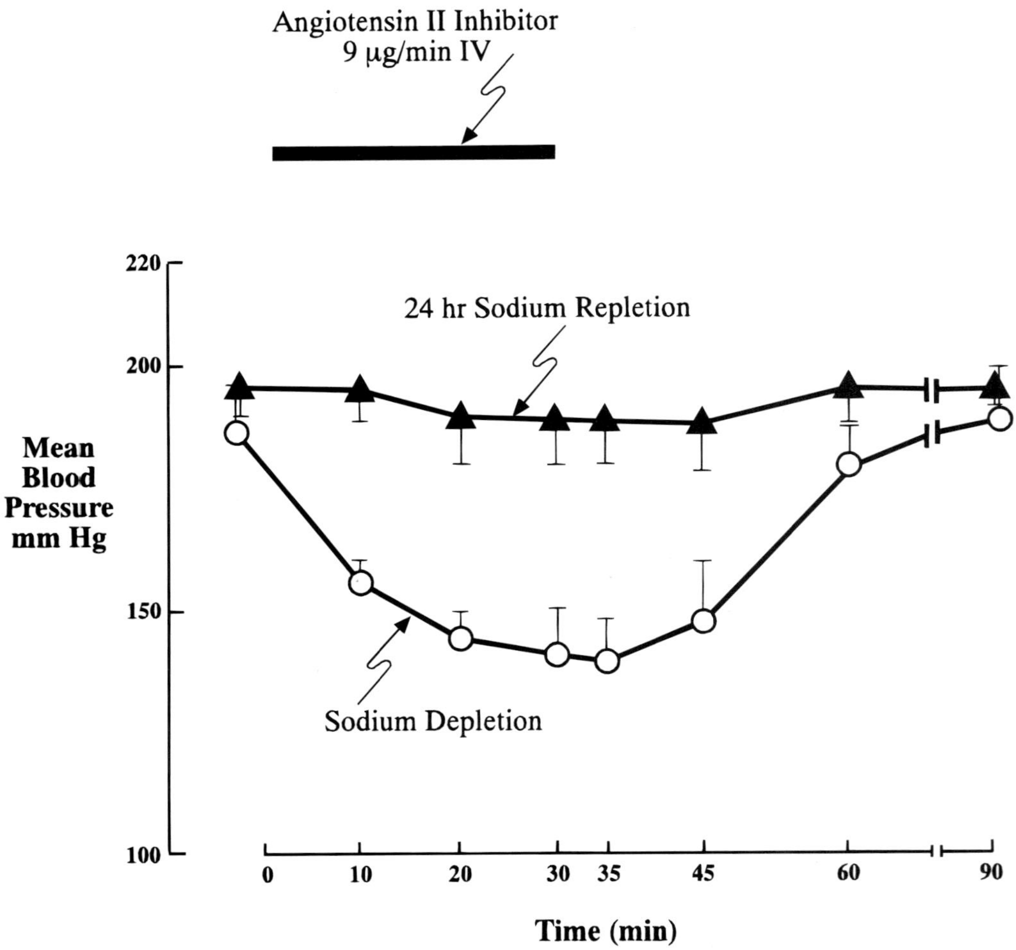

Figure 1–2. Effect of angiotensin II inhibition (angiotensin-converting enzyme inhibition) in sodium-repleted and sodium-depleted one-clip, one-kidney hypertension. Blood pressure elevation in one-clip, one-kidney hypertension is sodium dependent. Reprinted with permission from Gavras H, Brunner HR, Vaughan ED, Laragh JH. Angiotensin-sodium interaction in blood pressure maintenance of renal hypertensive and normotensive rats. Science 1973;180:1370.

portant experimental design to understanding renovascular hypertension in humans, results vary depending on the balance between the two clamps. As one might predict, the more equal the clamps restrict blood flow, the closer the model is to the one-clip, one-kidney model; the more divergent, the closer the result to the one-clip, two-kidney model.

RENIN ANGIOTENSIN SYSTEM

Although Goldblatt had some initial understanding of the human and animal renin angiotensin system, many details of this system are now much better understood. Renin is released in the kidney from cells of the juxtaglomerular apparatus, and forms of prorenin and preprorenin exist **(Fig. 1–3)**.

The relationship of preprorenin and prorenin, the work involved in their discovery and their pathways, has been summarized by Hsueh and Baxter.[10] Their review supports a system **(Fig. 1–3)** which begins with the primary translation product of renin messenger ribonucleic acid (RNA) as preprorenin. The messenger sequence directs insertion of the protein into the lumen of the rough endoplasmic reticulum where it is rapidly cleaved to form prorenin. This inactive prorenin passes through the rough endoplasmic reticulum and Golgi apparatus, leaves the Golgi and can then be sorted into one of three pathways.

First, a small amount of prorenin binds with mannose 6-phosphate at the carbohydrate moiety of prorenin and then binds to the mannose 6-phosphate receptors on lysosomes. Subsequent entry into the lysosomal compartment leads to degradation.

Second, an unregulated constitutive pathway delivers the prorenin to the cell surface at a constant rate. Studies have suggested that this transport is accomplished in clear membrane bound vesicles.[10]

Third, a regulated secretory pathway stores inactive prorenin and acutely releases the stores after stimulation by a secretagogue. The dense secretory granules mediate release of the stored renin and also serve as the site of the prorenin (molecular weight 45,000–50,000 daltons) to renin (36,000 daltons) conversion.[11]

Although the kidney processes prorenin to renin and is the major source of circulating renin in humans, it is also the major source of plasma prorenin. However, the identification and regulatory role of prohormone processing enzymes has not been fully worked out.[10]

Although Tigerstedt and Bergman had named a pressor extract of rabbit kidneys "renin,"[1] many years of laborious work were needed to identify the renin structure. The historical details of renin discovery have been described[2] as well as the details of the determination of the chemical sequence.[11,12] Renin is an aspartyl protease, activated from prorenin by cleavage of an arginine-leucine bond.[11] The release of renin is the rate-limiting step in the activation of the renin-angiotensin system. Although renin secretion is influenced by blood pressure, sympathetic nerves, salt intake, and hormones, the local control and fine modulation of release are still being detailed.[13] Endothelin,[14] prostacyclin,[15] and

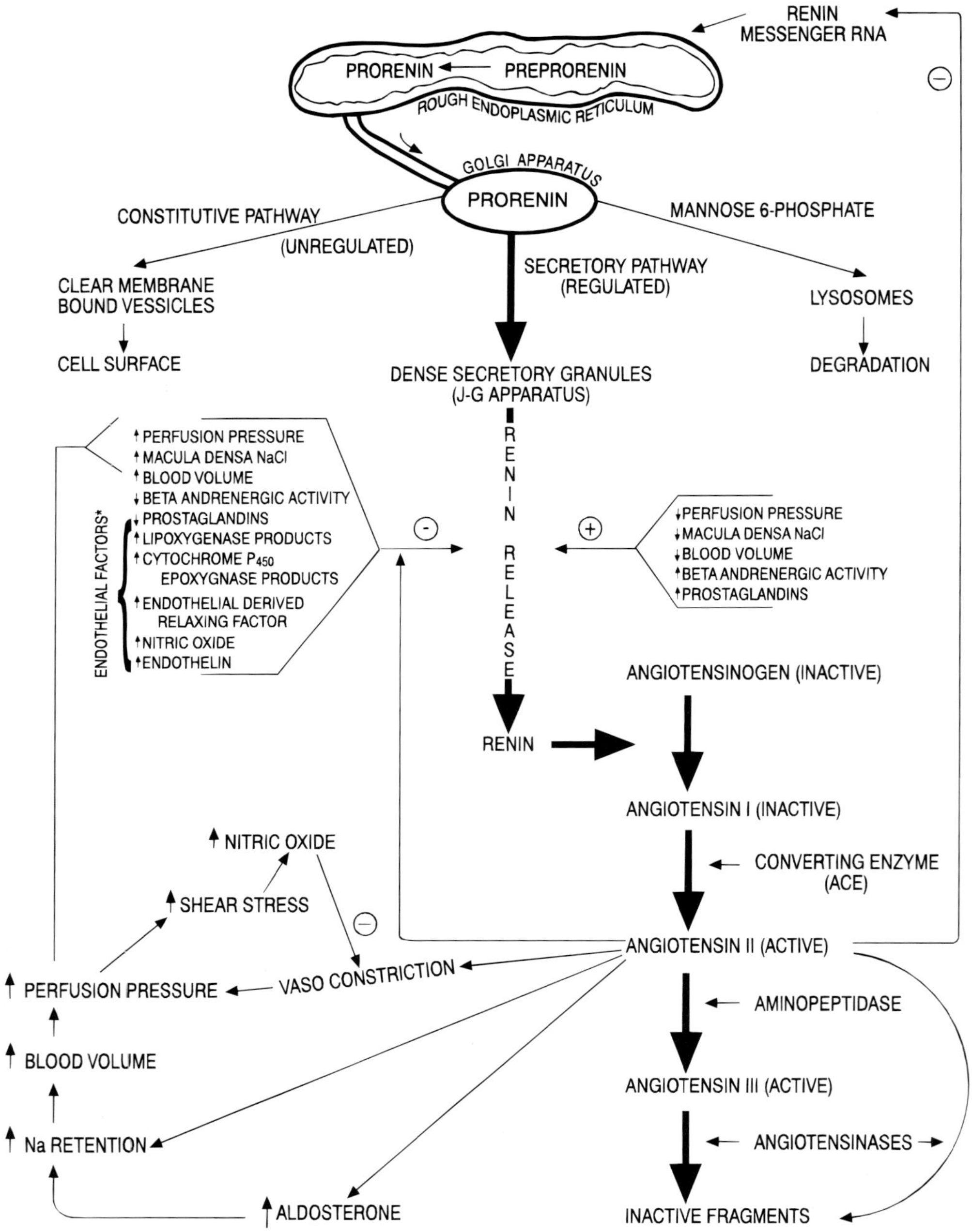

Figure 1–3. Overview of renin-angiotensin system and reported interactions. Heavy arrows = main pathway; + = positive feedback (increased effect or increased release); − = negative feedback (decreased effect or decreased release); J-G apparatus = juxtaglomerular apparatus; * = current best estimate of endothelial factor effects; Na = sodium; Na Cl = sodium chloride.

endothelin-derived relaxing factors (EDRF, which may include nitric oxide[16–17]) as well as many other local factors may influence renin secretion in vivo and in vitro.[13] One study appears to show that cyclic adenosine monophosphate stimulates renin secretion from juxtaglomerular cells and is modulated by endothelial cells and that endothelin, enthothelial-derived relaxing factor and postacycline may be oppositely acting autacoids mediating a tonical influence of the endothelium on juxtaglomerular cells.[18] The same paper also provides evidence that the endothelium could be an important modulator of renin secretion controlled by sympathetic nerve activity. Recent data suggest that prostaglandins and EDRF are required for the stimulation of renin secretion and renin gene expression in juxtaglomerular cells in response to hypoperfusion.[19]

Renin cleaves amino acids from angiotensinogen (an inactive tetradecapeptide) to form angiotensin I (an inactive decapeptide). Angiotensin converting enzyme (a zinc containing dicarboxypeptidase), which is present in the endothelium and other tissues, cleaves two amino acids from angiotensin I to form the active octapeptide angiotensin II.[20] Angiotensin II has multiple actions including vasoconstriction, increasing aldosterone release, increasing sodium retention, increasing blood volume, and increasing perfusion pressure, all of which decrease renin production. Although salt retention and increased perfusion pressure are well known effects of angiotensin II, many other effects of angiotensin II and many local effects may be important in modulation and control of the renin-angiotensin system. Angiotensin II has specific nuclear receptors that modulate transcription of messenger RNA, including specific messenger RNA for renin and angiotensinogen.[21] On a local level, interaction between angiotensin II and endothelin derived nitric oxide may be of major importance.[22] Thus in the one-clip, two-kidney model of hypertension, endothelin-derived nitric oxide synthesis increases in the non-clipped kidney, presumably related to increased shear stress, which counteracts the constrictor influence of elevated circulating angiotensin II.[22]

Angiotensin II, in turn, is converted to angiotensin III by an aminopeptidase, which while presently poorly understood, also appears to be active. Angiotensin III is subsequently degraded into inactive peptide fragments. An extensive review of the renin-angiotensin system and the effects of vasoactive peptides (including 1,010 references) is available for specific data.[23]

Clinical studies have been directed toward using this scheme to develop medications that block angiotensin-converting enzyme and thus prevent the formation of the active forms of angiotensin II and angiotensin III.[9] These drugs have both experimental implications for understanding the differences in the models of the one-kidney and two-kidney Goldblatt models as well as therapeutic implications in humans.

When Tigerstedt died in 1924, the list of his achievements did not mention renin.[2] In contrast, Goldblatt, who as noted earlier had done so much in regard to renovascular hypertension and attempts to isolate renin, was able at age 80, with J. Menard, to inject dogs with pure hog renin, thus helping to complete the circle of knowledge[12] and confirming the pathophysiology of renal artery stenosis.

PATHOPHYSIOLOGY OF HUMAN RENOVASCULAR HYPERTENSION

Although the human model of one-clip, one-kidney hypertension exists in humans, it is rare. It has been reported in patients with congenital solitary kidneys or after nephrectomy, and in patients who have undergone renal transplants. As in animals, this model appears to be related to increased renin production, but is subsequently maintained by fluid retention, which cannot be adequately regulated by the compromised kidney.

In humans, however, we are much more interested in the two-kidney models of hypertension, either unilateral stenosis or bilateral stenosis in the presence of two kidneys. Stenosis of only one of two renal arteries in humans is entirely analogous to the one-clip, two-kidney model. There is high plasma renin activity originating from one kidney and there is a prompt response to the administration of ACE inhibitors, but little change when sodium depletion is used.[24,25] Repair of the unilateral stenosis decreases blood pressure and sodium retention. These findings are analogous to what Goldblatt described with clamping and subsequent unclamping of a single renal artery **(Table 1–1)**.

The greatest problem is in human bilateral stenosis, in which both a renin effect and a volume effect exist, but the contribution of each varies depending on the degree and the symmetry of the stenoses. Because it is unusual in clinical situations to have equal bilateral stenoses, there is some similarity to the one-clip, two-kidney model in that renin activity increases and responds to ACE inhibitors, and blood pressure decreases with reversal of the stenosis. However, there is also a variable amount of sodium retention producing a volume component to the hypertension. Because there is a tremendous variability in the degree of stenosis bilaterally, there is commensurate variability in the contributions of renin and volume status to the hypertension in bilateral stenosis.[24]

Table 1–1. Comparison of Experimental Models of Renovascular Hypertension

Goldblatt Model	One-Clip, One-Kidney	Two-Clip, Two-Kidney	One-Clip, Two-Kidney
Human Equivalent	Stenosis in a Single Kidney	Bilateral Stenosis	Unilateral Stenosis
Plasma Renin Activity	Normal	High	High
Plasma Volume	High	High	Normal
Exchangeable Na	High	High	Normal
BP Response to Na Depletion	Decreases	Decreases	Little Change
BP Response to ACE I[a]	Little Change	Decreases	Decreases
Unclipping			
Effect on BP	Decreases	Decreases	Decreases
Effect on Na Excretion	Increases	Increases	Decreases

[a] ACE I = angiotensin converting enzyme inhibitors.

With an understanding of the renin angiotensin system and renin and volume-mediated contributions to the various Goldblatt models, the pathophysiology of human renovascular hypertension is understandable, and varying renin, aldosterone, and volume measurements in a particular patient can be interpreted.

REFERENCES

1. Tigerstedt R, Bergman PG. Niere und Kreislauf. *Scand Arch Physiol* 1898;8:223–271.
2. Peart WS. Evolution of renin. *Hypertension* 1991;18(suppl III): 100–108.
3. Goldblatt H, Lynch J, Hanzal RF, Summerville WW. Studies on experimental hypertension; production of persistent elevation of systolic blood pressure by means of renal ischemia. *J Exp Med* 1934;59: 347–380.
4. Goldblatt H. Studies on experimental hypertension; the pathogenesis of experimental hypertension due to renal ischemia. *Ann Intern Med* 1937;11:69–103.
5. Goldblatt H, Kahn JR, Lewis HA. Studies on experimental hypertension; experimental observations on hypertension associated with unilateral renal disease; effects of occlusion of the ureter on experimental hypertension due to unilateral renal ischemia. *Arch Surg* 1941;43: 327–340.
6. Goldblatt H. The renal origin of hypertension. *Physiol Rev* 1947;27: 120–165.

7. Brunner HR, Kirshman JD, Sealey JE, Laragh JH. Hypertension of renal origin: evidence for two different mechanisms. *Science* 1971; 174:1344–1346.
8. Gavras H, Brunner HR, Vaughan ED, Laragh JH. Angiotensin sodium interaction in blood pressure maintenance of renal hypertensive and normotensive rats. *Science* 1973;180:1369–1372.
9. Laragh JH, Sealey JE, Buhler FR, et al. The renin axis and vasoconstriction volume analysis for understanding and treating renovascular and renal hypertension. *Am J Med* 1975;58:4–13.
10. Hsueh WA, Baxter JD. Human prorenin. *Hypertension* 1991;17: 469–479.
11. Inagami T. Purification of renin and prorenin. *Hypertension* 1991; 18:241–251.
12. Corvol P, Menard J. Renin purification and cloning. *Hypertension* 1991;18:252–256.
13. Hackenthal E, Paul M, Ganten D, Taugner R. Morphology, physiology, and molecular biology of renin secretion. *Physiol Rev* 1990;70: 1067–1116.
14. Yanagisawa M, Kurihara H, Kimura S, Goto K, Masaki T. A novel potent vasoconstrictor peptide produced by vascular endothelial cells. *Nature (London)* 1988;332:441–415.
15. Lin L, Mistry M, Stier CT, Nasjletti A. Role of prostanoids in renin-dependent and renin independent hypertension. *Hypertension* 1991; 17:517–525.
16. Sigmon DH, Carretero OA, Beierwaltes WH. Plasma renin activity and the renal response to nitric oxide synthesis inhibition. *J Am Soc Nephrol* 1992;3:1288–1294.
17. Campbell WB, Henrich WL. Endothelial factors in the regulation of renin release. *Kidney Int* 1990;38:612–617.
18. Kurtz A, Kaissling B, Busse R, Baier W. Endothelial cells modulate renin secretion from isolated mouse juxtaglomerular cells. *J Clin Invest* 1991;88:1147–1154.
19. Schricker K, Hamann M, Kaissling B, Kurtz A. Renal autacoids are involved in the stimulation of renin gene expression by low perfusion pressure. *Kidney Int* 1994;46:1330–1336.
20. Bernstein KE, Shai SY, Howard T, Balogh R, Frenzel K, Langford K. Structure and regulated expression of angiotensin-converting enzyme and the receptor for angiotensin II. *Am J Kidney Dis* 1993; 21(suppl 1):53–57.
21. Eggena P, Zhu JH, Clegg K, Barrett JD. Nuclear angiotensin receptors induce transcription of renin and angiotensinogen m RNA. *Hypertension* 1993;22:496–501.
22. Sigmon DH, Beierwaltes WH. Renal nitric oxide and angiotensin II interaction in renovascular hypertension. *Hypertension* 1993;22: 237–242.
23. Ballermann BJ, Zeidel ML, Gunning ME, Brenner BM. Vasoactive peptides and the kidney. In: Brenner BM, Rector FR, eds. *The Kidney.* 4th ed. Philadelphia: W.B. Saunders, 1991;510–583.

24. Vaughan ED, Buhler FR, Laragh JH, Sealey JE, Baer L, Bard RH. Renovascular hypertension: renin measurements to indicate hypersecretion and contralateral suppression, estimate renal plasma flow, and score for surgical curability. *Am J Med* 1973;55:402–414.
25. Muller FB, Sealey JE, Case DB, et al. The captopril test for identifying renovascular disease in hypertensive patients. *Am J Med* 1986; 80:633–644.

Natural History of Renal Artery Stenoses and Aneurysms

2

James C. Stanley

Histologic and morphologic characterizations of renal artery stenoses and aneurysms are exceedingly important in understanding the natural history of these lesions and in making clinical treatment decisions. Renal artery stenoses represent a heterogeneous group of diseases occurring in differing age groups. A contemporary classification includes arteriosclerotic, fibrodysplastic, and developmental stenoses. Renal artery macroaneurysms are usually classified into true aneurysms and dissecting aneurysms. These entities are discussed separately in that their natural histories are different.

RENAL ARTERY ARTERIOSCLEROSIS

Arteriosclerotic stenoses are a frequent cause of renovascular hypertension. In an earlier necropsy study, moderate or severe renal artery arteriosclerosis was alleged to affect 49% of normotensive individuals and 77% of hypertensive patients.[1] The frequency of renovascular arteriosclerosis is regarded as age-dependent,[2] with men affected twice as often as women. Gender differences in renal artery arteriosclerosis are less apparent in elderly individuals.

Renovascular arteriosclerotic stenoses are located within the orifice as aortic spillover disease in 80% of cases **(Fig. 2–1)**, and as focal lesions in the proximal portion of the main renal artery in 15% of cases **(Fig. 2–2)**. The inferior and posterior arterial walls are most often affected with early lesions. More advanced disease appears concentric. Such lesions occasionally extend along the posterior vessel into segmental branches. Arteriosclerotic lesions limited to renal artery branches are uncommon, being observed in less than 5% of patients. Slightly more than 50% of individuals presenting with a hemodynamically important stenosis on one

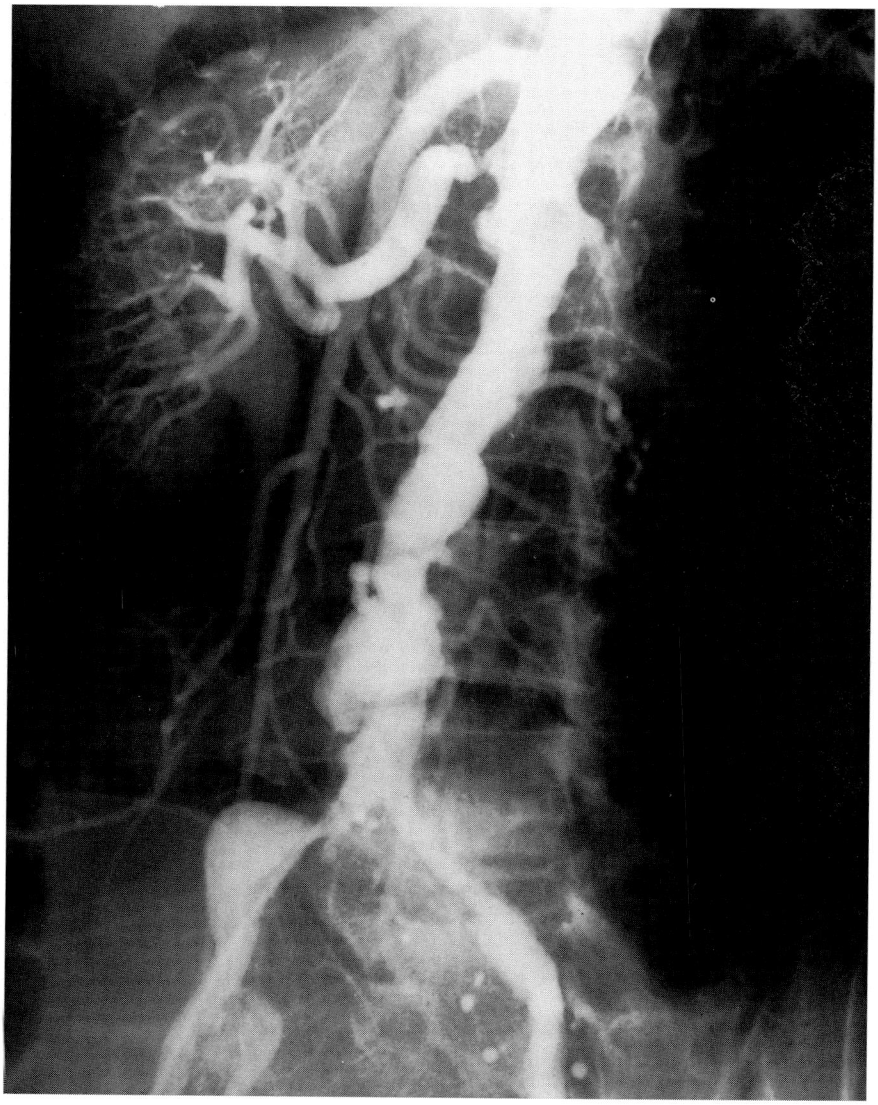

Figure 2–1. Aortic spillover renal artery arteriosclerosis. Extensive arteriosclerotic disease of the aorta with extension into origin of right renal artery and occlusion of left renal artery. Reprinted with permission from Stanley JC, Graham LM, Whitehouse WM Jr. Renovascular hypertension. In Miller TA, Rowlands BJ (eds), Physiologic Basis of Modern Surgical Care, pp 734–739, CV Mosby, St. Louis, 1988.

side have anatomic evidence of contralateral renovascular stenotic disease. Right-sided and left-sided lesions seemingly occur with equal frequency, although the left renal artery may be prone to more severe stenoses.

Early arteriosclerotic renal artery stenoses are characterized

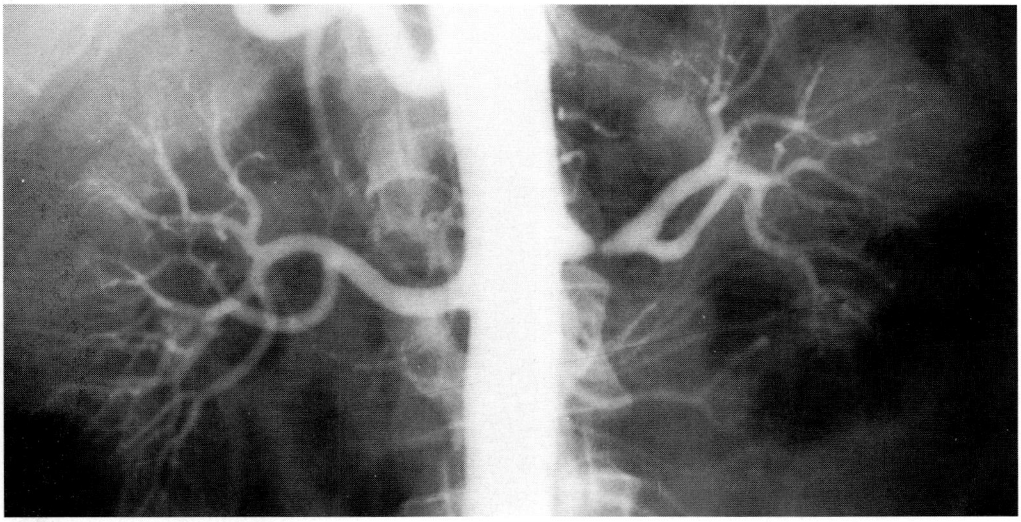

Figure 2–2. Intrinsic renal artery arteriosclerosis. Focal arteriosclerotic disease causing a concentric stenosis of the proximal renal artery. Reprinted with permission from Stanley JC. Morphologic, histopathologic and clinical characteristics of renovascular fibrodysplasia and arteriosclerosis. In Bergan JJ, and Yao JST (eds). Surgery of the Aorta and Its Body Branches, pp 355–376, Grune & Stratton, New York, 1979.

by subendothelial and medial cholesterol-laden cells. Fragmentation of the internal elastic lamina is common. Medial thinning becomes apparent with more extensive intimal lesions. Deposition of fibrous tissue, often with evidence of chronic inflammation, is a reflection of more chronic disease.

Advanced arteriosclerotic lesions frequently exhibit marked fibrosis, medial necrosis, and widespread calcification **(Fig. 2–3)**. Intramural hemorrhage, probably from vasa vasorum, may be conspicuous in areas of necrosis. Accumulations of neutral fats, cholesterol esters with crystalline clefts, and fatty acids are usually evident within fibrotic plaque tissues composed of collagen, elastin, abundant glycosaminoglycons, and glycoproteins. Intimal ulcerations with a platelet-fibrin coagulum on the surface are also often present in these vessels. Luminal thrombosis eventuating in total renal artery occlusion is a common event in patients with advanced renal artery arteriosclerosis.[3]

Approximately 85% of patients exhibiting advanced renal artery arteriosclerosis have clinically overt arteriosclerosis of the aorta and its major extrarenal branches. Occasional patients have clinically overt arteriosclerosis of the aorta and its major extrarenal branches. Patients without evidence of generalized arterio-

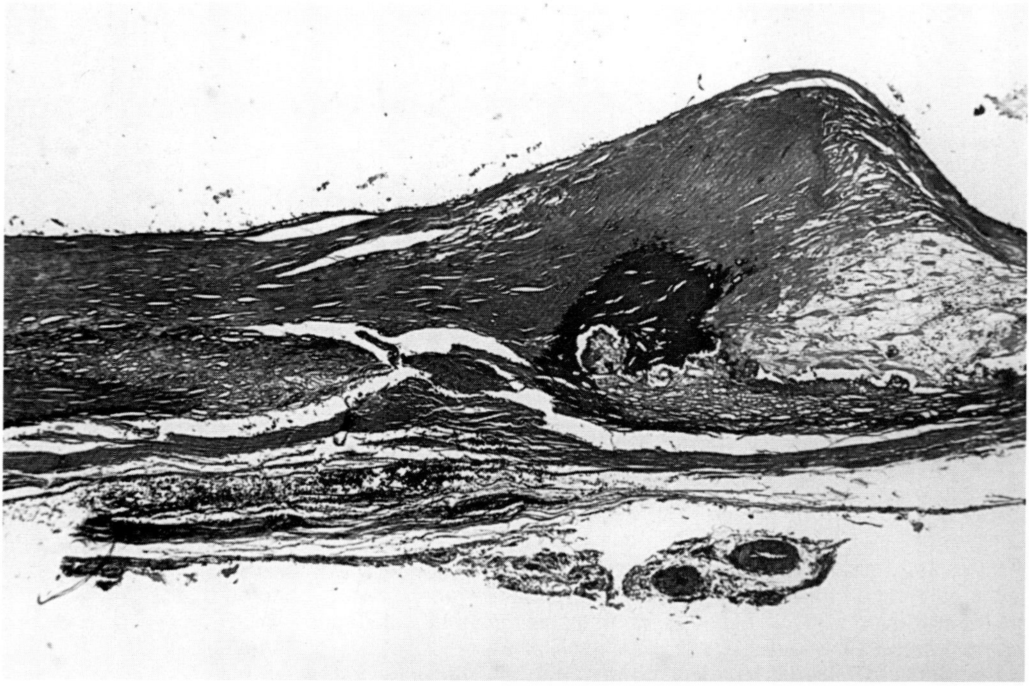

Figure 2–3. Renal artery arteriosclerosis. Complicated arteriosclerotic plaque. Medial necrosis, fibrosis, and calcification with accumulation of cholesterol esters characterize advanced renal artery arteriosclerotic stenoses. Hematoxylin and eosin stain, × 120. Reprinted with permission from Stanley JC. Morphologic, histopathologic and clinical characteristics of renovascular fibrodysplasia and arteriosclerosis. In Bergan JJ and Yao JST (eds). Surgery of the Aorta and Its Body Branches, pp 355–376, Grune & Stratton, New York, 1979.

sclerotic cardiovascular disease may evolve secondary renal arteriosclerosis in preexisting developmental or dysplastic stenoses.

Renal artery arteriosclerosis appears to progress in the same inexorable manner as arteriosclerosis elsewhere in the arterial circulation. Schreiber and associates reported on angiographic observations of 126 diseased arteries.[4] They documented progressive disease in 44%, with important differences ascribed to the initial degree of stenosis. Among stenoses less than 50% initially, 69% remained unchanged, 26% progressed to greater than 50%, and 5% became occluded. In contrast, among initial stenoses ranging from 75% to 99%, occlusion occurred in 39%. Progression of lesions in this series, regardless of initial degree of stenosis, appeared constant being 1.59% per month for stenoses less than 50%, 1.37% per month for 50–75% stenoses, and 1.77% per month for 75–99%

stenoses. These former progression rates were greater than the 0.38% per month reported by Tollefson and his colleagues in a study of 79 arteriosclerotic renal arteries.[5] An important finding from the later report was that no artery with less than a 60% initial stenosis progressed to occlusion within the follow-up period of the study. This is relevant in regard to deep abdominal ultrasonography as a means of assessing renal artery disease, where discrimination of the degree of a stenosis exceeding 60% proves difficult. Zierler and associates undertook ultrasonography of 139 arteries in 80 patients, and documented nearly twice the rate of progression in stenoses greater than 60%, compared with those less than 60%.[6] A survey report on the natural history of arteriosclerotic renal artery stenoses included in follow-up for 6 to 180 months suggested that progression occurs in 49%, and 14% of the lesions progress to occlusion.[7] More advanced renal artery arteriosclerosis must not be considered a quiescent, benign disease.

The predilection for plaque to occur in the ostia and proximal segments of the renal artery parallels the usual pathogenesis of arteriosclerosis. Abnormal blood flow with altered shear stresses and turbulence at such sites may cause endothelial injury, platelet deposition, migration of medial smooth muscle to intimal regions, and subsequent sequestration of intracellular lipids as precursors to arteriosclerotic disease.

RENAL ARTERY FIBRODYSPLASIA

The true incidence of renal artery dysplastic disease in the general population is unknown, but is less than 0.5%. Renal artery dysplasia is second only to atherosclerosis as the most common cause of surgically correctable hypertension. The specific types of renal artery fibrodysplasia warrant separate discussion.

Intimal Fibroplasia

Intimal fibroplasia of the renal artery affects both genders with equal frequency. This lesion accounts for approximately 5% of all dysplastic renal artery stenoses, being observed in infants, adolescents, and young adults more often than among the elderly. Primary intimal fibroplasia usually affects the main renal artery, usually occurring as a smooth focal stenosis **(Fig. 2–4)**. Segmental vessel involvement is an uncommon manifestation of intimal disease, usually presenting as a web-like lesion.[8]

Irregularly arranged subendothelial mesenchymal cells within a loose matrix of fibrous connective tissue characterize primary intimal fibroplasia **(Fig. 2–5)**. The internal elastic lamina, al-

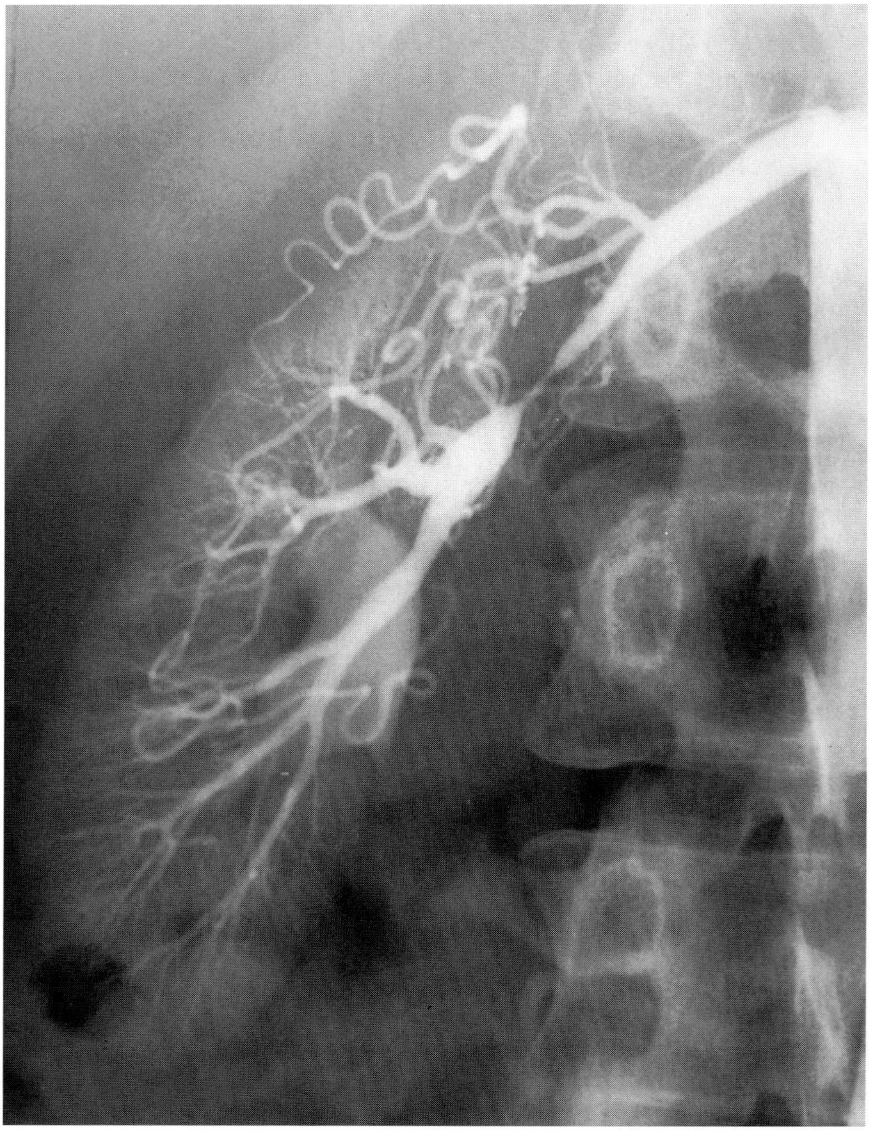

Figure 2–4. Primary intimal fibroplasia. Focal stenosis of main renal artery midportion in a young adult. Reprinted with permission from Stanley JC and Fry WJ. Renovascular hypertension secondary to arterial fibrodysplasia in adults. Criteria for operation and results of surgical therapy. Arch Surg 110: 922, 1975.

though occasionally disrupted, is always present. Medial and adventitial tissues are usually normal in these dysplastic vessels. The cause of primary intimal fibroplasia is unknown. In some cases it appears to represent persistent neonatal musculoelastic cushions, similar to the intimal cushions occurring at cerebral

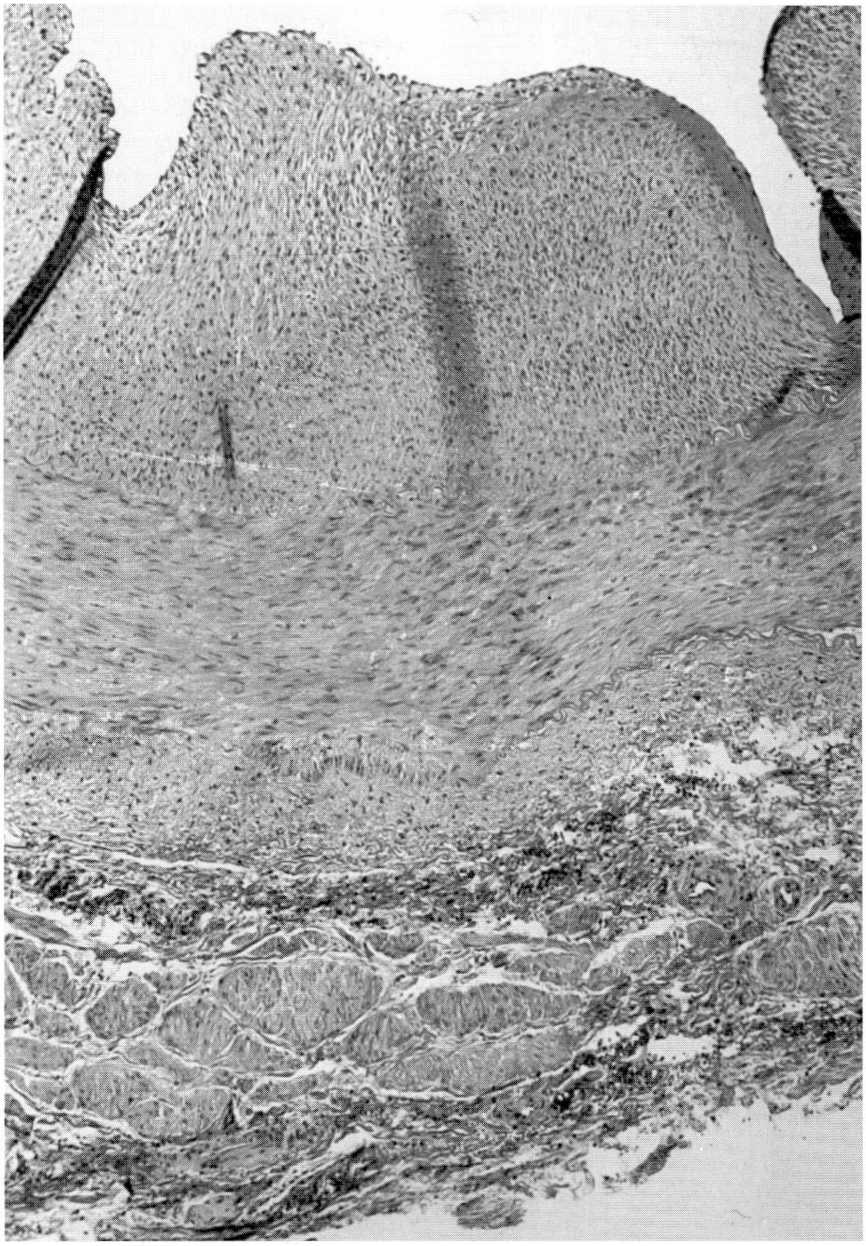

Figure 2–5. Primary intimal fibroplasia. Subendothelial mesenchymal cells within a loose fibrous connective tissue matrix are noted above an intact internal elastic lamina, normal media, and normal adventitial tissues. Luminal encroachments by this primary form of intimal fibroplasia are usually circumferential. Hematoxylin and eosin stain, × 100. Reprinted with permission from Stanley JC. Morphologic, histopathologic and clinical characteristics of renovascular fibrodysplasia and arteriosclerosis. In Bergan JJ and Yao JST (eds). Surgery of the Aorta and Its Body Branches, pp 355–376, Grune & Stratton, New York, 1979.

artery bifurcations in adults.[9] Secondary intimal fibroplasia is often difficult to differentiate from primary intimal disease. Certain secondary lesions occur with developmental ostial lesions. Blunt vascular trauma or intraluminal insults after thrombosis may contribute to other secondary lesions, with medial and adventitial structures in such cases appearing relatively uninvolved. Long tubular stenoses may be evidence of secondary disease, occurring as a consequence of recanalization of a previously thrombosed artery. In this regard certain cases of intimal fibroplasia have been suggested to represent a resolved arteritis, such as that due to rubella.[10] An infectious-immunologic etiology in certain cases has been supported by evidence of immunoglobulin deposition within the stenotic intimal tissues.[11]

Progression of intimal fibrodysplasia, once a hemodynamically important arterial stenosis develops, appears a likely consequence of abnormal surface blood flow, even if the initiating etiologic factors have resolved. The specific cellular messengers responsible for this proliferation have not been identified. Intimal lesions appear to progress at a much slower rate than do medial fibroplastic stenoses,[12] but reliable data on the natural history of this form of dysplasia are unavailable.

Medial Fibroplasia

Medial fibroplasia accounts for nearly 85% of dysplastic renovascular disease. More than 90% of patients with medial fibroplasia are women, with most being diagnosed during their fourth decade of life. Although medial fibroplasia is considered a systemic arteriopathy, clinically overt disease is usually limited to the renal, extracranial internal carotid, and external iliac arteries.

The morphologic appearance of renal artery medial fibroplasia ranges from a solitary focal stenosis to its more common presentation as a series of stenoses with intervening aneurysmal outpouchings **(Fig. 2–6)**. This classic "string of beads" appearance has not been encountered in men. The thin-walled mural aneurysms are usually evident grossly, as are distinct webs projecting internally. Medial fibroplasia most commonly affects the distal main renal artery, with extensions into first order segmental branches observed in approximately 25% of cases.

Progression of renal artery medial fibroplasia is less common than that associated with perimedial dysplasia.[13] Nevertheless, progression has been reported in from 12% to 66% of patients with main renal artery lesions.[4,12–16] In one study that included a dominant number of vessels with this form of dysplastic disease, progression over a 6-year period affected 83% of arteries to the right kidney and 54% of arteries to the left kidney.[14] This finding is similar to the predilection for greater involvement of disease

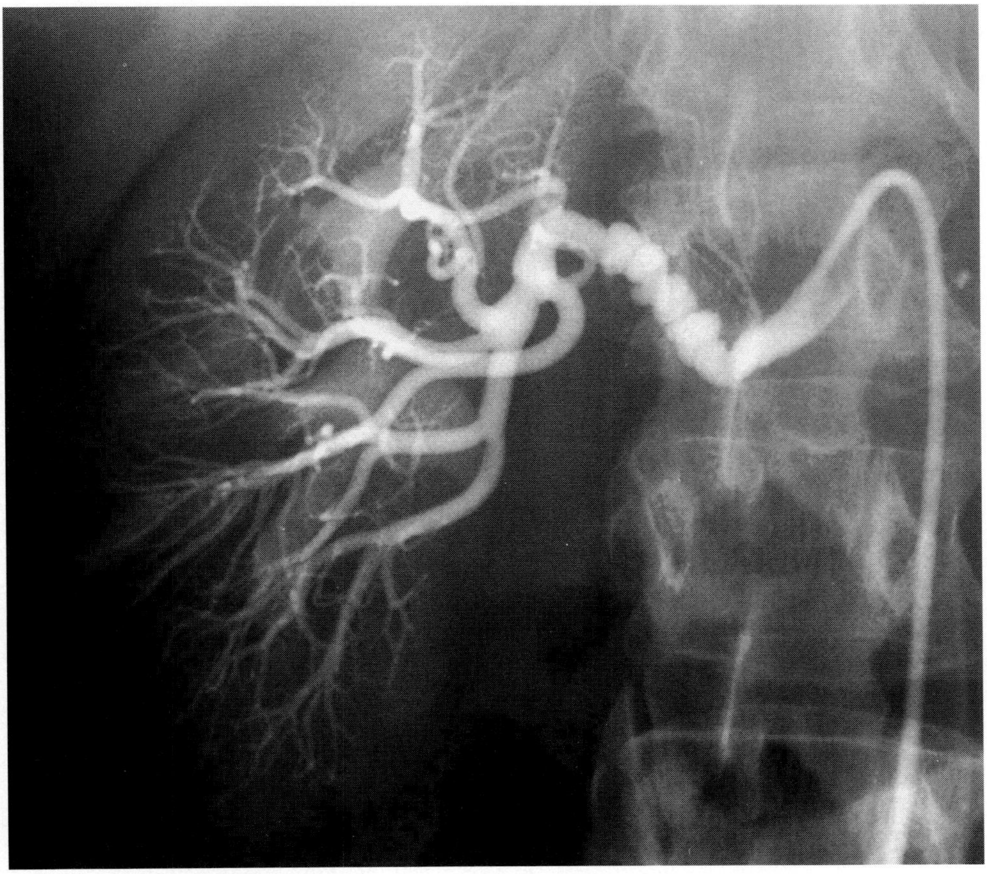

Figure 2–6. Medial fibroplasia. Serial stenoses alternating with mural aneurysms, producing a "string-of-beads" appearance in the midportion and distal main renal artery. Reprinted with permission from Stanley JC and Graham LM. Renovascular Hypertension. In Miller DC and Roon AJ (eds). Diagnosis and Management of Peripheral Vascular Disease, pp. 231–235, Addison-Wesley, Menlo Park, 1981.

on the right. Progression is thought to be more likely to affect premenopausal women, yet some have not noted age-related differences.[4] Among a group of 71 potential kidney donors with angiographic evidence of renal artery fibrodysplasia, hypertension developed in 26% over an average follow-up of 7.5 years.[17] Hypertension developed in only 6% of an age- and sex-matched group of control patients. Blood pressure increases in these instances were considered a reflection of progressive renal artery disease. Acute changes in fibrodysplastic renal vessels are relatively uncommon, although in one series 18% had progressed to complete occlusion.[19] This later experience is much worse than that reported by others, including a comprehensive study of 75 patients with fibrodysplasia, in whom 33% exhibited progression, but no case of occlusion was observed.[4]

Two histologic forms of renal artery medial fibroplasia are recognized. The first is evident by disease limited to the outer media (peripheral form). The second exhibits disease throughout the entire media (diffuse form). Gradations between these extremes may occur in the same vessel, supporting the tenet that they represent a common disease process. The peripheral form of medial fibroplasia is usually encountered in younger patients. With the passage of time, more advanced disease may evolve to affect the entire media.

Peripheral medial fibroplasia is characterized by compact fibrous connective tissue replacing smooth muscle in the outer media **(Fig. 2–7A)**, with moderate accumulations of collagen and ground substances separating disorganized smooth muscle within the inner media. Intimal tissues and the internal elastic lamina are rarely affected in these peripheral lesions. Although continuity of the external elastic lamina is frequently lost, the adventitia is usually normal. Certain peripheral forms of medial fibroplasia were previously classified as perimedial or subadventitial disease.[19–21]

Diffuse medial fibrodysplasia is characterized by more severe disorganization and disruption of normal smooth muscle architecture **(Fig. 2–7B)**. Excessive medial accumulations of fibrous tissue alternate with areas of marked medial thinning. In some cases the media is nearly absent, and these regions account for the mural aneurysmal dilations of the vessel. Internal elastic lamina fragmentation and subendothelial fibrosis may be evident, although such are usually considered secondary events in instances of more advanced medial fibroplasia. Adventitial tissues are uninvolved in medial fibroplasia.

Perimedial Dysplasia

Perimedial dysplasia is the dominant abnormality that affects approximately 10% of dysplastic renal arteries. Patients who exhibit perimedial dysplasia invariably have been women, usually in their fourth or fifth decades of life. These lesions present as either focal stenoses or multiple constrictions involving the midportion of the main renal artery without mural aneurysms **(Fig. 2–8A)**. Excessive elastic tissue at the junction of the media and adventitia is the distinguishing feature of perimedial dysplasia **(Fig. 2–8B)**, appearing as a homogenous collar of elastic tissue adjacent to the outer media. Minimal increases in medial ground substance surrounding intact smooth muscle cells, with little alteration of inti-

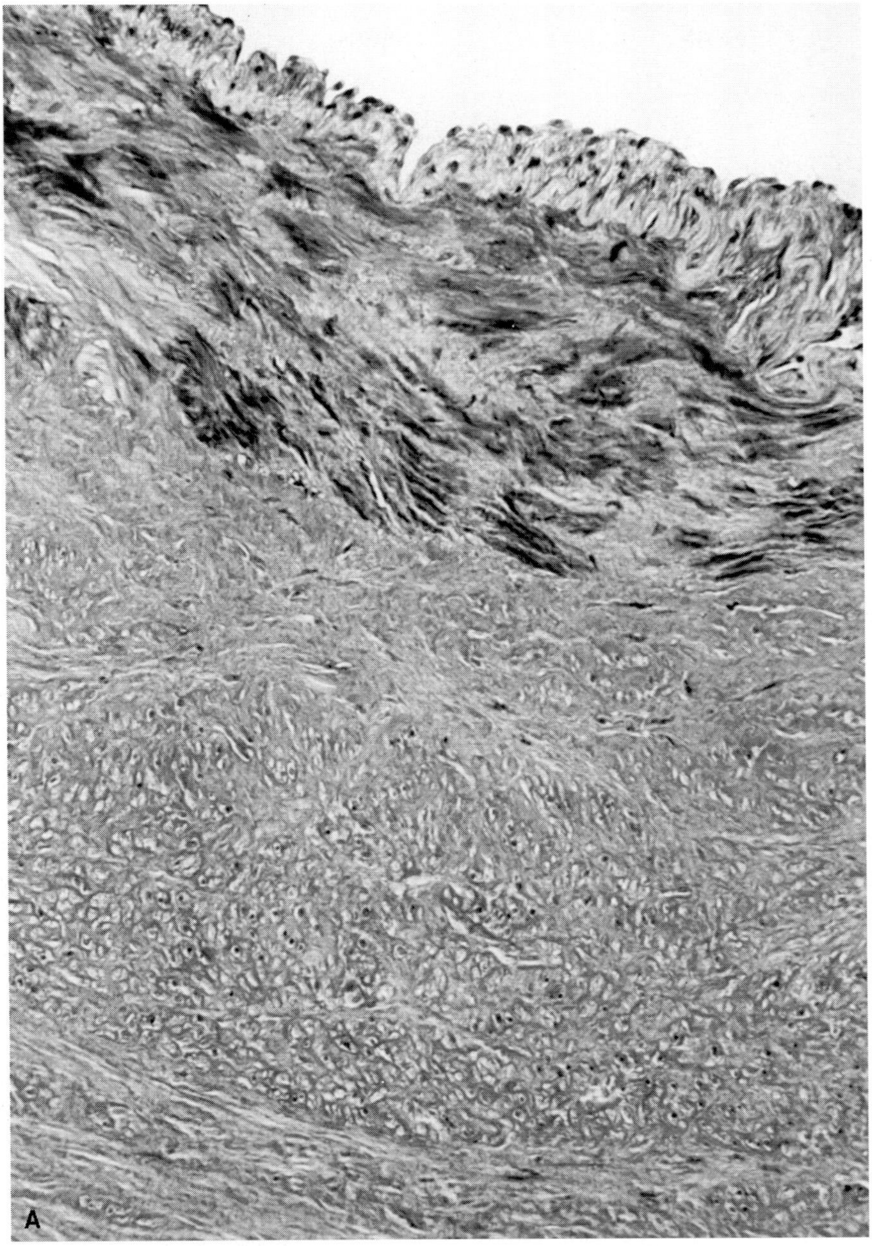

Figure 2–7. A. Peripheral form, medial fibrodysplasia, dense fibrous connective tissue in the outer media, with disordered inner medial smooth muscle, and normal intimal tissues. B. Diffuse form, medial fibroplasia. Total replacement of media by disorganized cellular tissue (myofibroblasts) surrounded by fibrous connective tissue. Masson stain, × 120. Reprinted with permission from Stanley JC. Morphologic, histopathologic and clinical characteristics of renovascular fibrodysplasia and arteriosclerosis. In Bergan JJ and Yao JST (eds). Surgery of the Aorta and Its Body Branches, pp 355–376. Grune & Stratton, New York, 1979. (Figure continues.)

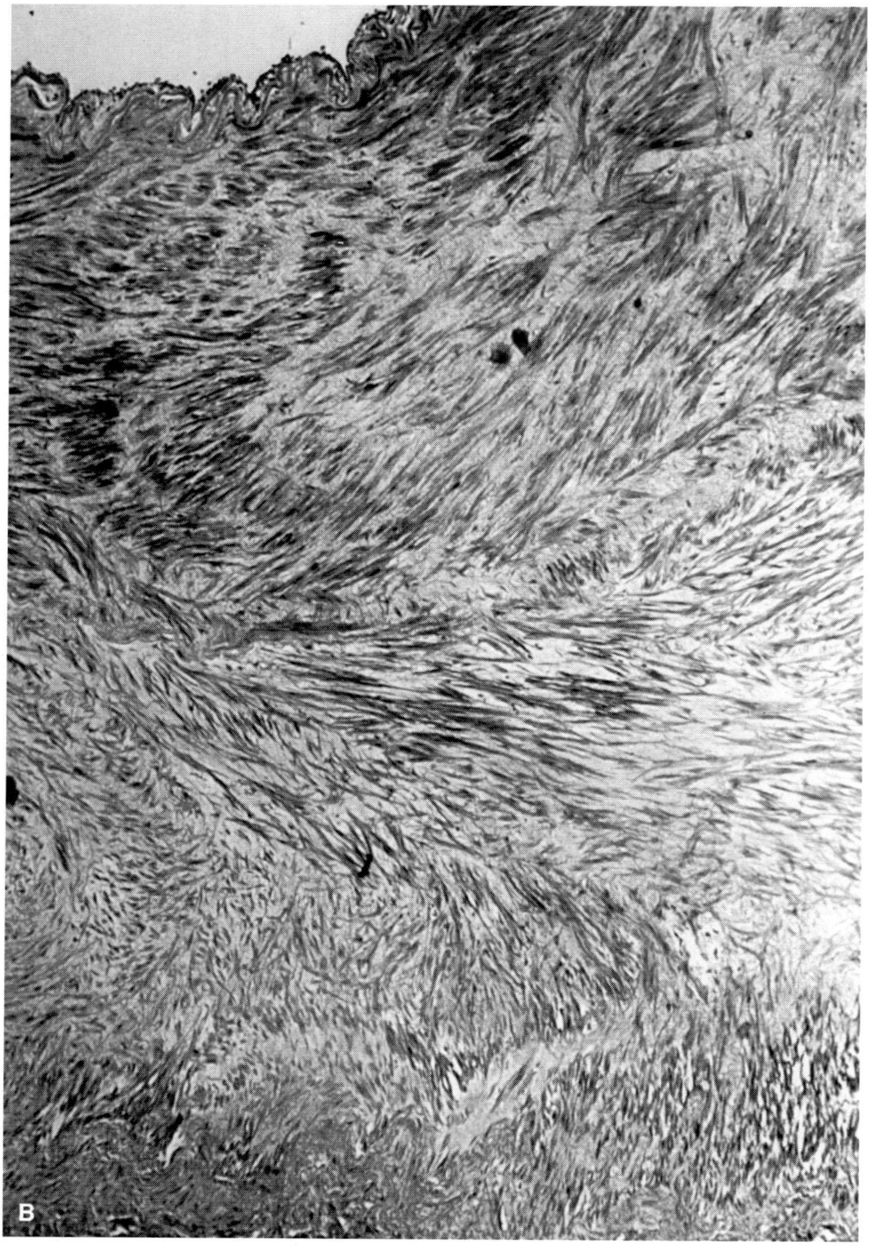

Figure 2–7. *(continued)*

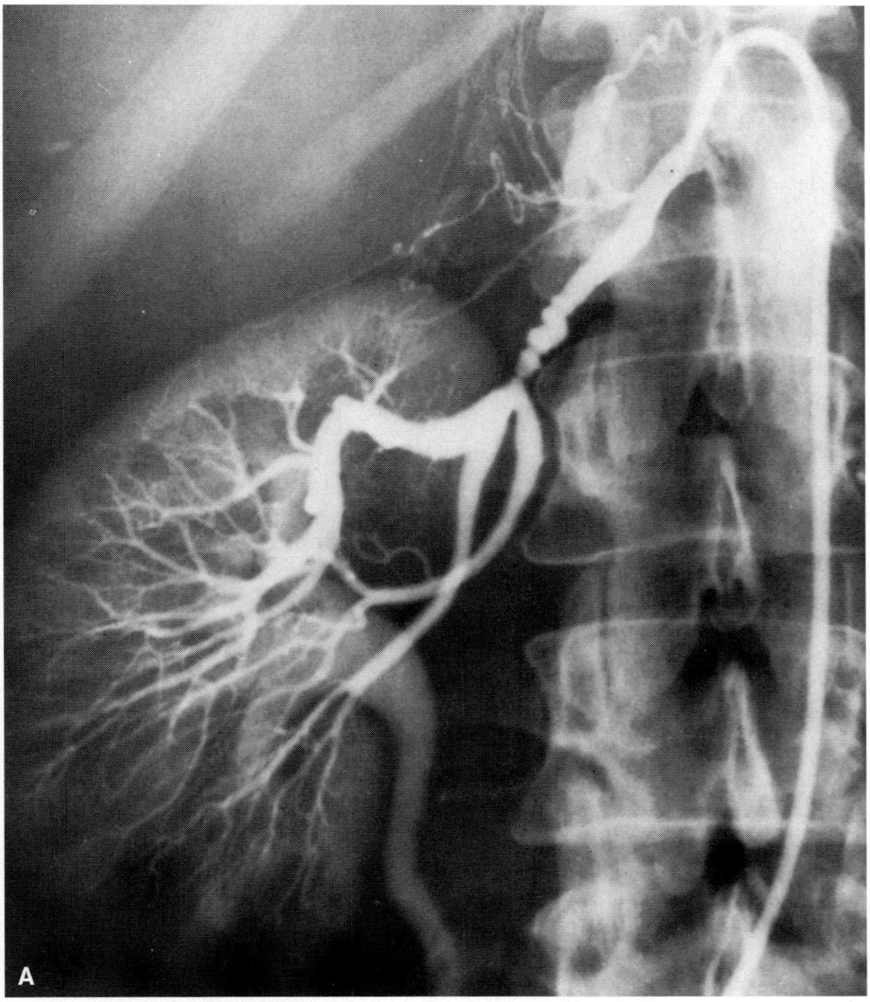

A

Figure 2–8. Perimedial dysplasia. A. Multiple stenoses without mural aneurysms in the midportion of the renal artery are characteristic of these lesions. B. These stenoses are due to excessive accumulations of elastic tissue at medial-adventitial junction. Verhoeff stain, × 120. Reprinted with permission from Stanley JC. Morphologic, histopathologic and clinical characteristics of renovascular fibrodysplasia and arteriosclerosis. In Bergan JJ and Yao JST (eds). Surgery of the Aorta and Its Body Branches, pp 355–376. Grune & Stratton, New York, 1979. (Figure continues.)

mal tissues, characterize inner portions of the vessel wall in many of these dysplastic lesions.

The pathogenesis of medial fibroplasia and perimedial dysplasia has been the subject of speculation.[8] Hormonal effects on smooth muscle, mechanical stresses on vessel walls, and the pecul-

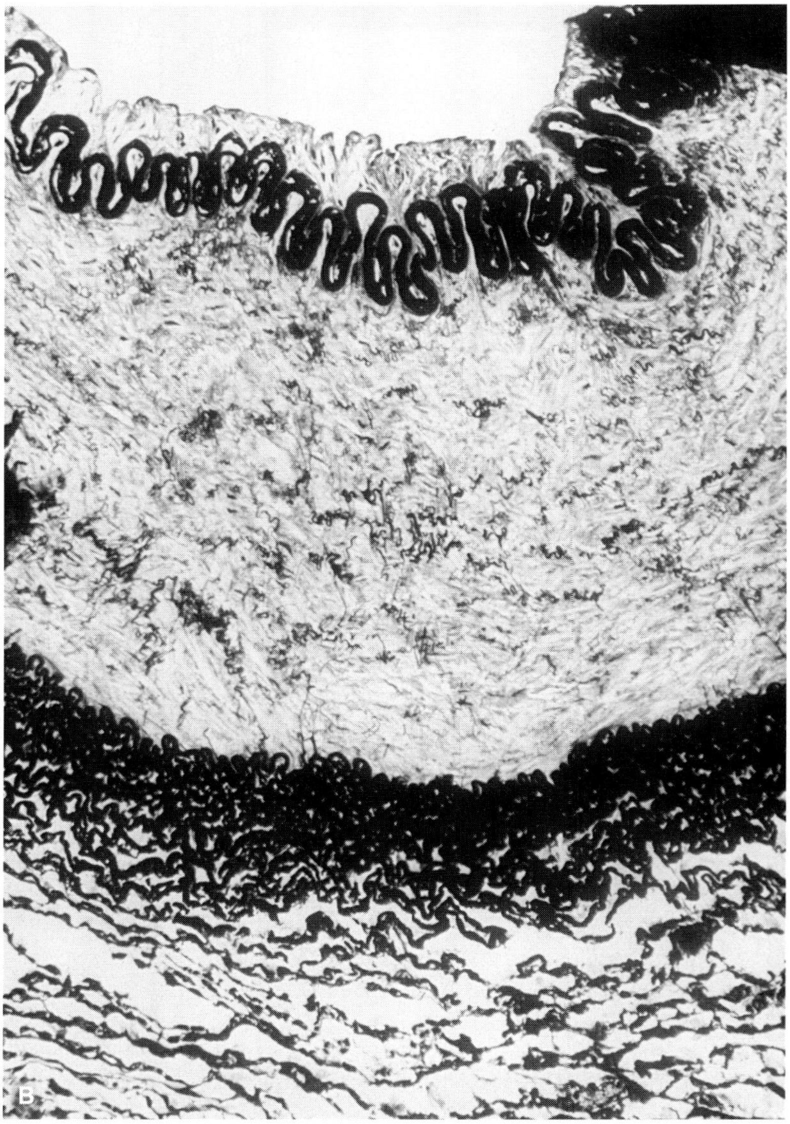

Figure 2–8. *(continued)*

iar distribution of vasa vasorum in arteries exhibiting these lesions are all considered contributing factors. The exact relation of these factors to each other, or their association with other unrecognized pathogenic mechanisms, remains unknown. Because of the familial nature of this disease, an autosomal dominant inheritance pattern etiology with incomplete penetrance has been suggested. However, confirmatory arteriographic or histologic evidence to firmly establish such a contention has not been presented.[22–26] In fact, the absence of a female gender predilection in the data generated by those touting a genetic etiology lessens the validity of their proposal.

Hormonal influences seem likely in view of arterial dysplasia's unusual female predilection. Pregnancy is not an obvious etiologic factor in arterial fibrodysplasia. The reproductive histories of patients in a large series of patients with this arteriopathy did not reveal gravity or parity rates different from the general population.[8] Antiovulants are also known to have a significant effect on the arterial wall. However, use of such drugs by less than half the University of Michigan series' female patients does not support an obvious cause and effect association of progesterins with arterial dysplasia.[8] A similar lack of association with oral contraceptives was reported in a case-control study.[26] On the other hand, certain smooth muscle cells and fibroblasts exposed to estrogens increase their synthesis of proteinaceous substances, including collagen. Physiologic preconditioning of vascular smooth muscle cells to a secretory state by normal circulating estrogens may account for the more frequent occurrence of medial dysplastic disease in women.

Unusual physical stresses due to ptosis of the kidneys may be associated with fibrodysplastic changes in the renal arteries. Comparable stretch or traction forces are less likely to occur in similar sized vessels unaffected by this disease. Ptotic kidneys are known to be common among patients with renal artery dysplastic lesions.[27,28] In some cases positional changes causing greater ptosis have been correlated with increases in blood pressure.[29] The fact that the right kidney is usually more ptotic than the left may account for the greater severity of right-sided disease in the majority of adults having bilateral medial fibroplasia. That women are more likely than men to have ptotic kidneys may also contribute to the observed gender difference. In addition, in the case of unilateral lesions, 80% involve the right renal arteries. Cyclic stretching of smooth muscle cells in tissue culture causes an unusually large synthesis of collagen and certain acid mucopolysaccharides.[30] Although existence of similar mechanisms in vivo are speculative, the predilection for dysplastic disease to occur most often in vessels subjected to peculiar mechanical forces may reflect an important etiologic phenomenon. However, in one recent case control study, renal mobility was not greater in patients with renovascular fibrodysplasia.[26]

A third etiologic factor may be related to mural ischemia in dysplastic arteries. Vasa vasorum of muscular arteries usually originate from branchings of parent vessels. The renal, extracranial internal carotid, and external iliac arteries are the three vessels most likely to develop medial fibrodysplasia. The latter two arteries, in particular, have few branches compared with similar sized vessels elsewhere. Compromised vasa vasorum in these vessels, where a sparsity of these nutrient channels may already exist, may lead to significant mural ischemia. Vasospasm may occur in these cases and further exacerbate vessel wall ischemia.[31,32] The concept that insufficient vessel wall nourishment causes dysplastic changes is supported by the common involvement of the outermost part of the media in peripheral medial fibroplasia. It is precisely this region where ischemia from inadequate vasa vasorum blood flow would be predictably greatest. Fibrodysplasia limited to the inner part of the media has never been reported. Vasa vasorum in these vessels have exhibited both dilation and isolation from adjacent medial smooth muscle cells.[33,34] Experimental occlusion of the vasa vasorum produces a dysplastic lesion in dogs similar to that seen in humans and supports the tenet that mural ischemia is a factor in the evolution of arterial dysplasia.[35]

DEVELOPMENTAL RENAL ARTERY STENOSES

Developmental renal artery stenoses represent a rare form of renal artery dysplasia. There is no apparent gender predilection for this entity. Nearly 40% of children with renovascular hypertension have developmental renal artery lesions.[36,37] Among adults with intimal fibrodysplastic renal artery disease, approximately 20% have stenoses that appear to represent growth or developmental defects. Similarly, certain adults with isolated renal artery arteriosclerosis may have had preexisting developmentally narrowed vessels. Thus developmental renal artery occlusive disease in adults appears to be uncommon, but not rare. Conversely, nearly 80% of patients with abdominal aortic developmental lesions have coexisting renal artery stenoses and renovascular hypertension.[38] Developmental stenoses of the renal arteries are usually hypoplastic in character, and as such have an external "hour-glass" appearance. Most developmental lesions occur at the origin of the renal artery **(Fig. 2–9)**.

The histologic character of the majority of these lesions includes abnormalities in all three layers of the vessel.[36,39,40] Sparse medial tissue and intimal fibroplasia with fragmentation and duplication of the internal elastic lamina and excesses in adventitial elastic tissue are common findings **(Fig. 2–10)**. Similarly, irregular deficiencies in medial tissue may be observed in these diminutive vessels.

Developmental renal artery narrowings appear related to certain in utero events. Under normal circumstances the paired dorsal aortae fuse and usually all but one of their lateral metanephric branches regress, leaving a solitary renal artery during the same

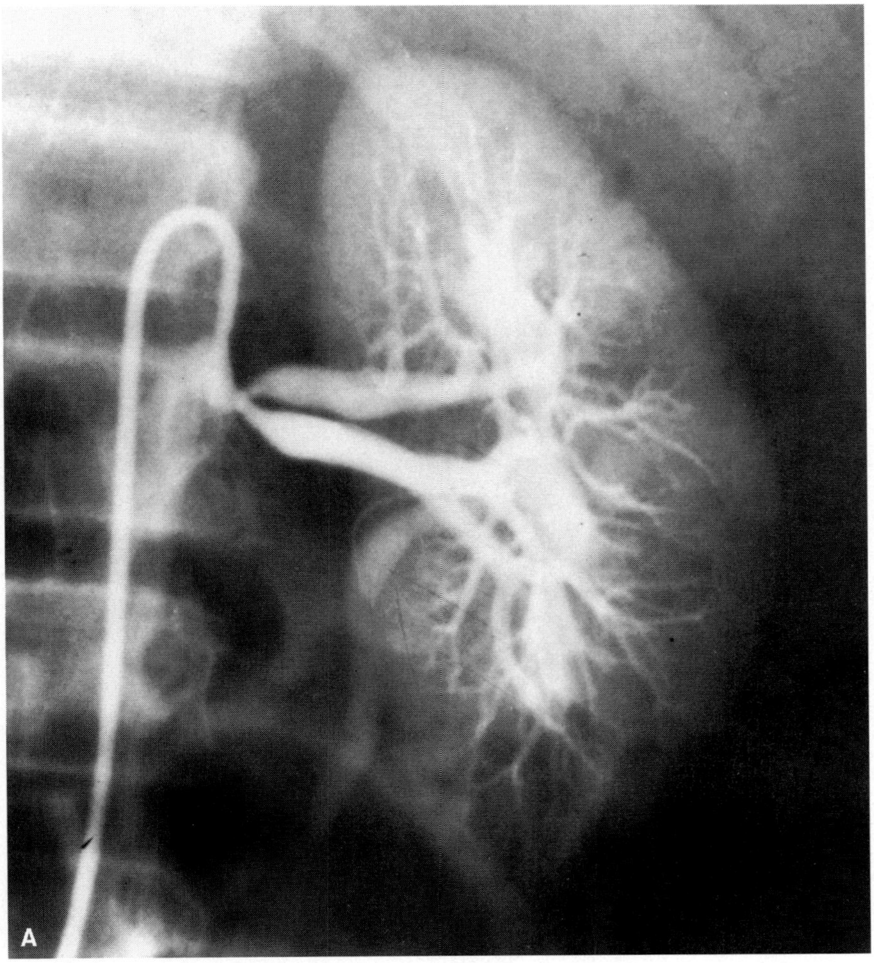

Figure 2–9. Developmental renal artery stenoses. A. Proximal lesion in a patient with neurofibromatosis. B. Multiple vessel stenoses in a patient with aortic hypoplasia. (A. Reprinted with permission from Stanley JC, Fry WJ. Pediatric renal artery occlusive disease and renovascular hypertension. Etiology, diagnosis and operative treatment. Arch Surg 116:669, 1984; B. Reprinted with permission from Graham LM, Zelenock GB, Erlandson EE, Coran, AG, Lindenauer SM, Stanley JC. Abdominal aortic coarctation and segmental hypoplasia. Surgery 86:519, 1979.) (Figure continues.)

period of embryonic development. Events that alter transition of mesenchyme to medial smooth muscle tissue at this time, or its later condensation and growth, may cause aortic or renovascular anomalies.

Several theories exist with regard to the cause of these lesions. One proposes that the constrictive lesions follow lack of, or un-

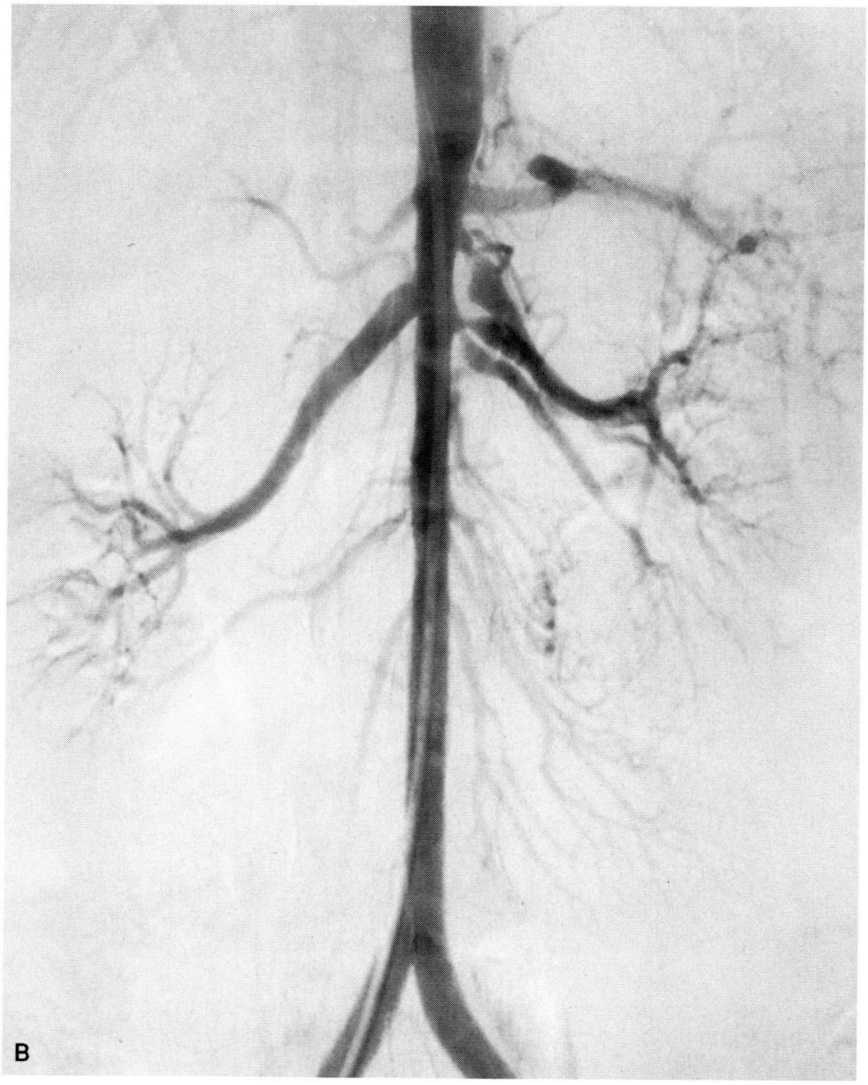

Figure 2–9. *(continued)*

Figure 2–10. Developmental, hypoplastic renal artery. A. Secondary intimal fibroplasia, fragmentation of the internal elastic lamina, and diminutions in medial tissue are typical features of this stenotic lesion. Greatest luminal dimension is 2 mm. Movat stain, × 80. B. Marked fragmentation and duplication of the internal elastic lamina and attenuation of medial tissues characterize this vessel. Intimal fibroplasia encroaches on the vessel lumen which is less than 1 mm in diameter. Adventitial elastic tissues appear excessive. Movat stain, × 100. Reprinted with permission from Stanley JC, Graham LM, Whitehouse WM Jr, Zelenock GB, Erlandson EE, Cronenwett JL, Lindenauer SM. Developmental occlusive disease of the abdominal aorta, splanchnic and renal arteries. Am J Surg 1981;142:190.

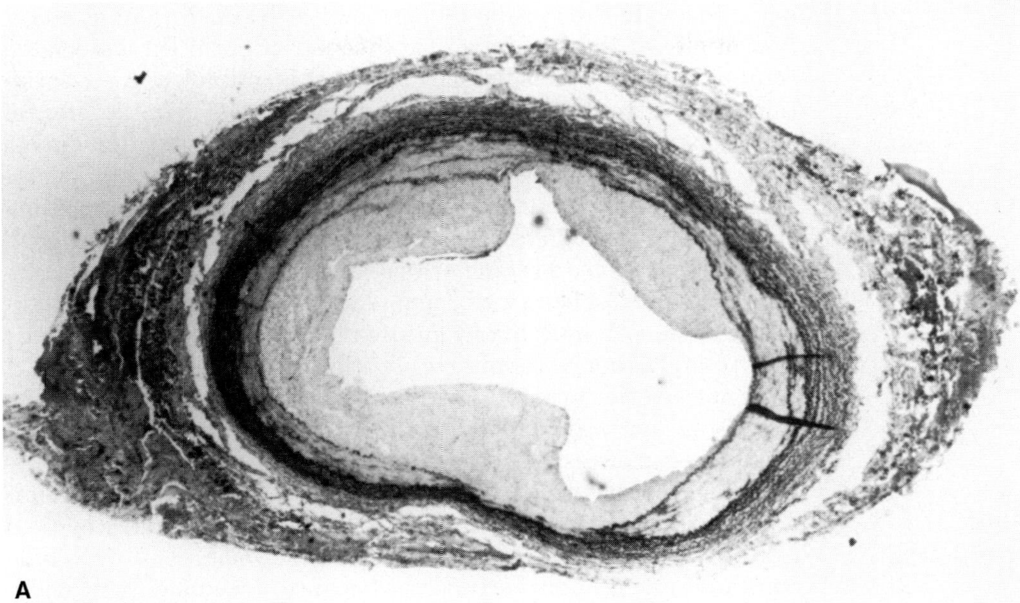

A

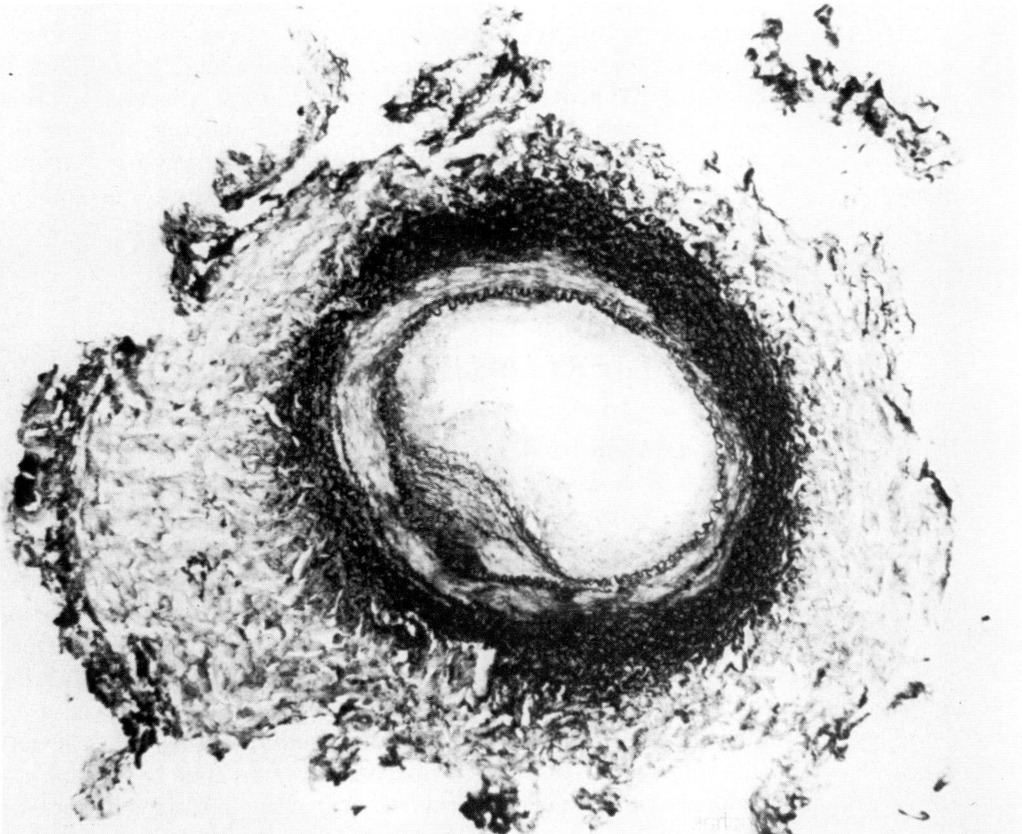

B

equal fusion of the two dorsal aortae,[41] with subsequent obliteration of one of these channels and constriction of the associated renal artery. The basis for such an event is unknown. An association with neurofibromatosis suggests a potential genetic defect of mesenchyme tissue.[42–45] An acquired insult in utero or during early life may arrest growth of an otherwise normal aorta in certain cases. This insult may be viral. Certain viruses, including rubella, are cytocidal as well as inhibitory to cell replication.[46] Aortic hypoplasia and renal artery stenosis associated with gestational rubella has been well documented.[47] In such instances inhibition of smooth muscle cell mitoses may preclude normal aortic growth and produce renal artery ostial stenoses.

Renal arteries originate within mesenchymal tissue about the two dorsal aortas. They are initially represented by a caudally located group of vessels to the mesonephros that are replaced during fetal growth with a more cephalic group of vessels to the metanephros. A solitary artery to the primitive kidney usually evolves from each of these lateral vessel groups. Development of a single dominant vessel apparently occurs because of its obligate hemodynamic advantage over adjacent vessels. Flow changes due to an evolving aortic coarctation in the region where single renal arteries might normally arise may give coexisting polar channels hemodynamic advantages that cause their persistence. In support of such a hypothesis of renal artery occlusive disease in this subgroup of patients is the fact that central abdominal aortic coarctation and hypoplasia are frequently associated with multiple stenotic renal arteries at least twice as often as the general population.[37,38,40]

RENAL ARTERY MACROANEURYSMS

Aneurysms of the renal artery represent unusual vascular lesions that have been described with increasing frequency.[48–53] Controversy persists concerning their natural history.[51–54] In part, this relates to the fact that complications of these aneurysms may be overestimated in reported series that usually represent surgical rather than population based experiences. Other misperceptions on the importance of these aneurysms reflect unrecognized differences among the four principal categories of these lesions: 1) true renal artery aneurysms, 2) dissecting renal artery aneurysms, 3) aneurysmal dilations occurring with medial fibrodysplastic disease, and 4) arteritis-related microaneurysms. The two renal artery macroaneurysms most important in clinical settings, true aneurysms and those associated with dissections, are presented individually.

True Renal Artery Aneurysms

The precise incidence of true renal artery aneurysms in the general population approaches 0.09%, a figure derived from incidental demonstration of these aneurysms in more than 8,000 patients subjected to arteriographic studies for nonrenal disease.[51] The reported frequency of these lesions depends on the patient population studied. Macroaneurysms were identified in 0.7% of arteriographic studies directed at renal disease,[55] in 2.5% of studies performed as part of a hypertension evaluation[51] and 9.2% of adults with renal artery fibrodysplasia.[8]

Women are affected with renal artery aneurysms 1.2 times more often than men, but when patients having arterial fibrodys-

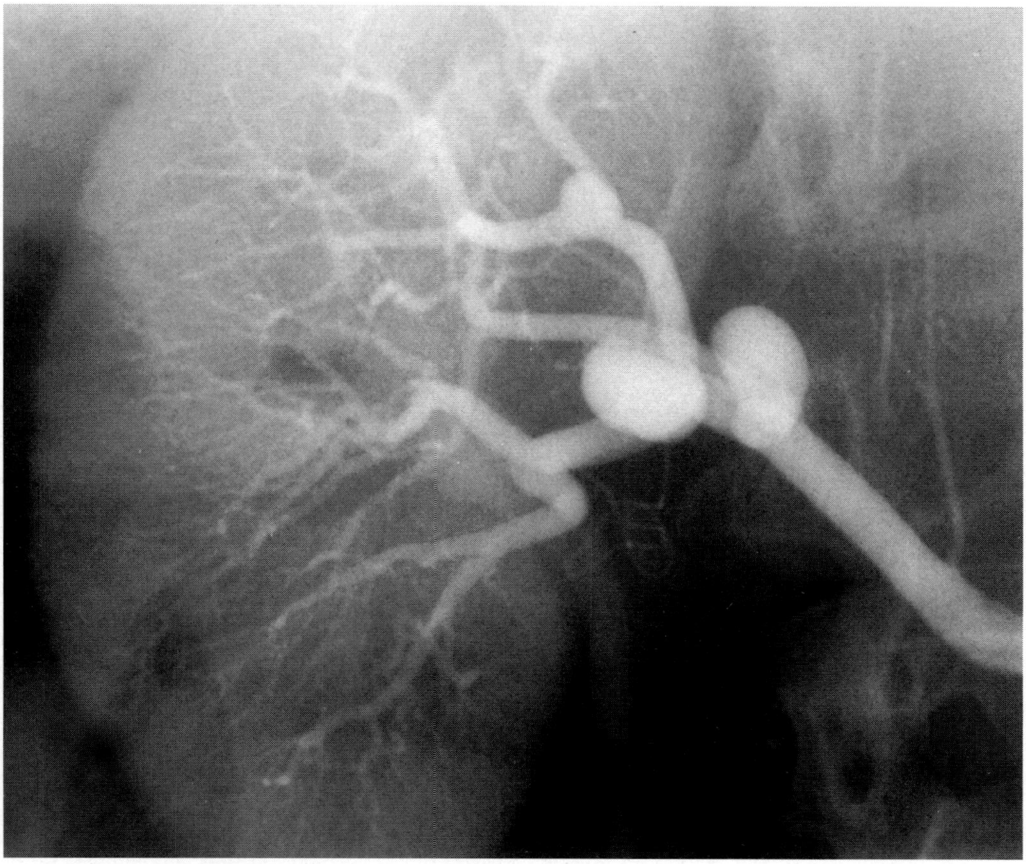

Figure 2–11. Renal artery aneurysms, at a second order branch. Reprinted with permission from Stanley JC, Rhodes EL, Gewertz BL, Chang CY, Walter JF, Fry WJ. Arch Surg 110:1327–1333, 1975.

plasia are excluded there appears to be no gender predilection. In regard to the latter, an apparent predisposition for these aneurysms to affect the right renal artery may reflect the greater incidence of right-sided fibrodysplastic disease.[8] Renal artery aneurysms are usually located at primary or secondary renal artery bifurcations **(Fig. 2–11)**. Most are saccular, and less than 1.5 cm in average diameter.[51] Extraparenchymal aneurysms are very common, accounting for more than 90% of these lesions.

Two distinct histologic categories of true renal artery aneurysms exist. The first type appears to be caused by a congenital defect or medial degenerative process **(Fig. 2–12)**. Internal elastic

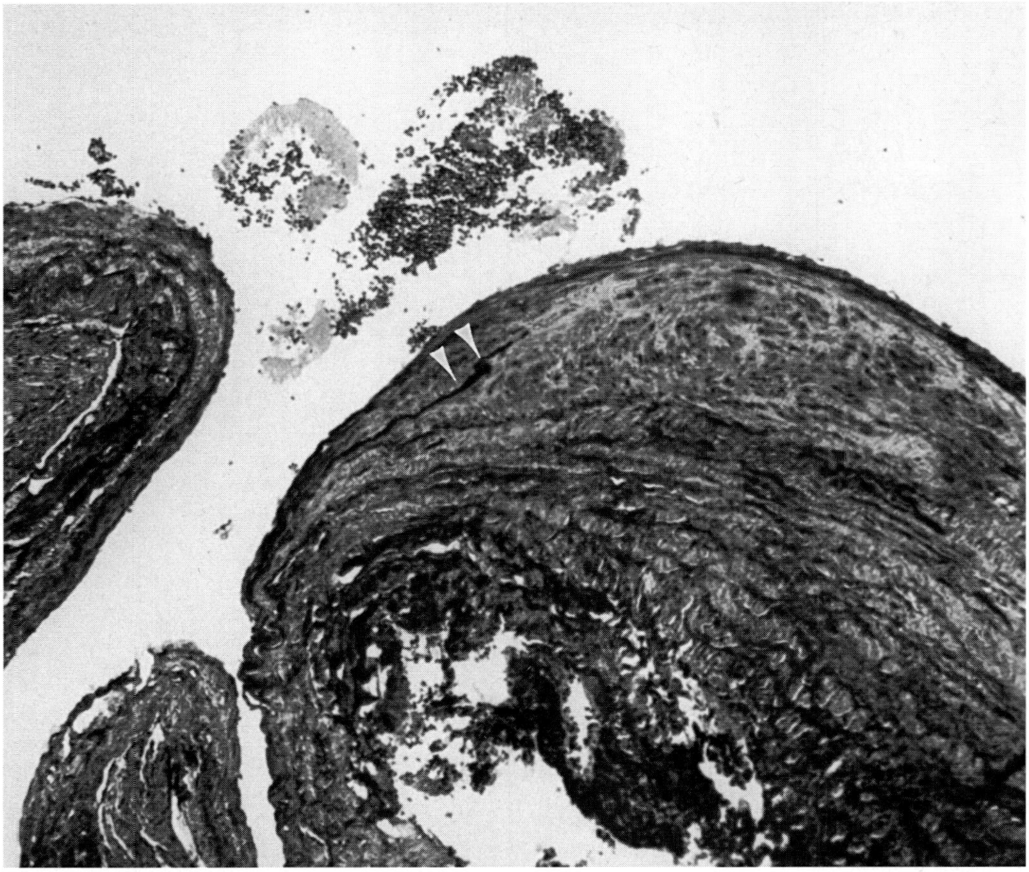

Figure 2–12. Renal artery aneurysm, of undetermined etiology. Interruption of internal elastic lamina (arrows) demonstrated at orifice of saccular renal artery aneurysm. Defects in elastic lamella have been related to the development of renal artery aneurysms (Movat stain × 60). Reprinted with permission from Stanley JC, Rhodes EL, Gewertz BL, Chang CY, Walter JF, Fry WJ. Arch Surg 110:1327–1333, 1975.

lamina fragmentation, excessive accumulations of collagen and other ground substances, with a paucity of elastic tissue and medial smooth muscle characterize these lesions. The second type of aneurysm exhibits arteriosclerosis **(Fig. 2–13)**. Hemorrhage, calcium deposition, collections of cholesterol, necrotic debris, and a matrix of fibrous tissue typify these lesions. Such atheromatous

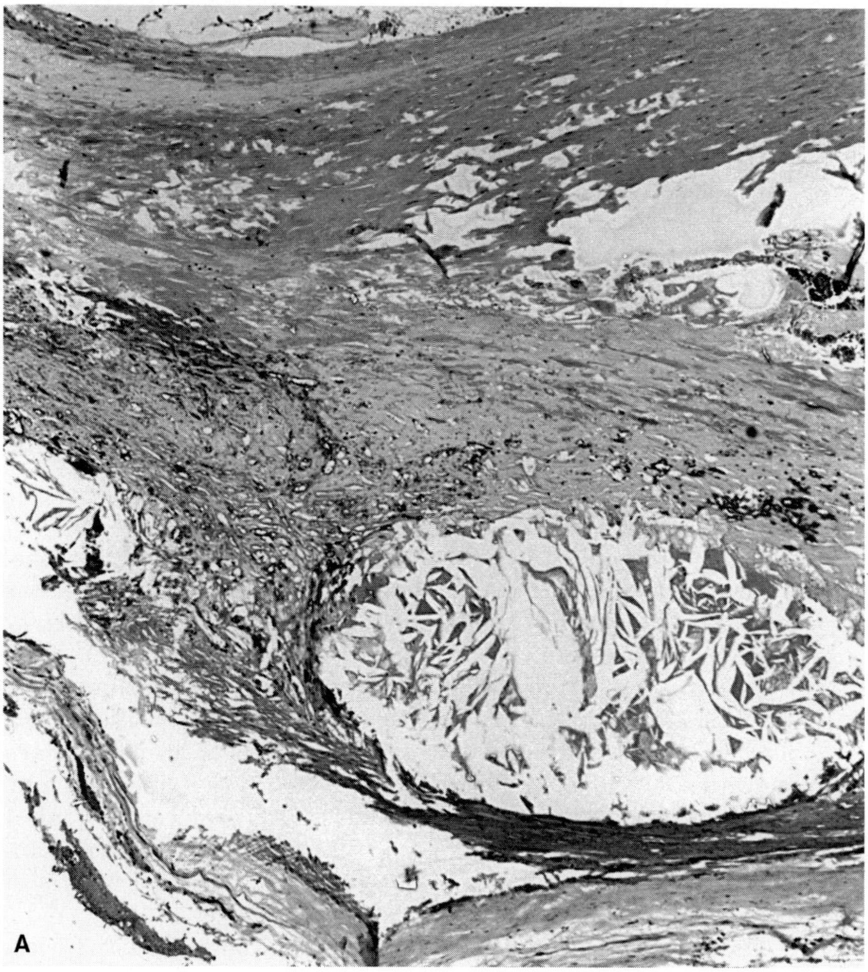

Figure 2–13. Arteriosclerotic renal artery aneurysm. A. Fibrocollagenous aneurysm walls, with loss of all normal architecture, frequently alternated with areas exhibiting arteriosclerotic changes Hematoxylin-eosin stain × 40. B. Calcium deposition and cholesterol clefts within matrix of fibrous tissue were typical of many larger arteriosclerotic aneurysms Hematoxylin-eosin stain × 40. Reprinted with permission from Stanley JC, Rhodes EL, Gewertz BL, Chang CY, Walter JF, Fry WJ. Arch Surg 110:1327–1333, 1975. (Figure continues.)

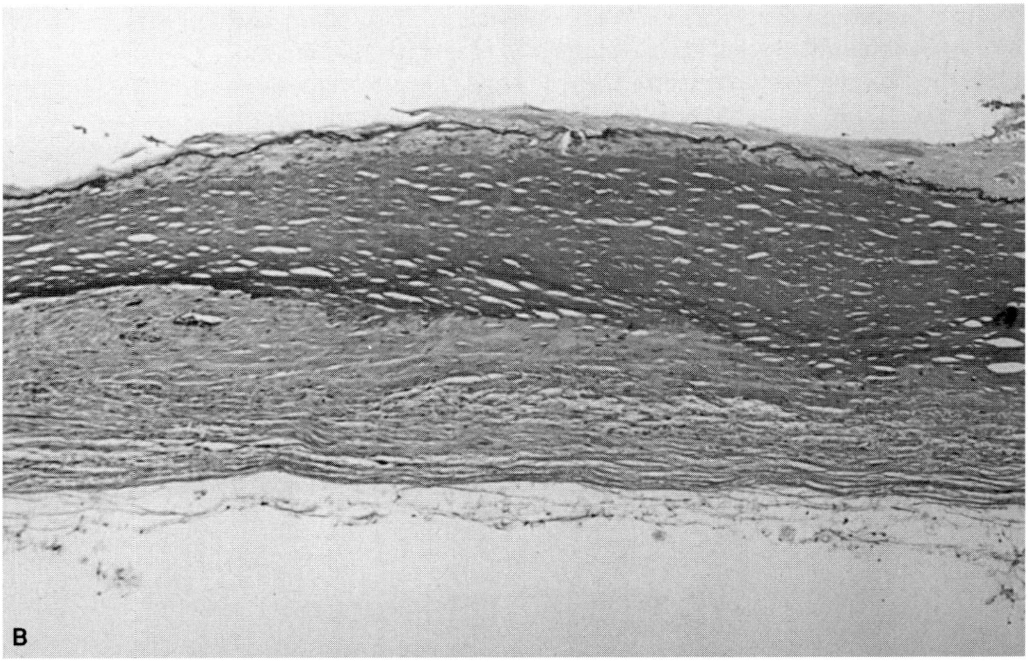

Figure 2–13. *(continued)*

changes often occur at irregular intervals in these aneurysms, with intervening areas composed of thin, collagenous acellular fibrous tissue. Severe arteriosclerosis of the adjacent renal artery in these cases is rare.

Both congenital and acquired factors appear to contribute to the formation of true renal artery aneurysms. Internal elastic lamina defects and deficiencies of smooth muscle cells at branchings are known to be common in nondiseased renal arteries, and such may contribute to the development of aneurysms considered congenital in origin. However, the reported increase in the prevalence of aneurysms with age suggests the presence of additional factors in aneurysm formation.[55]

The greater incidence of aneurysms among patients with hypertension secondary to dysplastic renal artery stenoses **(Fig. 2–14)**, in comparison to those with arteriosclerotic stenoses, supports the tenet that arterial fibrodysplasia is a direct contributor to aneurysmal changes.[51] Elevated blood pressure in 80% of patients with renal artery macroaneurysms may also play a role in aneurysm development. Increased mural tension in these cases may affect the structural integrity of the renal artery, especially in the presence of pre-existing medial defects at bifurcations.

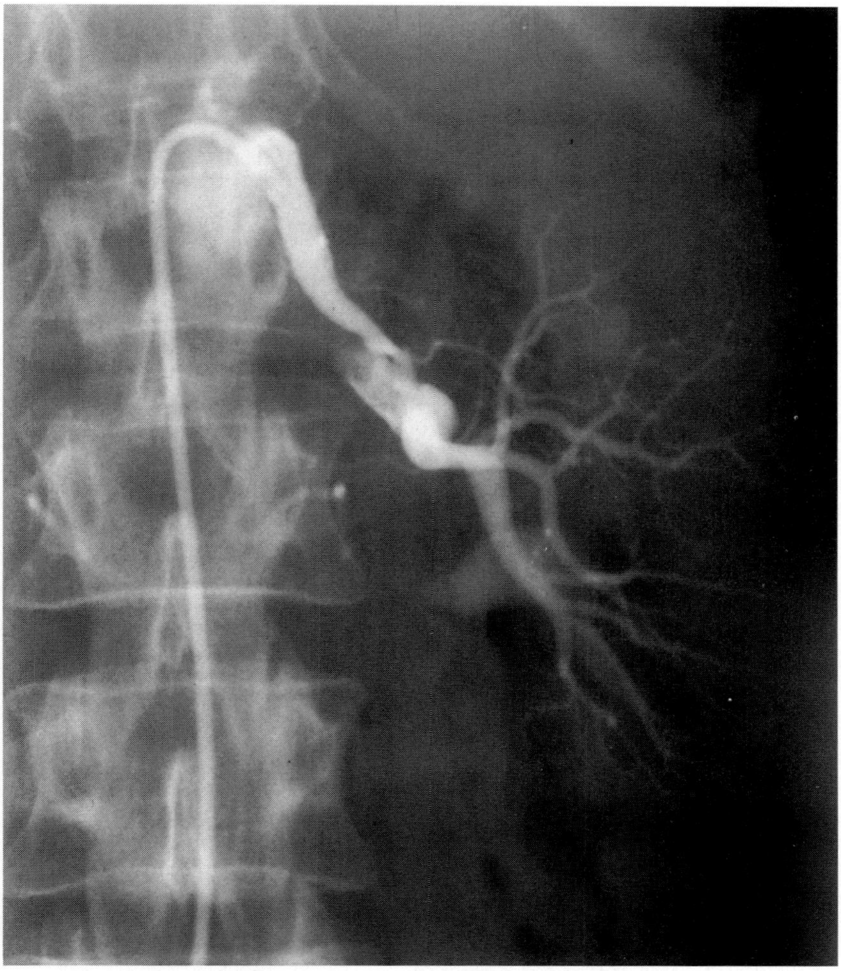

Figure 2–14. Saccular dissecting aneurysm of the main renal artery. Reprinted with permission from Gewertz BL, Stanley JC, Fry WJ. Renal artery dissections. Arch Surg 112:409–414, 1977.

Arteriosclerosis has been implicated as a cause of certain renal artery aneurysms. Medial thinning is a recognized part of the arteriosclerotic process and may serve as a precursor to aneurysmal dilation in rare cases. However, it is distinctly unusual for arteriosclerosis to affect the distal renal artery branchings where most macroaneurysms develop, and it is more likely to be a secondary event rather than a cause of these aneurysms. The fact that arteriosclerotic changes affect some but not all aneurysms in patients having multiple lesions, supports a nonarteriosclerotic cause of most renal artery aneurysms.[51–55]

The natural history of renal artery aneurysms is poorly defined. The majority of renal artery aneurysms are asymptomatic.[52–54] However, aneurysmal expansion, compression of nearby structures, and renal infarction from dislodged thrombus may occasionally be responsible for flank or abdominal pain. The potential for renal artery aneurysms to cause hypertension has been a subject of continued controversy.[50,56–58] Embolization of aneurysmal thrombus, or thrombotic occlusion of an adjacent artery may result in renal ischemia and renovascular hypertension. This is uncommon, being a clear cause of secondary hypertension in less than 3% of patients with renal artery aneurysms.[51] Atheromatous plaque ulceration within large aneurysmal sacs may predispose to this complication. Compression of a neighboring artery has been proposed as cause of renovascular hypertension, but such has rarely been documented.

Rupture is the most serious complication attending renal artery aneurysms. Exsanguinating hemorrhage from a ruptured renal artery aneurysm occurs less often than suggested in earlier reports. Mortality with rupture is approximately 10%. However, loss of a kidney is a near universal sequela of rupture.[51,58] Rupture among cases reported in the literature approaches 3%. Overt extraparenchymal rupture occurred in 2.8% of patients harboring these lesions, and covert rupture causing renal arteriovenous fistulas occurred in an additional 2.8% of one large series.[51] Higher frequencies of rupture, as noted in the earlier literature, have not been confirmed in more recent reports.[50,52,60] In fact, bland renal artery aneurysm rupture is likely to be considerably less common than previously thought. Aneurysmal rupture during pregnancy is an exception.[60–62] Rupture with pregnancy does not appear related to age, increased blood pressure, or number of pregnancies,[62] and unfortunately is responsible for fetal death in nearly 85% of cases, and is associated with a 55% maternal mortality.[61]

An increased risk of renal artery aneurysm rupture has been attributed to large size, absence of calcification, and elevated blood pressure. However, these factors are not always relevant. In fact, overt rupture often has been observed to occur in normotensive patients as well as with calcific atherosclerotic aneurysms.[51] Similarly, size is of limited value as an indicator of rupture potential, with the statistical validity of rupture occurring in larger aneurysms not forthcoming from the largest clinical experiences. Nevertheless, size remains a logical factor in assessing risk of rupture.

Dissecting Renal Artery Aneurysms

Isolated renal artery dissections causing aneurysms are rare.[48] Dissections are usually classified into two categories, including one group being due to blunt abdominal trauma or intraluminal catheter-induced injury, and a second group occurring spontaneously **(Fig. 2–14)**. Dissections of the renal artery affect men nearly ten times as often as women.[63] In part, this reflects the greater frequency of trauma-induced dissections in men. The predilection for right renal artery involvement may reflect ptosis-related physical stresses affecting the renal pedicle on that side. This may contribute to a greater likelihood for traumatic dissections, as well as development of fibrodysplasia which predisposes to spontaneous dissections. Approximately one third of renal artery dissections are bilateral. Factors contributing to dissecting aneurysms vary among the different categories of dissection. However, shear forces, and flow turbulence affect propagation of all dissections.

Two specific mechanisms contribute to renal artery dissections due to blunt abdominal trauma. The first is displacement of the kidney with deceleration causing marked stretching of the artery with fracture of the intima. The intima is the least elastic vessel wall component, and tears result in subintimal dissection. The second mechanism relates to the unyielding posteriorly located vertebral bodies. Direct trauma to renal arteries with compression against the vertebra may cause medial hemorrhage and false aneurysm formation due to rupture of vasa vasorum or actual vessel wall disruption.

Iatrogenic catheter-related renal artery dissections occurring during arteriography appears to be an uncommon cause of these lesions. In one series only four renal artery catheter dissections were encountered among more than 11,000 abdominal arteriographic examinations, including more than 2,200 selective renal arteriograms.[48] These iatrogenic dissections are more likely to occur in arteriosclerotic compared to dysplastic renal arteries, and are usually subintimal in location.

Primary or spontaneous dissections, causing pseudoaneurysms, affect the renal arteries more than any other peripheral artery. They may be related to coexistent arteriosclerotic or dysplastic renovascular disease.[51,64] Some have reported nearly a 9% incidence of dissections in patients with fibrodysplastic renal arteries,[65] yet others have encountered dissection in only 0.5% of similar patients.[48] Spontaneous dissections usually occur within the outer media adjacent to the external elastic lamina, and less commonly within the central media. This is in contradistinction to the inner location of traumatic dissections. In many instances these dissections have been attributed to rupture of abnormal vasa vasorum. The subsequent dissecting intramural hematoma may increase medial ischemia and contribute to further aneurysm formation. Spontaneous renal artery dissections usually affect proximal vessels, and terminate just proximal to sites of branching.

The natural history of renal artery dissections are poorly defined. Pain, hematuria, and elevated blood pressure frequently accompany acute dissections regardless of the cause.[48,66] Certain chronic renal artery dissections are associated with renovascular hypertension or impaired renal function. However, many dissections may be self-limited, asymptomatic, and of no functional importance.

REFERENCES

1. Holley KE, Hunt JC, Brown AL Jr, Kincaid OW, Sheps SG. Renal artery stenosis: a clinical-pathologic study in normotensive and hypertensive patients. *Am J Med* 1964;37:14.
2. Schwart CJ, White TA. Stenosis of renal artery. *Br Med J* 1964;2: 1415.
3. Whitehouse WM Jr, Kazmers A, Zelenock GB, Erlandson EE, Cronenwett JL, Lindenauer SM, Stanley JC. Chronic total renal artery occlusion. Effects of treatment on secondary hypertension and renal function. *Surgery* 1981;89:753–763.
4. Schreiber MJ, Pohl MA, Novic AC. The natural history of atherosclerotic and fibrous renal artery disease. *Urol Clin North Am* 1984; 383–392.
5. Tollefson DFJ, Ernst CB: Natural history of atherosclerotic renal artery stenosis associated with aortic disease. *J Vasc Surg* 1991;14: 327–331.
6. Zierler RE, Bergelin RO, Isaacson JA, Strandness DE Jr. Natural history of atherosclerotic renal artery stenosis: A prospective study with duplex ultrasonography. *J Vasc Surg* 1994;19:250–258.
7. Rimmer JM, Gennari FJ. Atherosclerotic renovascular disease and progressive renal failure. *Ann Intern Med* 1993;118:712–719.
8. Stanley JC, Gewertz BC, Bove EL, Sottiurai V, Fry WJ. Arterial fibrodysplasia. Histopathologic character and current etiologic concepts. *Arch Surg* 1975;110:561.
9. Wright I. Age changes in the peripheral arteries in man. *Cardiovasc Anat Pathol* 1964;11:157.
10. Stewart DR, Price RA, Nebesar R, Schuster SR. Progressing peripheral fibromuscular hyperplasia in an infant. A possible manifestation of the rubella syndrome. *Surgery* 1973;73:374.
11. Dornfeld L, Kaufman JJ. Immunologic considerations in renovascular hypertension. *Urol Clin North Am* 1975;2:285.
12. Meaney TF, Dustan HF, McCormack LJ. Natural history of renal arterial disease. *Radiology* 1968;91:881.
13. Goncharenko V, Gerlock AJ, Shaff MI, Hollifield SW. Progression of renal artery fibromuscular dysplasia in 42 patients as seen on angiography. *Radiology* 1981;139:45.
14. Lorelius LE, Hemmingsson A, Hagg A, Morlin C, Aberg A. Progres-

sive fibromuscular dysplasia of the renal artery. *Acta Radiol Diag* 1985;26:705–708.
15. Sheps SG, Kincaid OW, Hunt JC. Serial renal function and angiographic observations in idiopathic fibrous and fibromuscular stenoses of the renal arteries. *Am J Cardiol* 1972;30:55.
16. Stanley JC, Fry WJ. Renovascular hypertension secondary to arterial fibrodysplasia in adults: Criteria for operation and results of surgical therapy. *Arch Surg* 1975;110:922.
17. Cragg AH, Smith TP, Thompson BH, Maroney TP, Stanson AW, Shaw GT, Hunter DW, Cochran ST. Incidental fibromuscular dysplasia in potential renal donors: long-term clinical follow-up. *Radiology* 1989;172:145.
18. Ekelund L, Gerlock J, Molin J, Smith C. Roentgenologic appearance of fibromuscular dysplasia. *Acta Radiol [Diagn] (Stockh)* 1978;19:433.
19. Harrison EG, McCormack LJ. Pathologic classification of renal artery disease in renovascular hypertension. *Mayo Clin Proc* 1971;46:161.
20. McCormick LJ, Noto TJ Jr, Meaney TF, Poutasse EF, Dustan HP. Subadventitial fibroplasia of the renal artery: A disease of young women. *Am Heart J* 1967;73:602.
21. McCormack LJ, Poutasse EF, Meaney TF, Noto TJ, Dustan HP. A pathologic arteriographic correlation of renal arterial disease. *Am Heart J* 1967;73:602.
22. Gladstien K, Rushton AR, Kidd KK. Penetrance estimates and recurrence risks for fibromuscular dysplasia. *Clin Genetics* 1980;17:115.
23. Major P, Genest J, Cartier P, Kuchel O. Hereditary fibromuscular dysplasia with renovascular hypertension. *Ann Intern Med* 1977;86:583.
24. Morimoto S, Kuroda M, Uchida K, Funatsu T, Yamamoto I, Hashiba T, Kametani T, Takeda R, Matsubara. Occurrence of renovascular hypertension in two sisters. *Nephron* 1976;17:314.
25. Rushton AR. The genetics of fibromuscular dysplasia. *Arch Int Med* 1980;140:233.
26. Sang CN, Whelton PK, Hamper UM, Connolly M, Kadir S, White RI, Sanders R, Liang KY, Bias W. Etiologic factors in renovascular fibromuscular dysplasia. *Hypertension* 1989;14:472.
27. de Deeuw D, Donker AJM, Burema J, van der Hem GK, Mandema E. Nephroptosis and hypertension. *Lancet* 1977;1:213.
28. Kaufman JJ, Maxwell MH. Upright aortography in the study of nephroptosis, stenotic lesions of the renal artery, and hypertension. *Surgery* 1963;53:736.
29. Tsukamoto Y, Komuro Y, Akutsu F, Fujii K, Marumo F, Kusano S, Kikawada R. Orthostatic hypertension due to coexistence of renal fibromuscular dysplasia and nephroptosis. *Japan Circ J* 1988;52:1408.
30. Leung DYM, Glagov S, Matthews MB. Cyclic stretching stimulates synthesis of matrix components by arterial smooth muscle cells in vitro. *Science* 1976;191:475.

31. Fievez ML. Fibromuscular dysplasia of arteries: A spastic phenomenon? *Med Hypotheses* 1984;13:341.
32. Paulson GW. Fibromuscular dysplasia, antiovulent drugs, and ergot preparations. *Stroke* 1978;9:172.
33. Hata J-I, Hosoda Y. Perimedial fibroplasia of the renal artery. A light and electron microscopy study. *Arch Pathol Lab Med* 1979;103:220.
34. Sottiurai VS, Fry WJ, Stanley JC. Ultrastructure of medial smooth muscle and myofibroblasts in human arterial dysplasia. *Arch Surg* 1978;113:1280.
35. Sottiurai VS, Fry WJ, Stanley JC. Ultrastructural characteristics of experimental arterial medial fibrodysplasia induced by vasa vasorum occlusion. *J Surg Res* 1978;24:169.
36. Stanley JC, Fry WJ. Pediatric renal artery occlusive disease and renovascular hypertension. Etiology, diagnosis and operative treatment. *Arch Surg* 1981;116:669.
37. Stanley JC, Zelenock GB, Messina LM, Wakefield TW. Pediatric renovascular hypertension: A thirty-year experience of operative treatment. *J Vasc Surg* 1995;21:212–227.
38. Graham LM, Zelenock GB, Erlandson EE, Coran AG, Lindenauer SM, Stanley JC. Abdominal aortic coarctation and segmental hypoplasia. *Surgery* 1979;86:519.
39. Devaney K, Kapur SP, Patterson K, Chandra RS. Pediatric renal artery dysplasia. A morphologic Study. *Ped Pathol* 1991;11:609.
40. Stanley JC, Graham LM, Whitehouse WM Jr, Zelenock GB, Erlandson EE, Cronenwett JL, Lindenauer SM. Developmental occlusive disease of the abdominal aorta, splanchnic and renal arteries. *Am J Surg* 1981;142:190.
41. Maycock Wd'A. Congenital stenosis of the abdominal aorta. *Am Heart J* 1937;13:633.
42. Finley JL, Dabbs DJ. Renal vascular smooth muscle proliferation in neurofibromatosis. *Hum Pathol* 1988;19:107.
43. Halperin M. Currarino G. Vascular lesions causing hypertension in neurofibromatosis. *N Engl J Med* 1965;273:248.
44. Mena E, Bookstein JJ, Holt JF, Fry WJ. Neurofibromatosis and renovascular hypertension in children. *Am J Roentgenol* 1973;118:39.
45. Schurch W, Messerli FH, Genest J, Lefebvre R, Roy R, Cartier P, Rojo-Ortega JM. Arterial hypertension and neurofibromatosis: Renal artery stenosis and coarctation of abdominal aorta. *Can Med Assoc J* 1975;113:878.
46. Plotkin SA, Boue A, Boue JG. The in vitro growth of rubella virus in human embryo cells. *Am J Epideminol* 1965;81:71.
47. Siassi B, Glyman G, Emmanouilides GC. Hypoplasia of the abdominal aorta associated with the rubella syndrome. *Am J Dis Child* 1970; 120:476.
48. Gewertz BL, Stanley JC, Fry WJ. Renal artery dissections. *Arch Surg* 1977;112:409–414.
49. Hubert JP Jr, Pairolero PC, Kazmier FJ. Solitary renal artery aneurysm. *Surgery* 1980;88:557–565.

50. Martin RS III, Meacham PW, Ditesheim JA, Mulherin JL Jr, Edwards WH. Renal artery aneurysm: selective treatment for hypertension and prevention of rupture. *J Vasc Surg* 1989;9:26–34.
51. Stanley JC, Rhodes EL, Gewertz BL, Chang CY, Walter JF, Fry WJ. Renal artery aneurysms: significance of macroaneurysms exclusive of dissections and fibrodysplastic mural dilations. *Arch Surg* 1975; 110:1327–1333.
52. Henriksson C, Bjorkerud S, Nilson AE, Pettersson S. Natural history of renal artery aneurysm elucidated by repeated angiography and pathoanatomical studies. *Eur Urol* 1985;11:244–248.
53. Henriksson C, Lukes P, Nilson AE, Pettersson S. Angiographically discovered, non-operated renal artery aneurysms. *Scand J Urol Nephrol* 1984;18:59–62.
54. Tham G, Ekelund L, Herrlin K, Lindstedt EL, Olin T, Bergentz SE. Renal artery aneurysms. Natural history and prognosis. *Ann Surg* 1983;197:348–352.
55. Edsman G. Angiography and suprarenal angiography. *Acta Radiol* 1965;suppl 155:104–116.
56. Cummings KB, Lecky JW, Kaufman JJ. Renal artery aneurysms and hypertension. *J Urol* 1973;109:144–148.
57. Ruberti U, Miani S, Scorza R, Mingazzini P, Biasi GM. Aneurysm of the renal artery. *Int Angiol* 1987;6:407–414.
58. Vaughan TJ, Barry WF, Jeffords DL and Johnsrude IS. Renal artery aneurysms and hypertension. *Radiology* 1971;99:287–293.
59. Hageman JH, Smith RF, Szilagyi DE, Elliott JP. Aneurysms of the renal artery: Problems of prognosis and surgical management. *Surgery* 1978;84:563–572.
60. Burt RL, Johnson FR, Silverthorne RG, Lock FR, Dickerson AJ. Ruptured renal artery aneurysm in pregnancy: Report of a case with survival. *Obstet Gynecol* 1956;7:229–233.
61. Cohen JR, Shamash FS. Ruptured renal artery aneurysms during pregnancy. *J Vasc Surg* 1987;6:51–59.
62. Cohen SG, Cashdan A, Burger R. Spontaneous rupture of a renal artery aneurysm during pregnancy. *Obstet Gynecol* 1972;39:897–902.
63. Edwards BS, Stanson AW, Holley KE, Sheps SG. Isolated renal artery dissection: Presentation, evaluation, management and pathology. *Mayo Clin Proc* 1982;57:564–571.
64. Hare WSC, Kincaid-Smith P. Dissecting aneurysm of the renal artery. *Radiology* 1970;97:255–263.
65. Harrison EG Jr, Hunt JC, Bernatz PE. Morphology of fibromuscular dysplasia of the renal artery in renovascular hypertension. *Am J Med* 1967;43:97–117.
66. Rao CN and Blaivas JG. Primary renal artery dissecting aneurysm: A review. *J Urol* 1977;118:716–719.

3

Diagnosis of Renovascular Hypertension: An Overview

George H. Meier

Although hypertension remains common in Western society, renovascular disease accounts for less than 5% of these patients. Therefore, the goal of diagnostic testing is twofold: first, to screen a given population for the likelihood of renovascular disease; and second, to characterize the renovascular disease once diagnosed. These two goals of diagnosis require different approaches, with significant differences in risks and benefits.

The diagnosis of renovascular hypertension is difficult for many reasons. The anatomic definition of renovascular disease currently requires that angiography be used before planning any intervention. Angiography is an invasive procedure with slight but measurable risks.[1] The risk of most concern in renovascular disease is that of dye-induced renal dysfunction, which occurs in 11% of patients with a serum creatinine level of 1.5 mg/dl or greater.[2] Because many of these patients with renovascular disease have renal dysfunction at baseline, the added risk of renal compromise with angiography is a significant deterrent to its routine use. Before recommending angiography for the diagnosis of possible renovascular disease, some method of increasing the likelihood of a positive test is needed to minimize complications in those patients who do not benefit (i.e., when the test result is negative). Therefore, perhaps the major limitation of diagnostic testing in renovascular hypertension is the low prevalence of disease, particularly relative to the risk of angiography.

Two strategies exist for altering the risk–benefit ratio of a given diagnostic test, in this case angiography. The obvious first option is to lower the risk of the angiogram. Currently no other test exists that can provide the anatomic detail needed for most renovascular intervention. Nonetheless, numerous techniques are currently under investigation to lower the risk of testing and will be discussed in later sections. The second strategy for improving the risk–benefit ratio is to increase the potential benefit to the patient

Table 3–1. Predictive Value of Tests for Renovascular Hypertension

	Predictive Value	
Disease Prevalence	Positive (%)	Negative (%)
1	16	99.9
2	28	99.9
5	50	99.7
10	68	99.4
20	83	98.7

subjected to arteriography. Because the test has a predetermined usefulness in renovascular disease, the only method of increasing benefit is to increase the likelihood of renovascular disease in any given patient subjected to angiography. As most statisticians are aware, the prevalence of a disease process in a population to be diagnosed affects the predictive value of testing (also referred to as Bayes Theorem). If the disease is rare **(Table 3–1)**, then the positive test is more likely to be a false-positive than a true positive. With increasing disease prevalence, the positive predictive value improves. If 5% of hypertension is secondary to renovascular causes, then any diagnostic test is likely to have poor positive predictive value. Therefore, the population subjected to testing must be enriched prior to invasive diagnostic workup.

Increasing the prevalence of renovascular disease in a patient population undergoing testing can be accomplished in two ways. The simplest is the use of clinical criteria to help define patients at risk for renovascular disease.[3] Numerous clinical criteria have been used to define populations at increased risk for renovascular hypertension **(Table 3–2)**. These criteria provide a guideline for

Table 3–2. Clinical Clues Suggesting Renovascular Hypertension

Systolic/diastolic epigastric, subcostal or flank bruit
Accelerated or malignant hypertension
Unilateral small kidney discovered by any clinical study
Severe hypertension in child or young adult, or after age 50 years
Sudden development or worsening of hypertension at any age
Hypertension and unexplained impairment of renal function
Sudden worsening of renal function in hypertensive patient
Hypertension refractory to three-drug regimen
Impairment in renal function in response to angiotensin-converting enzyme inhibitor
Extensive occlusive disease in coronary, cerebral, and peripheral circulation

which patients should be subjected to further diagnostic testing.

The second method to enrich the population subjected to invasive diagnostic testing is the use of combinations of tests. This is often the next approach after screening for clinical criteria as outlined above. To effectively use this method, the specificity of the combined tests must remain high or conflicting data will result. Any conflicting data may then require additional testing to resolve. If the combined specificity is high, then the sensitivity of testing can usually be improved by using multiple tests prior to subjecting the patient to angiography.

A second major problem in diagnosing renovascular hypertension is the confounding relationships between renal physiology and renal anatomy. Although certain tests such as angiography are accurate at defining anatomy, the underlying physiology is the "gold standard" for determining the need for intervention. The relationship between end-stage renal parenchymal disease and physiology also clouds the diagnosis, since physiologic testing may be compromised in the presence of end organ renal damage. Finally, antihypertensive agents alter the physiology in unpredictable ways.[33] Some agents directly alter the levels of vasoactive substances while others simply alter the physiology by lowering blood pressure. The result of such alterations is similar: the value of the diagnostic test is compromised and the results may be confusing. Cessation of all antihypertensive therapy has been proposed to improve accuracy in this setting. This approach has an obvious negative impact on those patients with poor blood pressure control undergoing diagnostic testing. Furthermore, the modern long-acting antihypertensive agents require two or more weeks to clear, exposing the patient to prolonged risk from uncontrolled hypertension if these agents are stopped. The ideal diagnostic test should be independent of antihypertensive therapy to avoid this pitfall.

In a series of classic experiments originally published in 1934,[4] Goldblatt opened the modern era of renovascular physiology. In his model, partially occlusive clips were placed over one or both renal arteries in dogs. If a partially occlusive clip is placed in a dog with a normal contralateral kidney, hypertension develops rapidly. When the clip is removed, the hypertension resolves. This model is referred to as one-clip, two-kidney hypertension. The clinical implication is that repair of a unilateral renal artery stenosis should result in resolution of renovascular hypertension. These individuals have increased renin in the clipped kidney with suppression of the contralateral side, mild sodium retention, and increased sodium and water excretion by the contralateral kidney.[5] Elevated renin levels are found in this model in both the acute and chronic phases.[6] Despite these generalizations, with protracted occlusion, the renin levels decrease toward normal even in this hyperreninemic model.[7]

Because revascularization of the kidney was not yet feasible when Goldblatt described his models, early trials focused on nephrectomy to resolve the hypertension associated with unilateral renal artery stenosis.[8] Although these trials met with some success,[9] the high incidence of therapeutic failure led to limited use of nephrectomy for renovascular hypertension.[10]

The second Goldblatt model is both more intriguing and confusing. If a partially occlusive clip is placed on both renal arteries, hypertension also develops rapidly. In contrast to the first model, renin levels are increased only transiently.[11–13] If the clips are removed, the hypertension does not always improve. The implications of this two-clip, two kidney or one-clip, one-kidney hypertension are fundamentally different than those associated with the previous model. In this setting, hypertension will at some point become irreversible and therefore untreatable by revascularization.

The planning of diagnostic tests is influenced by the disease process undergoing evaluation. Two fundamental disease processes are responsible for the majority of the renovascular hypertension seen clinically. Most common in Western countries is atherosclerotic renovascular disease. Typically renal disease in this setting is an extension of generalized atherosclerosis elsewhere in the body. The pattern is often one of bilateral involvement, primarily of the main renal arteries. The incidence of renal dysfunction is high in these patients secondary to the diffuse involvement of both kidneys in many patients. This disease entity correlates well with Goldblatt's two-kidney, two-clip model.

The second common disease entity is that of fibromuscular dysplasia. Although this is actually a group of different disease entities, the overall characteristics are similar.[14] Typically these diseases involve younger patients, extending into middle age. The involvement in this disease group affects the branch vessels commonly as well as the main renal arteries. Bilateral involvement is possible, but unilateral disease is more common. These patients are more similar to Goldblatt's one-clip, two-kidney hypertension.

Although the definition of renovascular hypertension seems clear to most clinicians, the definition of what constitutes renovascular hypertension in research studies is much less clear. For example, some researchers define the coexistence of hypertension and renovascular disease as renovascular hypertension. In this setting, repair of the renovascular disease will not necessarily improve hypertension control. Alternatively, some studies define renovascular hypertension as the presence of hypertension, renovascular disease, and positive physiologic studies consistent with the diagnosis. With this definition, some patients with renovascular hypertension will not meet the criteria for diagnosis. Previous outcome studies after renal vein renin measurements have shown that up to 83% of patients without lateralizing renal vein renins will respond to surgical revascularization.[15,16] Therefore, this definition is too restrictive. A clearer definition is that renovascular hypertension exists when there is coexistence of hypertension and renovascular disease and repair of the renal artery disease results in improvement of hypertension control. When one reviews any clinical study, the definition used to define renovascular hypertension is critical to the interpretation of the results.

The diagnosis of renovascular hypertension must be a summation of both anatomic and physiologic data. No single diagnostic test is sufficient to warrant intervention in renovascular disease. The choice of what diagnostic testing is appropriate remains controversial and confusing. Nonetheless, certain generalizations arise. Prior to subjecting a patient with compromised renal perfusion to the risks of arteriography, some method of screening is essential. Even after subjecting a patient to anatomic definition via arteriography, additional testing may be needed to better define the underlying physiology responsible for hypertension.

Although much of this introductory discussion has centered on diagnosis in renovascular hypertension, additional complexities are added when intervention for renal dysfunction is included. The presence of significant renal impairment complicates the diagnosis by lowering the sensitivity and specificity of any diagnostic test. The salvage of renal function to preclude dialysis may require minimal functional renal parenchyma, yet the prediction of this residual is difficult. If the patient is at low risk for intervention, the clinician is often led to perform a therapeutic trial of intervention without a clear prediction of success. When the patient is at high risk, the decision-making concerning intervention for renal salvage can be extremely difficult. Nonetheless, suggestive signs for successful renal salvage are present in many patients and will be discussed in subsequent sections.

DIAGNOSTIC TESTS TO SCREEN FOR RENOVASCULAR DISEASE

History and Physical Exam

As previously outlined, the first clinical tool for the diagnosis of renovascular disease is the clinical history and physical findings of the patient presenting for diagnosis. While these criteria are helpful, none are foolproof, and some may even be misleading. Short duration or rapidly progressive hypertension are both relative terms that are difficult to quantitate. Similarly, poor control of blood pressure on multiple medications is as likely a result of poor patient compliance as renovascular hypertension. Extremes of age as a clinical indicator of renovascular disease is more reliable, yet excludes a number of patients, particularly those at risk for fibromuscular dysplasia.

What then is the ideal clinical scenario for renovascular hypertension? With atherosclerotic renovascular disease, the patient is typically older than 60 years, has poor blood pressure control on three or more medications, and has evidence of atherosclerosis in other vascular beds. Baseline tests reveal a normal or elevated serum creatinine level, a diastolic blood pressure of greater than 110 mm Hg, less than 500 mg per 24 hours of proteinuria, and a decreased renal size by ultrasound on at least one side. For fibromuscular dysplasia, rapid progression and poor blood pressure control predominate. The "typical" patient in either case is the exception, and the clinician is cautioned against the strict application of any specific clinical criteria.

Hypertensive Urography

In the 1970s, the intravenous pyelogram (IVP) was recognized as an important diagnostic test for renovascular disease in most medical centers.[17] The IVP remains one of the standard tests for the evaluation of renal abnormalities. Despite the retained utility in this group, the use of rapid sequence IVP in renovascular hypertension has been limited as newer tests have replaced it.

In a large cooperative trial in the 1970s, 1100 urograms were reviewed for diagnosis of renovascular hypertension.[18] From this large evaluation several signs were defined indicative of renovascular hypertension. The use of this test was severely limited in bilateral renovascular disease in this study, however. Virtually all signs of renovascular disease on the IVP rely on a comparison of one kidney relative to the other. In addition, segmental renal artery disease is poorly defined since the uptake in the kidney is generally viewed as a qualitative whole, preventing analysis of intra-renal differences. In spite of these limitations, the principles derived from rapid sequence IVP are important in the development of subsequent tests.

The most important sign from the rapid sequence IVP is a unilateral delay in the appearance of contrast medium on one side. After rapid injection of contrast, films are obtained at 1, 2, 3, 5, and 15 minutes. A difference of one or more minutes in the opacification of any calyx on the two sides is considered significant and indicative of a reduced blood flow to the delayed kidney. This is the single most valuable urographic feature of renovascular hypertension, seen in 2% of cases of essential hypertension, versus 59% in renovascular disease.[17]

A second finding indicative of renovascular disease on IVP is a difference of renal length of 1.5 cm or greater. The right kidney is usually slightly larger than the left.[19] Formulae for determining renal length disparity have been derived and provide some improvement over general qualitative analysis.[17] The final IVP finding suggestive of renovascular disease is that of contrast hyperconcentration on the abnormal side. The limited blood flow to an involved kidney leads to a unilaterally decreased GFR and delayed excretion of contrast in the tubules on late films. Bilateral hyperconcentration has also been shown to predict contrast induced renal dysfunction in patients following angiography.[20]

By combining these three signs, the largest series of rapid sequence IVPs revealed abnormal findings in 78% of patients with renovascular disease, versus 11% when the arteriogram was normal.[21] The overall positive predictive value in this population was 31%. As a result of this and other studies, alternative tests have replaced rapid sequence IVP as a diagnostic modality in renovascular disease.

Renal Scintigraphy

Radioisotope renal scintigraphy was first proposed in 1956 as a simpler method of screening for renovascular disease.[22] Initially, renal scintigraphy was used much as the rapid sequence intravenous pyelogram, evaluating differences in one kidney relative to the other. In this method, ^{131}I-hippuran is injected intravenously and monitored for renal uptake and excretion. Delayed uptake and delayed excretion with hyperconcentration are positive studies, similar to rapid sequence IVP. This technique of renal scintigraphy serves as an indirect measurement of effective renal plasma flow, producing analogous images to the rapid sequence intravenous pyelogram.[23] In multiple studies similar limitations were seen to those noted with conventional IVP.[24,25,26]

A significant advance in renal scintigraphy occurred in the late 1970s when the use of rapid sequence imaging with the tracer ^{99m}Tc-diethylenetriamine pentaacetic acid (DTPA) became common. At about the same time, computer analysis of the uptake and excretion of DTPA allowed accurate estimation of GFR.[27] The result of these two developments was a resurgence in the clinical use of renal scintigraphy in screening for renovascular disease. These advances allowed the independent assessment of each kidney with estimation of the contribution of each kidney to overall renal function. Segmental arterial disease could be assessed by computer analysis of different renal segments and abnormalities of GFR could be assessed in each kidney separately. Therefore, some of the limitations to conventional hippuran renography could be overcome. Collective results of three major series[25,28,29] suggest a combined sensitivity of about 86% and a specificity of 89%.

The use of renal scintigraphy in renovascular hypertension has expanded rapidly with the development of "stress" renal scintigraphy. In this method, captopril or exercise is used to induce a decrease in GFR which can be measured on each side independently. This technique will be discussed later in this chapter, both in its use as a screening test as well as role in defining renal physiology.

Duplex Ultrasonography

Duplex ultrasonography has advanced significantly in the past 20 years, and extensive experience has been acquired in renovascular disease. While a complete discussion of the use of ultrasound in renovascular disease is beyond the scope of this chapter, an overview is appropriate for a complete discussion of renovascular diagnosis. Ultrasound has virtually replaced IVP as the technique for sizing the kidneys. Gross anatomic details can easily be seen with ultrasound, allowing delineation of hydronephrosis and cysts. In any patient with renal dysfunction, ultrasound is often the initial test of choice to better define renal gross anatomy.

Modern ultrasound, however, goes beyond mere anatomic data. Most current hardware combines B-mode ultrasound with pulsed Doppler ultrasound, the combination commonly termed duplex ultrasound. As a result, anatomic detail can be obtained along with flow correlations to better define the physiology of renal blood flow. In screening for renovascular disease with ultrasound, recent series have demonstrated a sensitivity of 84 per cent with a specificity of 97 per cent, giving an overall accuracy of 93 per cent.[30] Unfortunately, these results are not duplicated in many centers. The use of an experienced, dedicated technologist is essential for consistent results in these time-consuming, tedious examinations. Until these screening results can be uniformly replicated, duplex ultrasound will occupy a limited role in renovascular diagnosis, restricted to those centers with demonstrated expertise.

Peripheral Renin Sampling

With the clinical introduction of plasma renin assays in the late 1960s, the hope for a blood test to define renovascular hypertension became closer to reality. Renin was first described by Tigerstadt and Bergmann in 1898.[31] Since that time its role in renovascular hypertension was suspected but poorly defined. With the development of angiotensin converting enzyme inhibitors in the early 1970's[32] significant insight into the renal physiology underlying renovascular hypertension was finally realized. Therefore, the next logical step was the use of renin assays to help define the presence or absence of renovascular hypertension.

Early use of peripheral renin sampling was based on the theoretical relationship between renal vein renin production and peripheral renin levels.[33] As further experience with renal revascularization accrued, it became apparent that a large percentage of patients with normal peripheral renin levels were cured of hypertension by renal revascularization.[15] From this experience, numerous causes for alteration of renin levels were defined. The most significant of these related the plasma renin level to the individual's sodium balance.[34] As urinary excretion of sodium (and therefore sodium intake) goes down, renin levels go up. Therefore, using a ratio of peripheral renin level to urinary sodium excretion improves diagnostic accuracy, identifying 80% of patients with unilateral renovascular disease (as defined by improvement by renal revascularization).[35]

A second major limitation of peripheral renin measurement became apparent at about the same time. Virtually every antihypertensive medication in use has some effect on peripheral renin levels.[33] Thus, all antihypertensives must be stopped for at least two weeks prior to peripheral renin sampling to maximize reproducibility. The implications of this maneuver in the severely hypertensive patient are clear and often dramatic.

The Captopril Test

When saralasin became available as the first experimental angiotensin II inhibitor, early experience demonstrated augmentation of renin secretion with angiotensin inhibitors or angiotensin converting enzyme inhibitors in renovascular disease.[36] Therefore, proponents of peripheral renin sampling began using oral captopril to stimulate renin levels prior to testing. Using this protocol, patients were maintained on a normal or high sodium diet to minimize false positive tests and most antihypertensive medications were withdrawn for two weeks. This method improved diagnostic accuracy significantly compared with most other screening tests.[37] Nonetheless, the severe changes in pre-test blood pressure medications as well as the difficulty in controlling the methodology has limited the usefulness of this test to a few centers with extensive experience.[38]

DIAGNOSTIC TESTS FOR RENAL PHYSIOLOGY

Although the detection of renal artery disease is an important first step in the treatment of renovascular disease, the significance of any arterial disease to the kidney resides in the physiologic importance of such disease. Previous studies have confirmed the possibility of significant renovascular disease coexisting with normal blood pressure.[39] In addition, the identification of curable renovascular hypertension remains more art than science.[40] If a procedure to revascularize the kidney could be done without morbidity or mortality, then the physiology behind renovascular disease would be less important than the anatomic presence of disease. However, many of these patients have multisystem disease and are at high risk for surgical or endovascular intervention. This results in an ongoing quest for renal physiologic confirmation before vascular intervention.

Split Renal Function Studies

The earliest attempts to assess individual differences in renal physiology originated in the 1950s with the use of ureteral catheters to quantitate individual kidney urine output and quality.[41] With reduction in renal blood flow, the affected kidney compensates by increasing the concentration of the urine being produced, in an effort to increase intravascular volume. The result is that the involved kidney produces less urine, excretes less sodium, and excretes a higher creatinine concentration (due to increased water resorption) than the normal kidney.[42]

Because renal functional assessment in this method samples the kidney as a whole, significant limitations exist. Specifically, segmental renal arteries or bilateral disease can yield erroneous results using this method. To improve this technique, modifications have been proposed.[43] Despite these and other modifications, the value of the test in predicting reversible renovascular hypertension is limited.[42]

The current role of split renal function measurements is in conjunction with renal vein renin assessments. If the renal vein renins are indeterminate, then split renal function may be helpful. Split renal function provides an accurate assessment of the reversibility of renovascular disease when combined in this manner.[44,45] Finally, the uncommon need to determine residual renal function remains an occasional indication for split renal function measurement.[46]

Early experience with captopril administration while measuring split renal function documented a decrease in GFR with captopril when an inflow stenosis was present.[47] Although this will be discussed more completely in the stress renal scintigraphy section, this change is predictive of a physiologically significant renal artery stenosis and reversible renovascular hypertension.[48]

Selective Renal Vein Renin Sampling

Because the determinations of renin levels in the peripheral circulation were unsatisfactory in diagnosing renovascular hypertension, a more selective method of renin determination was used in the early 1970s. Specifically, selective measurement of renal vein renin levels seemed a logical means of detecting Goldblatt's one-clip, two-kidney hypertension. In this technique, the level of renin excretion by each kidney is measured and compared. A positive result is generally considered to be a renin ratio of 1.5 or greater compared to the contralateral kidney.[4] Early results using this method described satisfactory results when revascularization was limited to these patients.[49] Despite these reports, additional experience suggested that significant numbers of patients with non-lateralizing renal vein renins also benefited from renal revascularization.[32,15] As a result, further refinements of selective renal vein renin sampling were undertaken to standardize testing. Methods have been defined to improve the determination in bilateral disease as well.[50]

Numerous factors influence the levels of renin measured. Of major importance, most antihypertensive agents have an influence on renin levels.[51] Volume status and sodium intake similarly alter renin excretion.[33,52] Postural changes, particularly on awakening, also can increase the renin measured.[53] As a result of these variations, extensive protocols have evolved to better standardize renin measurements.[49,54] Nonetheless, proponents of selective renal vein renin assays readily admit the limited usefulness of this testing modality in bilateral disease or in segmental artery disease.[53]

The use of selective renal vein renin determinations is useful in selected clinical scenarios. This is particularly true relative to the patient with an occlusion contralateral to a stenosis. The question of revascularization versus nephrectomy in this setting may be aided by the lateralization of the selective renal vein renins. If the renal vein renins are non-lateralizing or lateralize to the stenotic side, then revascularization is warranted to improve hypertension control. If on the other hand the measurements lateralize to the occluded side, then nephrectomy (or bypass of the occluded renal artery) may be necessary to provide this improvement.

The fastest-growing segment of patients having renal revascularization are those who undergo the procedure for renal salvage, either alone or in combination with renovascular hypertension.[55] In the setting of operation for renal salvage, selective renal vein renin measurements have little use. The variability introduced by bilateral disease associated with renal dysfunction makes the determinations confusing at best. Therefore, the use of selective renal vein renin sampling is limited to patients being investigated for renovascular hypertension alone.

Stress Renal Scintigraphy

As computer analyzed renal scintigraphy became widely available in the 1980s, the limitations of diagnosis using this test were rapidly reached. Renal scintigraphy could accurately estimate GFR,[26] but this loss of GFR could be due to either loss of renal plasma flow from renovascular disease or loss of glomerula from end stage parenchymal disease. Although the decrease in renal function was equivalent, the ability to treat the underlying causes was quite different. Therefore, efforts to uncover renal changes suggestive of in-flow stenosis were undertaken.

At about the same time, a series of reports began to appear in the European literature documenting renal dysfunction induced by the use of captopril.[56,57] As further evaluation of these patients was done, the presence of bilateral renovascular disease or unilateral disease in a solitary kidney appeared to be the common denominator.[58] Further investigation using split renal function studies documented a reversible decrease in renal function induced by the administration of captopril.[59] This change appeared to be independent in each kidney; that is, if in-flow stenosis was present, renal function often decreased in response to captopril administration. This explained the normal renal function after captopril seen with unilateral renal artery stenosis: the normal kidney maintained GFR unless it, too, was diseased.

In 1987, the first reports of exercise-induced renal dysfunction in normal hypertensive patients appeared.[60] Further evaluation revealed the correlation of an absence of this response to the presence of renal artery disease.[61] With these sets of observations stress renal scintigraphy became a viable modality for the diagnosis of renovascular hypertension, both using pharmacologic stress and exercise.

Captopril

Because the initial experience with stress renal scintigraphy was with captopril, this modality was the obvious choice for early evaluation. With physiologic studies the mechanism behind the renal dysfunction began to be better defined. In the normal setting, transglomerular filtration is maintained by regulation of in-flow pressure by the afferent arteriolar sphincter and out-flow pressure by the efferent sphincter **(Fig. 3–1)**. With significant renal artery in-flow disease, the afferent sphincter remains maximally vasodi-

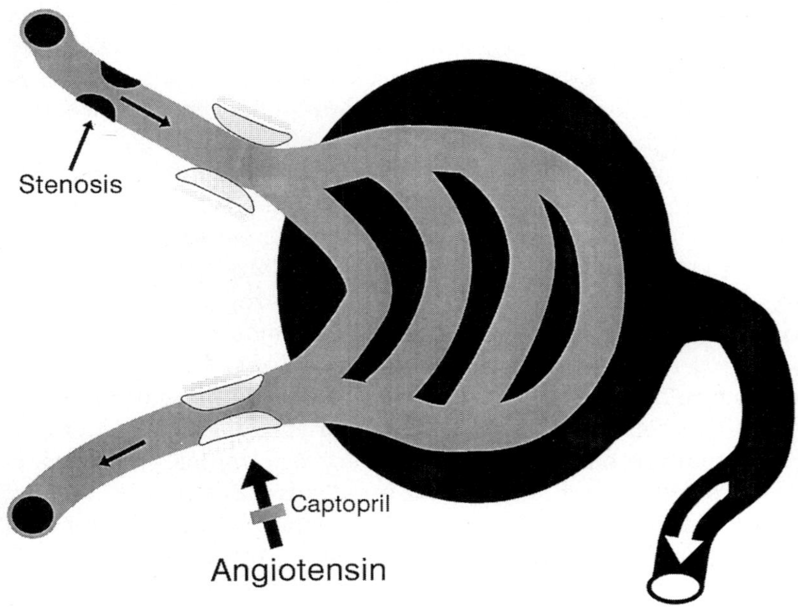

Figure 3–1. The effect of captopril with renal artery stenosis. In the presence of an inflow stenosis, the efferent sphincter is maximally dilated. The tone of the afferent sphincter is increased to maintain transglomerular filtration. Captopril blocks the effect of angiotensin within the kidney, resulting in loss of filtration and therefore loss of GFR.

lated. To maintain transglomerular filtration pressure, the efferent sphincter must be more vasoconstricted. This action is dependent on angiotensin, acting within the kidney. Captopril causes loss of efferent sphincter tone, reducing transglomerular filtration and therefore GFR. In normal kidneys, the tone in both sphincters is lost together after captopril, resulting in no net change to GFR. Therefore the challenge is the determination of unilateral loss of renal function following captopril administration.

With modern computerized DPTA renal scintigraphy, the assessment of serial renal function measurements in each kidney independently was readily available at most medical centers. From the combination of this technique with captopril administration, stress renal scintigraphy was developed. To perform this test, all angiotensin converting enzyme inhibitors are withheld for 7 to 14 days. On the day of the examination, a standard DPTA renogram with computer estimation of GFR is done as a baseline. A dose of 50 mg of captopril is given, followed by a repeat renal scintigram. Two types of positive results are sought: first, any significant asymmetry in blood flow in the baseline scan suggests the presence of renovascular disease. Second, any increase in accumulation of radioactive tracer in either kidney after captopril suggests in-flow stenosis. This increase is most commonly associated with the time to peak activity of the renal uptake curve. Normally, the time to peak activity is less than 11 minutes. If this increases to greater than 11 minutes, then a captopril-induced change is present. In this way, baseline renal scintigraphy is augmented by physiologic stress to improve the diagnostic accuracy.[60]

Initial experience with captopril renal scintigraphy as a screening modality for renovascular hypertension suggested high sensitivity and specificity.[62,63] **Table 3–3** summarizes the results of captopril renal scintigraphy as the initial test for screening for renovascular hypertension. These results can be maintained in the setting of renal dysfunction or bilateral disease.[64] Captopril renal scintigraphy provides effective screening for renovascular hypertension,[65–70] but its use in renal salvage is limited.

An additional insight into renal physiology is obtained from the evaluation of captopril-induced changes in the renal scintigram. When the renogram changes from normal pre-captopril to abnormal post-captopril, the kidney is angiotensin dependent for maintenance of GFR. Evaluation of revascularization in these patients suggests that this change predicts reversibility of renovascular hypertension[47,71] with a high sensitivity and specificity. Theoretically, this correlates with the stage prior to Goldblatt's irreversible one clip, one kidney hypertension. While Goldblatt's observations did not include prediction of this reversibility, this has been recognized clinically.[72] The prediction of the transition from reversible to irreversible one clip, one kidney hypertension has been impossible until captopril stress scintigraphy became widely available. Captopril-induced change appears to predict reversal of one clip,

Table 3–3. Results of Captopril Scintigraphy

Author	Reference Number	Number of Patients	Number with Renal Artery Disease	Sensitivity	Specificity
Elliott, 1993	70	150	59	91	91
Frommei, 1991	69	424	230	84	92
Svetkey, 1991	68	140	31	74	44
Setaro, 1991	63	94	44	91	94
Chen, 1990	62	50	23	91	93
Dondi, 1989	61	105	50	92	97
Kremer-Hovinga, 1989	67	15	15	86	—
Sfakianakis, 1988	66	31	16	71	—
Maher, 1988	65	44	13	85	72

two kidney (high renin) as well as of one clip, one kidney (low renin) hypertension. If further study supports this observation, then the evaluation prior to treatment of renovascular hypertension will by necessity include captopril renal scintigraphy. If a captopril-induced change in the renogram occurs, then treatment of that kidney by revascularization will be warranted; in the absence of such changes, revascularization would primarily be indicated for renal salvage.

EXERCISE

A transient, postural and exercise mediated change in baseline renograms has been noted and evaluated in Germany.[59] Specifically, *o*-iodohippurate scintigraphy is commonly abnormal after exercise in patients with essential hypertension,[73] a change which is not seen in normotensive patients. In patients with renovascular disease, both normal and abnormal responses are seen.[60] When revascularization is performed, abnormal exercise renograms (similar to the scans of patients with essential hypertension) correlate strongly with irreversible hypertension. Similarly, normal preoperative exercise renograms suggest reversible hypertension in patients with renal artery disease. The implications of these observations remain confusing. Further work to define the physiology associated with exercise induced renal perfusion changes in patients with essential hypertension will be needed before the implications of this observation can be fully understood. Furthermore, the relationship of this observation is unclear relative to the better understood changes associated with captopril in renal artery disease. In atherosclerosis, its use is obviously limited by the extensive extra-renal disease, commonly with associated claudication and coronary disease. In this setting exercise stress is often ill-advised.

RENAL BIOPSY

Although renal biopsy has been done for years, its utility lies in the benefit of the biopsy relative to its risk. The benefit of biopsy relies on the demonstration of normal glomerular architecture on histologic staining. If the sampling of glomerula is representative of the kidney as a whole, then end-organ damage can be accurately assessed. Unfortunately, biopsies may correlate poorly with overall renal parenchymal disease, depending on the region sampled. The risk of renal loss is the major concern relative to biopsy, but generally appears unjustified.[74] Histologically, renal biopsy segments are examined for the presence of glomerular disease, usually glomerulosclerosis. In the presence of isolated renovascular disease, glomerular damage would be unusual. Therefore, the absence of glomerular damage might logically predict which kidneys to revascularize to salvage renal function.

If this were the only issue, then biopsies would be clearly useful. However, the risk of biopsy is not minor, with evidence of hematoma by CT scan in up to 90% of patients.[75] The addition of ultrasound guidance has improved the overall results, but the risk of bleeding remains similar.[76] The major risk is bleeding which occurs as gross hematuria in about 10%.[77] Newer techniques of percutaneous transvenous needle biopsy may reduce the risk[78] while allowing improved renal sampling. Further experience is needed before biopsy will again be considered valuable.

DIAGNOSTIC TESTS FOR RENAL ANATOMY

In preparation for revascularization, anatomic information is needed to plan the procedure. Currently, no single test provides the anatomic detail needed for intervention, while at the same time defining the underlying physiology. As a result, the current method of evaluation requires combining tests to provide both physiologic as well as anatomic data.

The current standard for anatomic testing is angiography, which has been in use for many years. Newer modalities such as magnetic resonance angiography hold the promise of changing the diagnostic workup of renovascular disease, but require further improvement before these can replace angiography as the standard.

Angiography (Conventional and Carbon Dioxide)

The use of angiography in renovascular disease is important to the effective diagnosis and treatment of renal artery disease. Currently it remains unequalled in defining the anatomy associated with renal artery disease. The addition of digital subtraction techniques has decreased the amount of contrast required, lowering the risk of dye-induced renal dysfunction. Current angiographic techniques are both safe and effective diagnostic tools.[79]

Conventional angiography is associated with problems that limit its effectiveness and continue the search for a more ideal diagnostic test. The obvious limitation in patients with renal artery disease is the nephrotoxicity associated with the use of conventional iodinated contrast. This limitation is particularly problematic in those patients being evaluated for salvage of renal function. In these patients, the serum creatinine level is usually elevated at baseline, increasing the risk of dye-induced renal dysfunction. Newer contrast agents with decreased osmolarity have not dramatically reduced the incidence of dye-induced renal dysfunction.[80–82] As a result, other techniques have been used to lower renal toxicity. The most commonly used technique is carbon dioxide angiography.[83] While a complete discussion of this is beyond the scope of this chapter, the use of carbon dioxide gas lowers both resolution and renal toxicity. Nonetheless, in certain clinical settings this technique can prove useful.

An additional limitation of angiography is the difficulty in defining anatomy at the renal artery origin. The anatomic detail in this region often requires multiple series of films, exposing the patient to added risk with each additional contrast injection. Success in defining the renal artery anatomy relies on the experience and expertise of the angiographer. Therefore, the technique is operator dependent in "real" time; that is, the operator must make decisions concerning the anatomy and the adequacy of the films during the procedure, with no opportunity for post-procedure data processing.

Finally, angiography remains an invasive procedure requiring the insertion and manipulation of catheters. This is always a disadvantage both in terms of cost and risk.

Spiral Computed Tomography

Conventional computed tomography (CT) of the abdominal aorta provides limited resolution of renal and visceral arteries due to loss of registration between tomographic slices, as well as loss of resolution due to motion during the acquisition of the images. As a result, its utility in renal artery disease has been quite limited. Recently, however, a new technique has overcome some of the technical limitations of conventional CT scans. Called spiral CT, this study involves continuous tube rotation with continuous table feed. The result is rapid acquisition of images, usually requiring less than a minute for a typical abdominal CT.[84] With this rapid image acquisition the issue of motion is reduced or eliminated. In addition, the combination of high dose, short duration contrast with this technique allows a spiral CT angiogram to be performed.[76] With advanced computer processing, three dimensional surface mapping as well as maximum intensity projections can be derived to produce high quality images of the abdominal aorta and its branches.

Early experience with this technique is promising.[85,86] Specifically, a sensitivity of 92% with a specificity of 83% was obtained when compared to conventional renal arteriography.[78] The limitations of this technique are the post-processing image analysis techniques and the need for doses of contrast similar to those used for conventional arteriography.[77] The post-processing techniques will improve as new software allows better analysis of the images captured. The need for contrast remains a concern in patients with pre-existent renal dysfunction. Therefore the role for spiral CT currently remains limited to research studies until additional data concerning its efficacy is available.

Magnetic Resonance Arteriography

Nuclear magnetic resonance has been used as an experimental tool for research in chemistry and physics for at least 40 years. Advances in technology have allowed the computer analysis necessary for imaging in three dimensions. As a result, clinical experience with magnetic resonance imaging (MRI) is limited to the past ten years in this rapidly evolving technique.

Magnetic resonance imaging relies on the analysis of radiofrequency resonation in unpaired protons (usually hydrogen) exposed to pulsed magnetic field gradients. When these unpaired protons are subjected to a external magnetic field, they align themselves along the axis of the primary magnetic field. With the application of a radiofrequency pulse a secondary magnetic field is created which tips the axis away from the primary magnetic field. The rotation of these tipped magnetic dipoles generates a radiofrequency signal, whose frequency is dependent on the strength of the magnetic field. By varying the magnetic gradient in defined ways, spatial orientation in three dimensions can be determined. In addition, the magnetic gradients can be varied in any plane, allowing reconstruction of the radiofrequency signal in any two dimensional plane. For a more complete explanation of MRI, the reader is referred to recent review articles.[87,88,89]

To provide better blood flow data, MRI has been modified to examine the patterns of blood flow directly, visually representing the MR data similar to an angiogram. In order to allow vessel reconstruction, the most common technique, referred to as the "bright blood" technique, provides saturation pulses in the plane of imaging, allowing in-flowing blood which has not been saturated to remain bright. By stacking multiple thin slices on top of each other, a two or three dimensional reconstruction can be made to provide an anatomic outline similar to an angiogram. One of the limitations in this technique is the artifact introduced by this stacking process: if the scanned segments are not aligned, there will be an artifact generated by the misalignment. These limitations appear to be addressed by the three-dimensional technique.[90,91,92]

The MRA signal strength does not require injection of contrast, but relies on the flow of blood to provide the contrast necessary for the image. Nonetheless, multiple other mechanisms can induce the loss of MRA signal. The most common is the loss of flow associated with a stenosis, resulting from the slowing of blood before and after a stenosis. At slow flow rates, the blood becomes saturated and does not flow quickly enough to bring high-signal blood into the segment being studied. In this setting, a stenosis may appear to be a complete occlusion, overestimating the degree of stenosis. Similarly, turbulent flow around the area of a stenosis may cause signal dropout from the summation of multiple vectors to a net vector of zero. The result is that differentiation of high grade stenoses from complete occlusions can be difficult.

In the renal arteries, additional technical restrictions exist which limit the quality of magnetic resonance imaging. The major problem in renal MRA is the application of the second magnetic field. Usually this field is best when applied at 90° to the direction of blood flow. In the case of the renal arteries, the arteries run perpendicular to the primary magnetic field. Application of a secondary magnetic field perpendicular to the axis of the renal artery is difficult. Therefore, this secondary magnetic field is oblique to the direction of renal artery blood flow, as well as the primary magnetic field. This results in diminished signal strength and thus the quality of renal artery imaging can be compromised.

Early results from renal MRA document the promise of this technique.[93–96] In addition, recent evidence supports the use of this modality as a screening tool for renovascular disease.[97,98] Renal MRA is undergoing numerous technical modifications and the standard technique is currently evolving. Nonetheless, this method of evaluation holds the most promise of any renal diagnostic modality.

CURRENT RECOMMENDATIONS

The evaluation of a patient with poorly controlled hypertension for renovascular causes is an inexact science, subject to personal preference and intrinsic bias. Nonetheless, several generalizations can be made. First, the selection of patients for further workup of renovascular disease is made by clinical criteria applied by an experienced observer. This leads the clinician to a suspicion of renovascular disease, enriching the population subjected to screening. As a single step, this is perhaps the most important to providing effective diagnosis of renovascular disease.

Second, a screening test is applied to the enriched population of patients. This screening modality is perhaps the most variable segment of evaluation. Centers with great expertise with the captopril test prefer this modality, while others prefer captopril stress scintigraphy. Some centers have gained sufficient expertise with alternative diagnostic tests to prefer these to more conventional tests. The important issue is that a screening test be applied to an enriched population, varying the specific test with the expertise of the center involved. Ideally, the screening modality should have a high sensitivity, with equal or lower specificity. In this manner, all patients at risk are captured, further enriching the screened population.

Finally, a definitive anatomic test is performed on a further enriched cohort. This test remains angiography at most centers in spite of the potential renal toxicity. In the future, magnetic resonance angiography may replace conventional angiography, but MRA is currently limited to research settings.

Additional testing will always be needed in special circumstances. Additional definition by selective renal vein renins can be quite useful in renal artery occlusions, particularly with bilateral renal artery disease. Ultrasound measurement of renal span and cortical thickness can help guide decisions concerning potential salvage of a diseased kidney. Nonetheless, these tests often provide secondary information in the assessment of risk and benefit for a given patient and as a result are not used in the initial diagnosis of renovascular disease.

The diagnosis of renovascular hypertension is often more straightforward than the diagnosis of renal dysfunction due to renovascular disease. The patient with renal dysfunction is often at an advanced stage of disease, with extensive extra-renal atherosclerosis. Often these patients have already started dialysis, limiting the potential benefit of renovascular diagnosis. If not yet on dialysis, then the risk of acute renal failure after angiography often prohibits complete diagnosis. As a result, many of these patients proceed undiagnosed to chronic dialysis.

CONCLUSIONS

The diagnosis of renovascular disease remains an art, rather than a science. Because no ideal test exists, the combination of clinical expertise with a battery of diagnostic tests is necessary to effectively diagnose this disease. Further refinements in technology promise improved noninvasive diagnosis in the future. Magnetic resonance imaging holds the promise of both physiologic and anatomic diagnosis in a single modality.

With the aging population in the United States, more advanced atherosclerotic disease is inevitable. Therefore, renovascular disease is expected to increase in frequency as well. The diagnosis of these diseases will also change as the incidence in the general population changes. As a result, the diagnostic path for renovascular disease will change as experience and expertise change. Although no one can fully anticipate the innovations to come, improvements and altered diagnostic pathways are guaranteed by the level of research ongoing in this difficult entity.

REFERENCES

1. Reiss MD, Bookstein JJ, Bleifer KH. Radiologic aspects of renovascular hypertension. Part IV. Arteriographic complications. *JAMA* 1972; 221:374–378.
2. Solomon R, Werner C, Mann D, D'Elia J, Silva P. Effects of saline, mannitol, and furosemide on acute decreases in renal function induced by radiocontrast agents. *N Engl J Med* 1994;331:1416–1420.
3. Working group on renovascular hypertension. Detection, evaluation, and treatment of renovascular hypertension. Final report. *Arch Int Med* 1987;147:820–829.
4. Goldblatt H, Lynch J, Hanzel RF, Summerville WD. Studies in experimental hypertension. I. The production of persistent elevation of systemic blood pressure by means of renal ischemia. *J Exp Med* 1934; 59:347–79.
5. Gross F. The renin-angiotensin system in hypertension. *Ann Intern Med* 1971;75:777–787.
6. Möhring J, Möhring B, Naumann HJ, et al. Salt and water balance and renin activity in renal hypertension of rats. *Am J Physiol* 1975; 288:1847–1855.
7. Gavras H, Brunner HR, Thurston H, Laragh JH. Reciprocation of renin dependency with sodium volume dependency in renal hypertension. *Science* 1975;188:1316–1317.
8. Leadbetter WF, Burkland CE. Hypertension in unilateral renal disease. *J Urol* 1938;39:611–626.
9. Boyd CH, Lewis LG. Nephrectomy for arterial hypertension. Preliminary report. *J Urol* 1938;39:627–635.
10. Smith HW. Unilateral nephrectomy in hypertensive disease. *J Urol.* 1956;76:685–701.
11. Ayers CR, Harris RH, Lefer LG. Control of renin release in experimental hypertension. *Circ Res* 1969;24(5 Suppl):103–112.
12. Bianchi G, Tenconi LT, Lucca R, et al. Effect in the conscious dog of constriction of the renal artery to a sole remaining kidney on hemodynamics, sodium balance, body fluid volume, plasma renin concentration and pressor responsiveness to angiotensin. *Clin Sci* 1970;38: 741–766.
13. Liard JF, Cowley AW, McCaa RE, Guyton AC. Renin, aldosterone, body fluid volumes, and the baroreceptor reflex in the development and reversal of Goldblatt hypertension in conscious dogs. *Circ Res* 1974;34:549–560.
14. Youngberg SP, Sheps SG, Strong CG. Fibromuscular stenosis of the renal arteries. *Med Clin North Am* 1977;61:623–641.

15. Marks LS, Maxwell MH. Renal Vein Renin Value and Limitations in the Prediction of Operative Results. *Urol Clin North Am* 1975;2: 311–325.
16. Marks LS, Maxwell MH, Varady PD, Lupu AN, Kaufman JJ. Renovascular hypertension: does the renal vein renin ratio predict operative results? *J Urol* 1976;115:365–368.
17. Russell RP. Renal hypertension. *Surg Clin North Am* 1974;54: 349–361.
18. Bookstein JJ, Abrams HL, Buenger RE, et al. Radiological aspects of renovascular hypertension. Part I: The role of urography in unilateral renovascular disease. *JAMA* 1972;220:1225–1230.
19. Moell H. Size of normal kidneys. *Acta Radiol* 1956;46:640–645.
20. Boijsen M, Granerus G, Jacobsson L, Bjorneld L, Aurell M, Tylen U. Glomerular filtration rate estimated after multiple injections of contrast medium during angiography. *Acta Radiol* 1988;29:669–674.
21. Maxwell MH, Bleifer KH, Franklin SS, Varady PD. Cooperative study of renovascular hypertension: demographic analysis of the study. *JAMA* 1972;220:1195–1204.
22. Winter CC. A clinical study of a new renal function test. The radioactive diodrast renogram. *J Urol* 1956;76:182–196.
23. Britton KE and Maisey MN. Renal radionuclide studies. In Maisey, Britton KE, and Gilday DC(eds.): Clinical Nuclear Medicine. Philadelphia, W.B. Saunders Co, 1983, p93.
24. Burbank MK, Hunt JC, Tauxe WN, Maher FT. Radioisotope renography: diagnosis of renal arterial disease in hypertensive patients. *Circulation* 1963;27:328–338.
25. Giese J, Mogensen P, Munck O. Diagnostic value of renography for detection of unilateral renal or renovascular disease in hypertensive patients. *Scand J Clin Lab Invest* 1975;35:307–310.
26. Arlart L, Rosenthal J, Adam WE, Bargon G, Franz HE. Predictive value of radionuclide methods in the diagnosis of unilateral renovascular hypertension. *Cardiovasc Radiol* 1979;1:115–125.
27. Gates GF. Glomerular Filtration Rate: Estimation from Fractional Renal Accumulation of 99m Tc-DTPA (stannous). *Am J Roentgenol* 1982;138:565–570.
28. McAfee JG, Thomas FD, Grossman Z, Streeten DH, Dailey E, Gagne G. Diagnosis of angiotensinogenic hypertension: the complementary roles renal scintigraphy and the saralasin infusion test. *J Nucl Med* 1977;18:669–675.
29. Chiarini C, Esposti ED, Losinno F, et al. Renal scintigraphy versus renal vein renin activity for identifying and treatment of renovascular hypertension. *Nephron* 1982;32:8–13.
30. Taylor DC, Kettler MD, Moneta GL et al. Duplex ultrasound in the diagnosis of renal artery stenosis: a prospective evaluation. *J Vasc Surg* 1988;7:363–369.
31. Tigerstadt R and Bergman PG. Niere und kreislauf. *Skandin Arch F Physiol* 1898;8:223–271.
32. Brunner HR, Kirshman JD, Sealey JE, Laragh JH. Hypertension of

renal origin: evidence for two different mechanisms. *Science* 1971; 174:1344–1346.
33. Sealey JE, Buhler FR, Laragh JH, Vaughan ED. The physiology of renin secretion in essential hypertension: estimation of renin secretion rate and renal plasma blood flow from peripheral and renal vein renin levels. *Am J Med* 1973;55:391–401.
34. Laragh JH, Baer L, Brunner HR, Buhler FR, Sealey JE, and Vaughan ED. Renin, angiotensin and aldosterone system in pathogenesis and management of hypertensive vascular disease. *Am J Med* 1972;52: 633–652.
35. Pickering TG, Sos TA, Vaughan ED, et al. Predictive value and changes of renin secretion in hypertensive patients with unilateral renovascular disease undergoing successful renal angioplasty. *Am J Med* 1984;76:398–404.
36. Case DB, Laragh JH. Reactive hyperreninemia in renovascular hypertension after angiotensin blockade with saralasin or converting enzyme inhibitor. *Ann Intern Med* 1979;91:153–160.
37. Muller FB, Sealey JE, Case DB, et al. The captopril test for identifying renovascular disease in hypertensive patients. *Am J Med* 1986; 80:633–644.
38. Dean RH. Functional significance of renal arterial occlusive disease. In: Ernst CB, Stanley JC, eds. *Current Therapy in Vascular Surgery.* Second edition. Philadelphia: B.C. Decker; 1991, pp 827–831.
39. Eyler WR, Clark MD, Garman JE, Rian RL, Meininger DE. Angiography of the renal areas including a comparative study of renal arterial stenosis in patients with and without hypertension. *Radiology* 1962; 78:879–892.
40. Foster JH, Maxwell MH, Franklin SS, et al. Renovascular occlusive disease: Results of operative treatment. *JAMA* 1975;231:1043–1048.
41. Connor TB, Berthrong M, Thomas WC, Howard JE. Hypertension due to unilateral renal disease with a report on a functional test helpful in diagnosis. *Bull Johns Hopkins Hosp* 1957;100:241–276.
42. Howard JE and Connor TB. Use of differential renal function studies in the diagnosis of renovascular hypertension. *Am J Surg* 1964;107: 58–66.
43. Maxwell MH, Lupu AN, Kaufmann JJ. Individual kidney function tests in renal arterial hypertension. *J Urol* 1968;100:384–394.
44. Dean RH, Lawson JD, Hollifield JW, Polterauer P, Rhamy RK. Revascularization of the poorly functioning kidney. *Surgery* 1979;85: 44–52.
45. Schaeffer AJ, Fair WR. Comparison of split function ratios with renal-vein renin ratios in patients with curable hypertension caused by unilateral real artery stenosis. *J Urol* 1974;112:697–701.
46. Vaughan ED, Buhler FR, Laragh JH, Sealey JE, Gavras H, Baer L. Hypertension and unilateral parenchymal renal disease: evidence for abnormal vasoconstriction-volume interactions. *JAMA* 1975;233: 1177–1183.
47. Miyamori I, Yasuhara S, Takeda Y, et al. Effects of converting en-

zyme inhibition on split in renovascular hypertension. *Hypertension* 1986;8:415–421.

48. Meier GH, Sumpio B, Setaro JF, Black HR, Gusberg RJ. Captopril renal scintigraphy: a new standard for predicting outcome after renal revascularization. *J Vasc Surg* 1993;17:280–287.
49. Winer BM, Lubbe WF, Simon M, Williams JA. Renin in the diagnosis of renovascular hypertension. *JAMA* 1967;202:121–128.
50. Vaughan ED, Buhler FR, Laragh JH, Sealey JE, Baer L, Bard RH. Renovascular hypertension: renin measurements to indicate hypersecretion and contralateral suppression, estimate renal plasma flow, and score for surgical curability. *Am J Med* 1973;55:402–414.
51. Johnston CI. Effect of antihypertensive drugs on the renin-angiotensin system. *Drugs* 1976;12:274–291.
52. Strong GG, Hunt JC, Sheps SG, Tucker RM, Bernatz PE. Renal venous renin activity: enhancement of sensitivity of lateralization by sodium depletion. *Am J Cardiol* 1971;27:602–608.
53. Cohen EL, Rovner DR, Conn JW. Postural augmentation of plasma renin activity. Importance in diagnosis of renovascular hypertension. *JAMA* 1966;197:973–978.
54. Dean RH. Functional significance of renal arterial occlusive disease. In Ernst CE and Stanley JC (eds), Current Therapy in Vascular Surgery, Second edition. B.C. Decker, Philadelphia, Pennsylvania, 1991, 827–831.
55. Dean RH, Lawson JD, Hollifield JW, Shack RB, Polterauer P, Rhamy RK. Revascularization of the poorly functioning kidney. *Surgery* 1979;85:44–52.
56. Collste P, et al. Reversible renal failure during treatment with captopril. *Br Med J* 1979;279:612.
57. Farrow PR, Wilkinson R. Reversible renal failure during treatment with captopril. *Br Med J* 1979;279:1680.
58. Hricik DE, et al. Captopril-induced functional renal insufficiency in patients with bilateral renal artery stenoses or renal artery stenoses in a solitary kidney. *NEJM* 1983;308:373–376.
59. Miyamori I, et al. Effects of Converting Enzyme Inhibition on Split Renal Function in Renovascular Hypertension. *Hypertension* 1986; 8:415–421.
60. Clorius JH, Schmidlin P. The exercise renogram: a new approach documents renal involvement in systemic hypertension. *J Nucl Med* 1983;24:104–109.
61. Clorius JH, Allenberg J, Hupp T, et al. Predictive value of exercise renography for presurgical evaluation of nephrogenic hypertension. *Hypertension* 1987;10:280–286.
62. Dondi M, Franchi R, Levorato M, et al. Evaluation of hypertensive patients by means of captopril enhanced renal scintigraphy with technicium-99m DTPA. *J Nucl Med* 1989;30:615–621.
63. Chen CC, Hoffer PB, Vahjen G, et al. Patients at high risk for renal

artery stenosis: a simple method of renal scintigraphic analysis with Tc-99m DTPA and captopril. *Radiology* 1990;176:365–70.

64. Setaro JF, et al. Simplified captopril renography in diagnosis and treatment of renal artery stenosis. *Hypertension* 1991;18:289–298.
65. Maher ER, Othman S, Frankel AH, et al. Captopril-enhanced 99m-TC DTPA scintigraphy in the detection of renal-artery stenosis. *Nephrol Dial Transplant* 1988;3:608–611.
66. Sfakianakis GN, Jaffe DJ, Bourgoignie JJ. Captopril scintigraphy in the diagnosis of renovascular hypertension. *Kidney Int* 1988;34: 142–144.
67. Kremer-Hovinga TK, de Jong PE, Piers DA, Beekhuis H, van der Hem GK, de Zeeuw D. Diagnostic use of angiotensin converting enzyme inhibitors in radioisotope evaluation of unilateral renal artery stenosis. *J Nucl Med* 1989;30:605–614.
68. Svetkey LP, Wilkinson R, Dunnick NR, et al. Captopril renography in the diagnosis of renovascular disease. *Am J Hypertens* 1991;4: 711S–715S.
69. Frommei E, Mezzasalma L, Ghione S, et al. European captopril radionuclide test multicenter study. Preliminary results: inspective renographic analysis. *Am J Hypertens* 1991;4:690S–697S.
70. Elliott WJ, Martin WB, Murphy MB. Comparison of two noninvasive screening tests for renovascular hypertension. *Arch Int Med* 1993; 153:755–764.
71. Setaro JF, Saddler MC, Chen CC, et al. Simplified captopril renography in diagnosis and treatment of renal artery stenosis. *Hypertension* 1991;18:289–298.
72. Laragh JH. On the mechanisms and clinical relevance of one-kidney, one-clip hypertension. *Am J Hypertens* 1991;4:541S–545S.
73. Clorius JH, Mann J, Schmidlin P, Strauss LG, Saur T, Irngartinger G. Clinical evaluation of patients with hypertension and exercise-induced renal dysfunction. *Hypertension* 1987;10:287–293.
74. Schow Da, Vinson RK, Morrisseau PM. Percutaneous renal biopsy of the solitary kidney: a contraindication? *J Urol* 1992;147:1235–1237.
75. Ralls PW, Barakos JA, Kapstein EM, et al. Renal biopsy-related hemorrhage: frequency and comparison of CT and sonography. *J Comput Assist Tomogr* 1987;11:1031–1034.
76. McDonald MW, Sosnowski JT, Mahin EJ, Willard DA, and Lamm DL. Automatic spring-loaded biopsy gun with ultrasonic control for renal transplant biopsy. *Urology* 1993;42:580–582.
77. Sweet M, Brouhard BH, Ramirez-Seijas F, Kalia A, and Travis LB. Percutaneous renal biopsy in infants and young children. *Clin Nephrol* 1986;26:192–194.
78. Mal F, Meyrier A, Callard P, Kleinknecht D, Altmann JJ, Beaugrand M. The diagnostic yield of transjugular renal biopsy. Experience in 200 cases. *Kidney Int* 1992;41:445–449.
79. AbuRahma AF, Robinson PA, Boland JP, et al. Complications of arte-

riography in a recent series of 707 cases: factors affecting outcome. *Ann Vasc Surg* 1993;7:122–129.

80. Davidson CJ, Hlatky M, Morris KG, et al. Cardiovascular and renal toxicity of a nonionic radiographic contrast agent after cardiac catheterization: a prospective trial. *Ann Intern Med* 1989;110:119–124.
81. Barrett BJ, Parfrey PS, Vavasour HM, et al. Contrast nephropathy in patients with impaired renal function: high versus low osmolar media. *Kidney Int* 1992;41:1274–1279.
82. Gomes AS, Lois JF, Baker JD, McGlade CT, Bunnell DH, Hartzmann S. Acute renal dysfunction in high-risk patients after angiography: comparison of ionic and nonionic contrast media. *Radiology* 1989; 170:65–68.
83. Seeger JM, Self S, Harward TR, Flynn TC, Hawkins IF. Carbon dioxide gas as an arterial contrast agent. *Ann Surg* 1993;217:688–697.
84. Rubin GD, Dake MD, Napel SA, McDonnell CH, Jeffrey RB. Three-dimensional spiral CT angiography of the abdomen: initial clinical experience. *Radiology* 1993;186:147–152.
85. Galanski M, Prokop M, Chavan A, Schaefer CM, Jandeleit K, Nischelsky JE. Renal arterial stenoses: spiral CT angiography. *Radiology* 1993;189:185–192.
86. Rubin GD, Dake MD, Napel S, et al. Spiral CT of renal artery stenosis: comparison of three-dimensional rendering techniques. *Radiology* 1994;190:181–189.
87. Horowitz AL. *MRI Physics for Physicians.* New York: Springer-Verlag, 1989.
88. Morris PG. *Nuclear Magnetic Resonance Imaging in Medicine and Biology.* Oxford: Clarendon, 1986.
89. Valk J, MacLean C, and Alara PR. *Basic Principles of Nuclear Magnetic Resonance Imaging.* Amsterdam: Elsevier, 1985.
90. Keller P, Drayer B, Fram E, et al. MR angiography with two-dimensional acquisition and three-dimensional display: Work in progress. *Radiology* 1989;173:527–32.
91. Masaryk TJ, Modic MT, Ruggieri PM. Three-dimensional (volume) gradient-echo imaging or the carotid bifurcation: preliminary clinical experience. *Radiology* 1989;171:801-6.
92. Dumoulin C, Cline HE, Souza S, et al. Three-dimensional time-of-flight magnetic resonance angiography using spin saturation. *Magn Reson Med* 1989;11:35–46.
93. Debatin JF, Spritzer CE, Grist TM, et al. Imaging of the renal arteries: value of MR angiography. *Am J Roentgen* 1991;157:981–990.
94. Lewin JS. Time-of-flight magnetic resonance angiography of the aorta and renal arteries. *Invest Radiol* 1992;27(2 Suppl):S84–89.
95. Hertz SM, Holland GA, Baum RA, Haskal ZJ, Carpenter JP. Evaluation of renal artery stenosis by magnetic resonance angiography. *Am J Surg* 1994;168:140–143.
96. Vock P, Terrier F, Wegmuller H, et al. Magnetic resonance angiography of abdominal vessels: early experience using the three-dimensional phase-contrast technique. *Br J Radiol* 1991;64:10–16.

97. Servois V, Laissy JP, Feger C, et al. Two-dimensional time-of-flight magnetic resonance angiography of renal arteries without maximum intensity projection: a prospective comparison with angiography in 21 patients screened for renovascular hypertension. *Cardiovasc Inter Radiol* 1994;17:138–142.
98. Loubeyre P, Revel D, Garcia P, et al. Screening patients for renal artery stenosis: value of three-dimensional time-of-flight MR angiography. *Am J Roentgen* 1994;162:847–852.

4

Diagnosis of Renal Artery Stenosis: Ultrasound and Arteriography

Brian Johnson and
D. Eugene Strandness, Jr.

Renal artery stenosis (RAS) is a cause of hypertension that can be ameliorated or cured by surgery or percutaneous transluminal angioplasty.[1,2] Untreated it can lead to deterioration in renal function, loss of renal mass, and, in extreme cases, complete occlusion of the renal artery.[1,3,4] The diagnosis of high blood pressure secondary to RAS (renovascular hypertension, RVH) is thus very important.

Hypertension is a major public health problem with 10 to 15% of United States citizens, or about 30 million people, requiring treatment.[5] Only 1% of these individuals and certainly no more than 5% will have hypertension primarily due to renal artery stenosis.[6] This estimate agrees well with the prevalence of 3% for RVH among a hypertensive hospital outpatient population.[7]

The main cause of RAS is atherosclerosis (75%) and fibromuscular dysplasia (FMD) is responsible in most of the remainder (20%). Other causes include trauma, arteritis (polyarteritis nodosa, systemic lupus erythematosis, scleroderma and Takayasu's disease) and extrinsic compression by fibrous bands or tumor.[8] Atherosclerosis is the usual cause in elderly patients, while FMD and congenital causes are most common among children and young adults. Atherosclerotic narrowing is usually located at the origin and in the proximal one third of the renal artery, is often accompanied by aortic disease, and may be bilateral in about one third of cases.[9,10] FMD usually affects the middle and distal thirds of the renal artery, as well as the branch arteries near the hilum of the kidney, is largely confined to females and is bilateral in up to 45% of cases.[10] Medial fibrodysplasia is the most common type of FMD and accounts for 85% of cases. The degenerative changes in the media allow for aneurysmal dilatation alternating with fibrous constriction. Intimal fibroplasia accounts for many of the remainder and causes intermittent constricting bands alternating with areas of normal caliber wall, without the tendency to aneurysm formation. The cause of FMD is unknown, but intrauterine viral infections and repeated minor trauma have been suggested.[10]

Attention was focused on the association between RAS and hypertension by Goldblatt in 1934 in a series of canine experiments which demonstrated that persistent hypertension would develop by inducing RAS. Translumbar aortography in the assessment of occlusive vascular disease was popularized in 1929 by dos Santos and one consequence was the first diagnostic test to permit detection of renal artery lesions.[8] Initially, nephrectomy was performed to remove the responsible organ, but a review of the published data to 1956 showed that only 26% patients so treated had better control of their hypertension.[11] The first report of relief of hypertension after revascularization of a kidney was by Freeman et al, but experience over the first 10 years with operations to improve arterial inflow revealed a success rate of only 50%.[1,12]

Attention was turned to degree of stenosis as the important determinant for RVH by the experimental findings of Hamovici and Zinicola in a canine model.[13] They demonstrated that a pressure drop would develop distal to a 60% or greater diameter reduction (representing an 84% decrease in cross-sectional area). About that time, however, Holley et al performed a postmortem study that demonstrated that although 77% patients with a history of hypertension had RAS of >25% and 56% had RAS of >50%, normotensive individuals also had similar degrees of renal artery narrowing in 49% and 17% of cases, respectively.[9] Thus, the association between renal artery narrowing and hypertension is not always a certain one. Essential hypertension is a risk factor for atherosclerosis, and atherosclerosis is the most common cause of RAS. Also, when only one renal artery is significantly narrowed, the gradual development of hypertensive glomerulosclerosis in the contralateral kidney that is "unprotected" from the high perfusion pressure will prevent alleviation of hypertension by surgical correction of the originally responsible RAS.[14]

It is therefore important to demonstrate a causal effect for stenosis of the renal artery in the pathogenesis of hypertension. The criteria that should be met for a firm diagnosis of RVH are: 1) a lesion should be present, 2) it should be hemodynamically significant, and 3) repair of the lesion should be associated with amelioration of hypertension. This implies three stages of assessment: diagnosis, assessment of technical success (a completion study), and postintervention follow-up.

Diagnosis: Clinical Evaluation

The low prevalence of RVH among the general hypertensive population dictates a low predictive value for most diagnostic tests according to Bayes theorem and even a highly specific diagnostic test would result in a considerable number of false positive results and unnecessary interventions.[15,16] Effective antihypertensive drugs, the small but existent mortality of angioplasty and surgery (0.5–1.0% in the best hands) and significant morbidity, which includes early and late failures, demand efficient screening for those patients who will benefit from interventional therapy.[1–2]

Diagnostic accuracy can be improved by selecting subgroups of patients with a greater prevalence of RVH. Clinical factors associated with an increased prevalence of RVH were identified in the Cooperative Study of Renovascular Hypertension but no single factor can be applied with certainty.[17] The available information has been distilled by Gifford and five criteria recommended which increase the likelihood of hypertension being of renovascular origin:[6]

1. A systolic-diastolic bruit in the epigastrium or flank
2. Abrupt onset or exacerbation of hypertension with rapid progression
3. Age of onset of hypertension less than 30 years or more than 55 years
4. Accelerated hypertension (retinopathy grade III or IV)
5. Arteriopathic retinal vascular changes

The greater the number of positive criteria, the greater the likelihood of RVH and the prevalence in such selected populations is often as high as 33%.[18] Severity of hypertension as the sole discriminating factor has been found to be useful by some workers. Dean reported 0 of 102 patients with diastolic blood pressures of less than or equal to 115 mm Hg had RVH, whereas 9 of 35 (26%) patients with diastolic blood pressures of >115 mm Hg had RVH.[19] This same study suggested that racial differences existed and that RVH was predominantly a problem of the white race, but another study that selected patients on the basis of all clinical parameters, rather than the level of diastolic hypertension, did not show a statistical difference between the African American and white races.[20] Ying et al investigated a group of patients with refractory hypertension and found that 39 of 106 (37%) patients had RVH, and when refractory hypertension was associated with an element of renal failure, 10 of 21 (48%) patients had RVH.[21]

Diagnosis: Arteriography and Physiological Tests

Abdominal aortography, using the Seldinger technique via the femoral or brachial route and modern fine bore catheters has few technical complications.[22] However, atheroembolic disease may complicate injection of contrast into the abdominal aorta, especially when there is severe accompanying aortic atheroma and this can cause impaired renal function and accelerated hypertension.[23]

More commonly, impaired renal function related to contrast load in a dose-dependent manner can complicate up to 11% of all examinations, and this figure increases to 42% in the presence of preexisting impaired renal function, with 8% requiring dialysis.[24] Although adverse reactions with newer non-ionic contrast media can be reduced by a factor of 4 or 5, the risk is not insignificant.[25]

Standard aortograms with cut films give a good demonstration of atherosclerotic lesions in the aorta, renal artery origins, and proximal one third of the renal arteries **(Fig. 4–1)**. However, the "string of beads" appearance of medial fibrodysplasia in the distal renal and branch arteries is especially difficult to classify in terms of degree of stenosis from a single frontal view after aortic injection.[3] To better demonstrate the distal renal and branch arteries,

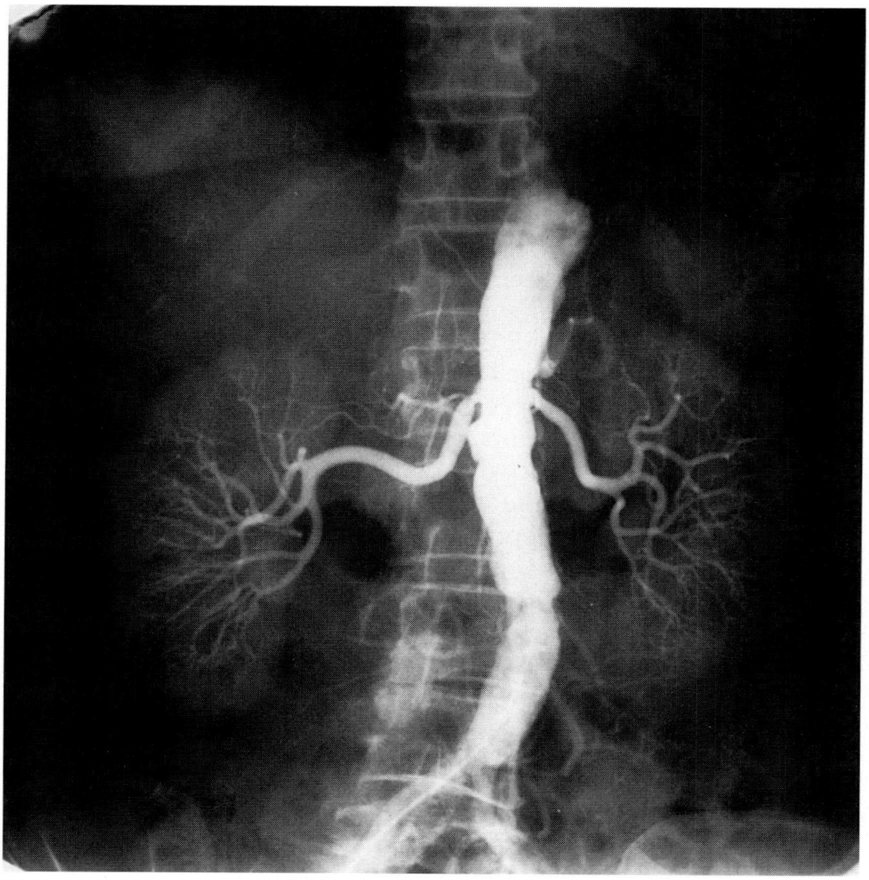

Figure 4–1. Standard cut film frontal aortogram via the right transfemoral approach showing a stenosis in the proximal right renal artery.

bilateral selective renal artery injections with oblique views will improve the diagnostic accuracy, as well as demonstrate parenchymal abnormalities.[10] These manipulations increase the risk from contrast dose and atheroembolism.

Digital subtraction arteriography (DSA) subtracts background bony structures and reduces the concentration of contrast material required. This allows for intravenous injection of the contrast (IVDSA), avoiding arterial puncture, but due to dilution during circulation, the total dose of contrast required is not reduced. Reported sensitivity and specificity in detecting significant RAS is high at 90% but technical factors such as patient movement or bowel gas movement with peristalsis render 7–25% of studies uninterpretable.[14,26] Intraarterial injection for DSA reduces the contrast load, but results in less spatial resolution and therefore loss of image quality, a problem which is shared by IVDSA.[10]

Newer arteriographic methods such as those obtained by computerized tomography (CT) and the more recent development of spiral CT angiography combines intravenous injection with good image quality. There are advantages in that parenchymal disease is easier to detect, but expense and contrast load remain limiting factors. Magnetic resonance arteriography (MRA) is proving to be useful in imaging of the visceral arteries and is non-invasive. However, the long-term safety of MR imaging is not established and improved image quality and contrast techniques are needed before this modality is ready to replace more conventional arteriography.

To determine if an angiographically demonstrated stenosis is responsible for hypertension, and thereby reduce the number of unnecessary interventions, adjunctive tests of the functional significance of the lesion have been used. These tests make use of impaired renal perfusion, or the physiological renin response to impaired perfusion.[14] Rapid sequence intravenous urography, split renal function tests and isotope renography suffer from relatively low sensitivity (70–80%) and specificity (85%) or their invasive nature, and exposure to contrast injection and ionizing radiation have limited their applicability.[10] Improved results can be achieved by stopping antihypertensive medication prior to the test, but this is rarely practicable when hypertension which is difficult to control is the prime indication. Plasma renin activity can be measured either in the peripheral blood as an office procedure, or in renal vein effluent (RVR) during central venous cannulation. The sensitivity and specificity of these tests are similar to those reported for tests of renal perfusion, but their performance can be improved in conjunction with captopril, an angiotensin converting enzyme (ACE) inhibitor drug, with sensitivities >80% and specificities >90%.[14] However, in the presence of RAS, ACE inhibitors can cause worsening of renal function and should be used with caution when RVH is suspected.

If split renal function tests and RVR are positive, then a good blood pressure response to successful operation can be expected in 95% cases.[1] However, even in the absence of lateralization with RVR, 50% of patients with RVH respond to surgical correction of RAS.[27] A major drawback of function tests is their inability to demonstrate the anatomy of the vascular lesion.[10] Their performance is also impaired in the presence of bilateral RAS and renal failure, which may be present in 30–50% patients. Even when these tests are negative, if the clinical evidence is overwhelmingly in favor of RVH, physicians who have a special interest in RVH will still resort to arteriography.[19]

Duplex ultrasound has the advantage of being able to provide physiological data related to accurately localized sites in the renal arteries and is rapidly gaining acceptance as a useful modality to screen patients before arteriography.[1,28]

Duplex Ultrasound in RVH

Duplex ultrasound is able to provide both anatomic and physiologic information in the same test. It has the potential to detect renal artery stenosis and renal parenchymal abnormalities.

Technically, renal artery duplex requires the highest degree of skill and adequate time (1–2 hr). Patient factors that interfere with the examination and prevent adequate visualization are bowel gas, obesity and recent surgical scars. Only the first of these is controllable to any degree and examination early in the morning after an overnight fast helps to avoid interference from bowel gas. With appropriate scheduling 90% examinations can be completed at the first attempt.[28,30–31] Some workers have not enjoyed such success but with repeat preparation for those incomplete studies, a satisfactory examination is often achieved at the second attempt.[29,32]

The availability of low frequency transducers, color imaging, and better scanhead design facilitate the examination. Two complimentary approaches are used, a midline epigastric approach with the patient lying supine and a flank approach with the patient in the lateral decubitus position. With the patient supine, and the scanhead just below and to the left of the xiphisternum, a longitudinal view of the aorta is obtained. This allows visualization of the celiac and superior mesenteric arteries. By rotating the scanhead 90 degrees counter clockwise and angling it inferiorly, the left renal vein can be seen crossing the aorta and the renal arteries identified arising from the lateral sides of the aorta. The right is usually anterior to and the left posterior to the mid-coronal plane of the aorta. Color flow imaging can be very helpful to identify the origin and course of the renal arteries, especially on the right where it passes behind the inferior vena cava. This is the best approach to visualize and record Doppler spectral data from the origin, proximal and mid renal artery. The flank approach with either lateral or posterior imaging of the kidney allows measurement of renal size and spectral traces to be obtained from the renal parenchyma, hilum and the distal, mid and proximal renal artery to be recorded. These last recordings can serve as a useful check for those velocities recorded from the anterior approach, as it can be difficult to be certain of the angle of the Doppler beam used for data collection from these deeply placed arteries.

The Doppler spectral waveform of the renal artery is characteristic with no reverse flow and a high end diastolic velocity, similar to the internal carotid arterial waveform as the kidney, like the brain, offers low vascular resistance. This feature helps to identify the renal artery. It is ten years since Norris et al. documented waveform changes, notably spectral broadening and an increased peak systolic velocity (PSV) with duplex Doppler assessment of RAS.[34] To avoid loss of the Doppler signal due to respiratory movement, a larger sample volume is used which encompasses the entire renal artery. This results in spectral broadening of the waveform, a feature which in the center stream of the carotid artery would indicate turbulent flow due to disease, but in the renal artery waveform obtained in this way may be normal. In our laboratory, spectral broadening is not used to assess disease in the renal artery. The most important parameter is the PSV and its change over the length of the renal artery. With the velocity waveform taken at a Doppler angle of 60 degrees it has been shown that a focal PSV >180 cm/s is consistent with the presence of at least minimal disease[28] **(Fig. 4–2)** This finding alone is not used to detect those lesions that are hemodynamically significant.

It is the degree of stenosis that determines hemodynamic significance as shown by the experiments of Hamovici and Zinicola.[13] When comparing Doppler spectral criteria with arteriographically determined stenosis, Avasthi et al found that a PSV of 100 cm/s differentiated a <50% stenosis from one of >50%, whereas Miralles et al found a PSV >210 cm/s determined a >60% stenosis.[33,35] The inherent error of velocity calculation from Doppler spectra with linear array scanheads was demonstrated by Daigle et al but maintaining an angle of 60 degrees or less minimizes this error.[36]

We have used two approaches to overcome the problems inherent in using absolute PSV data to classify stenosis in this location. The first is to always take measurements as close to a 60 degree Doppler angle as possible, and the second strategy is to use the patient as their own control by calculating a ratio of the maximum renal artery peak velocity to the maximum aortic peak velocity, the renal aortic ratio (RAR). The aortic velocity spectrum is taken at a 60 degree Doppler angle from the region of the superior mesenteric artery in the longitudinal scan at the beginning of the examination. The PSV in the aorta may be reduced by aneurysmal

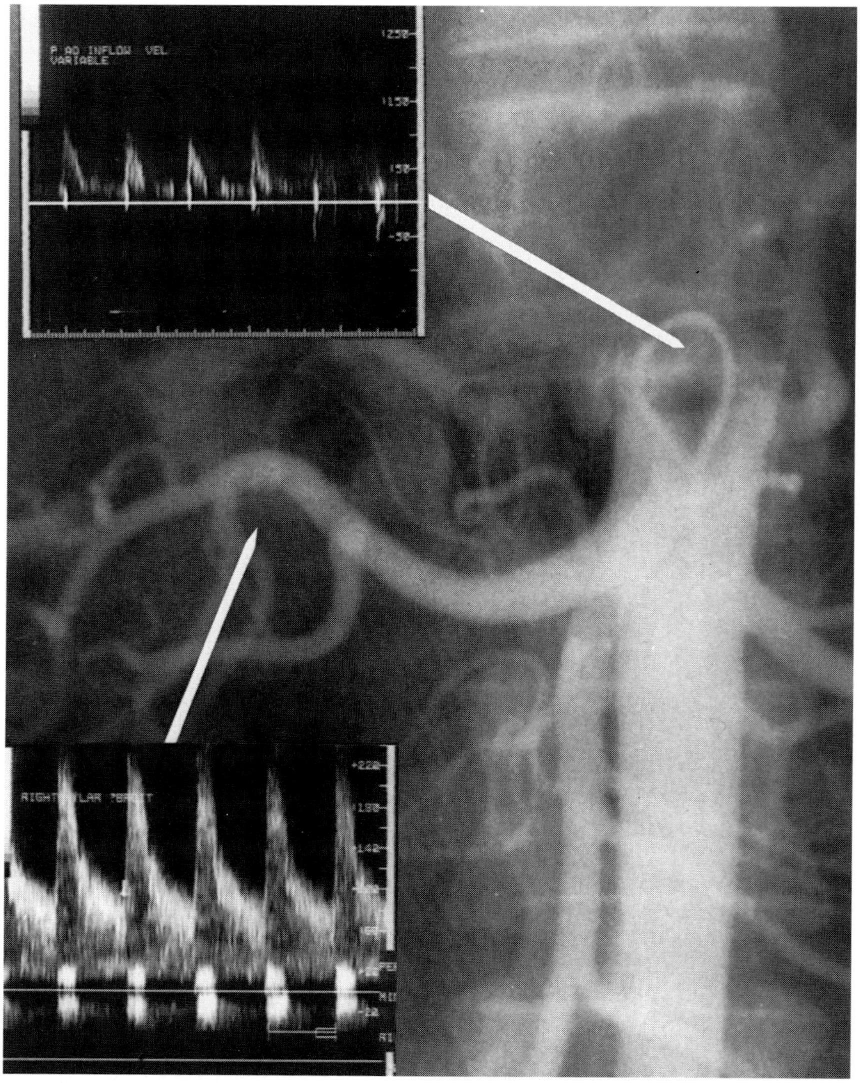

Figure 4–2. Fibromuscular dysplasia in a distal right renal branch artery, which is difficult to classify on the arteriogram. Peak systolic velocity of 230 cm/sec confirms the presence of disease, but RAR is <3.5.

dilatation, although this cause will be evident from the B mode scan, and the aortic PSV also declines with age.[30] However, as long as the aortic PSV is >40 cm/s the RAR has been found to be reliable. RAR has been correlated with angiographic stenosis, and a ratio of >3.5 predicts a >60% stenosis of the renal artery, with a sensitivity of 89% and a specificity of 97% and an overall agreement of 93%.[30,37] Variance of the degree of stenosis as assessed by two radiologists examining the same radiograph is of the same order as the disagreement between RAR and arteriography.[28]

Renal artery occlusion is important to recognize and is suggested by complete absence of a flow signal in the renal artery. Indirect confirmation of occlusion may be necessary in difficult cases, such as extreme obesity and in the immediate post-operative period, using renal length measurements and renal parenchymal flow signals. With the patient in the lateral position, renal length measurements are a good indicator of patency, as a renal length of <9 cms suggests renal artery occlusion **(Fig. 4–3)**. When the renal artery is occluded, flow throughout the cortex and medulla is usually <10 cm/s. Untreated 60–99% RAS is associated with deterioration of renal function and a progressive loss of renal

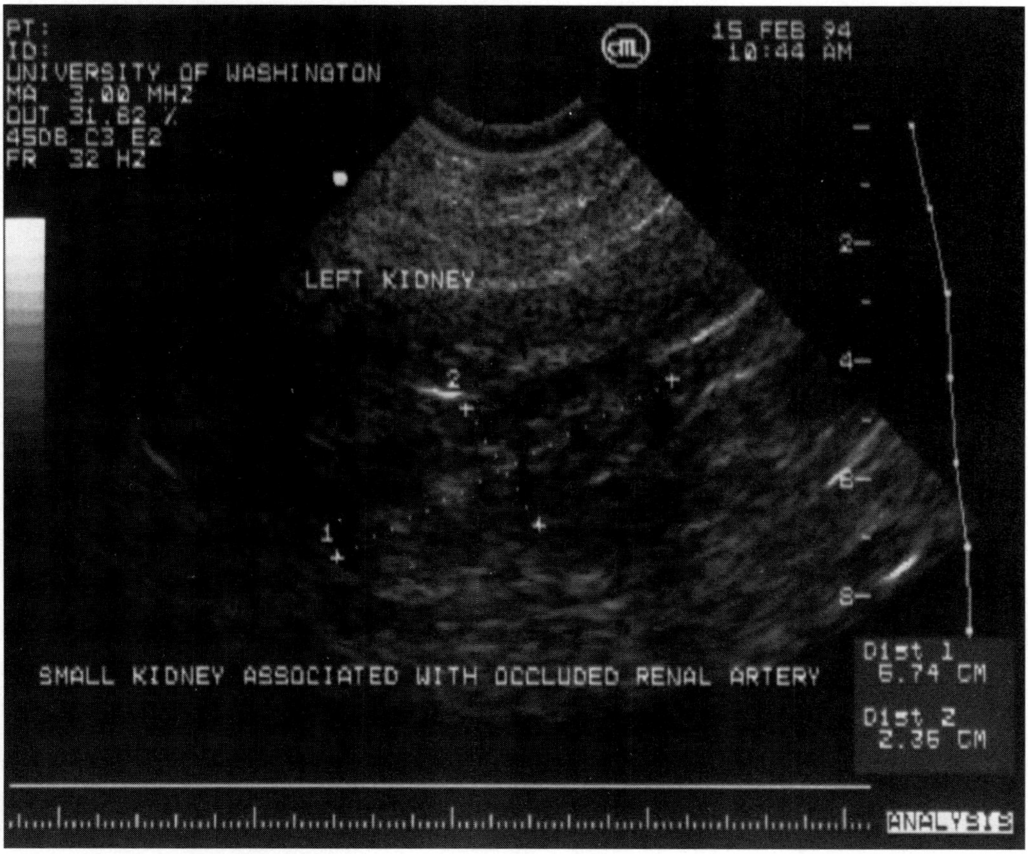

Figure 4–3. B-mode image of a small kidney from a flank approach. This was associated with an occluded renal artery.

mass as evidenced by a significant reduction in renal size over a 1-year period.[3]

The flank approach allows parenchymal Doppler signals to be recorded from the cortex and medulla, the distal renal artery and its branches in the hilum. The mid and proximal renal artery can also be scanned from this approach and traced back to the aorta. This serves as a double check for the proximal and mid-renal artery and helps to avoid errors from misdirection of the Doppler angle cursor.

The kidney is more readily imaged from the flank and almost all studies from this aspect will be technically complete. In view of this, attention has turned to the value of hilar signals in assessing proximal stenosis. Distal to significant arterial narrowing, the increase time of the pulse is delayed and the peak velocity achieved is attenuated. This clinical observation has been applied to the slow rise and diminished peak of the Doppler spectral waveform—so called tardus and parvus waveform.[38] Applying this to the renal artery, an acceleration index derived from the distal renal artery waveform was able to diagnose a >75% RAS in children with a high degree of accuracy.[39] However, another group found that objective criteria were not useful and resorted to loss of early systolic peak in hilar vessels to discriminate between significant RAS and lesser narrowing.[40] In the largest series examined thus far, Kliewer et al assessed 118 renal arteries and were unable to differentiate >50% stenosis from <50% stenosis in the renal artery using distal renal artery waveform indices and changes in the early systolic peak alone, although severe stenosis (80–99%) could be differentiated from non-hemodynamically significant (<50%) stenosis.[41] Our current view is that hilar signals provide adjunctive evidence, when used in conjunction with Doppler in the renal artery, of a >60% stenosis in the renal artery if the acceleration time of the waveform exceeds 100ms, but cannot be used to determine if lesser degrees of stenosis exist **(Fig. 4–4).**

Hypertension after renal transplantation has many possible causes and peak velocity in the transplant renal artery has been found to be useful in demonstrating transplant RAS.[42] The major difference is that iliac velocities tend to be higher than aortic velocities and a ratio of 2.5 has maximum accuracy for determining hemodynamically significant lesions.

High-end-diastolic flow has already been noted as a characteristic by which to recognize the renal artery because the kidney normally offers low vascular resistance. By injecting gel microspheres into canine renal arteries to increase the vascular resistance, Norris et al demonstrated that the end-diastolic flow and its ratio to peak systolic flow, the end-diastolic ratio (EDR), were reduced when the vascular resistance increased.[34] Normal healthy adults have an EDR of 0.33 to 0.35, and a reduced EDR was correlated (in the absence of significant RAS) with an increase in serum cre-

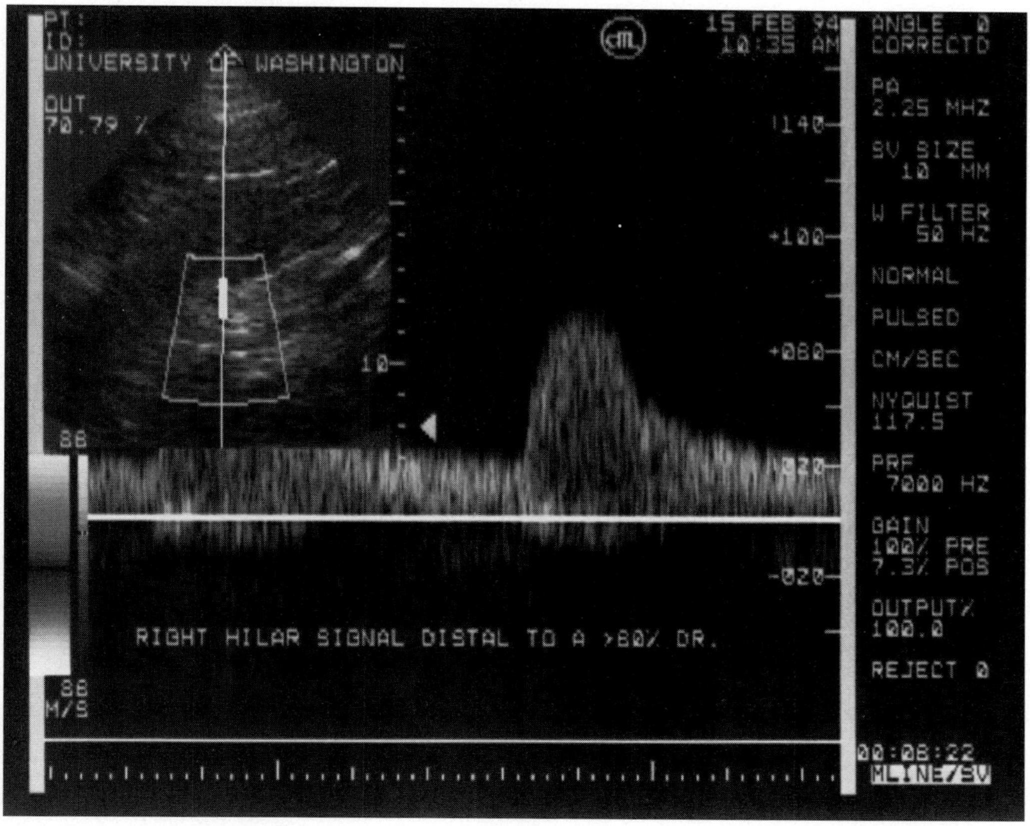

Figure 4–4. A Doppler spectral waveform taken from the hilum of a kidney distal to a >80% renal artery stenosis. Increased sweep speed of the display enables accurate calculation of the acceleration time which is 160 msec, corresponding to 4 small divisions of the scale.

atinine[30] levels **(Fig. 4–5)**. The Pourcelot index ([PSV-EDV]/PSV), a reciprocal of EDR, has also been used in this regard, especially in transplant studies.[43] Renal transplant rejection is associated with edema and cellular infiltration in the kidney parenchyma, and several workers have shown altered pulsatility in vessels at the hilum or from interlobar and interlobular arteries running through the parenchyma of the transplant, which reflect increased vascular resistance.[43–45] A reduced EDR is highly specific for renal transplant rejection, but not very sensitive for it, although spectral criteria were superior to morphologic B-mode criteria in diagnostic accuracy.[43]

Detection of renal parenchymal disease is important in the assessment of RVH because it is a potential cause of failure to ameliorate hypertension after technically successful treatment of

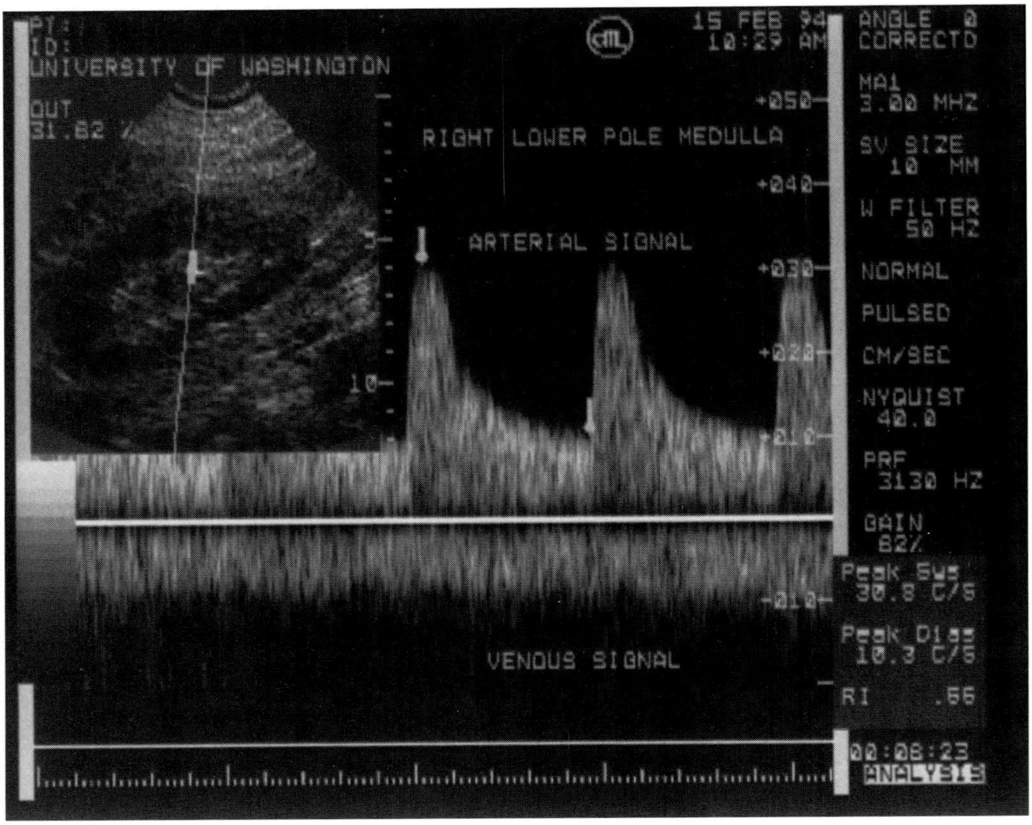

Figure 4–5. Doppler spectral waveform from the interlobar vessels of the medulla. The arterial signal is above the zero line with a venous signal below the baseline from flow in the opposite direction. The trace and EDR are normal. Cortical signals from interlobular vessels are similar but small in amplitude.

RAS. The work in kidney transplants has stimulated interest in the assessment of native renal disease. One study compared resistance index with histology of native kidneys obtained at percutaneous needle biopsy immediately after duplex scan.[46] This study showed that increased vascular resistance positively correlated with histologic changes of the intrarenal vasculature, namely arteriolosclerosis, glomerulosclerosis, arteriosclerosis, focal interstitial fibrosis, and edema. Although these are nonspecific histological findings and there was no correlation with the tissue diagnosis, this avenue of research may provide a noninvasive answer to the question of why some patients do not respond to revascularization.

One major drawback for Duplex assessment in renal artery stenosis is the consistent inability to recognize accessory renal arteries. Postmortem studies indicate that 12 to 25% kidneys have multiple renal arteries although arteriography may not identify all of these because in our study only 7 of 85 (8%) kidneys had multiple renal arteries.[9,28,47] However, none of these accessory vessels was detected by duplex ultrasound. With greater experience and diligent scanning of the abdominal aorta throughout its length in addition to the adjunctive use of color, this situation may be redressed.

Completion Studies after Revascularization

Completion arteriography is the standard for documenting technical success at the end of the procedure for peripheral arterial reconstructions.[48] The problem with its use in renal revascularization include the necessity of a suprarenal aortic clamp while the contrast is being injected and the film taken, limitation to a single projection on the operating table and artifacts of intrarenal vasospasm as well as the potential nephrotoxic effects of x-ray contrast medium. At the time of surgery duplex sonography can be performed expeditiously and has an advantage over continuous wave Doppler in that the sample volume can be placed accurately at the site of a B-scan defect.[49] By applying this technique, Okuhn et al. demonstrated a 90% sensitivity for abnormalities and achieved 99% patency at discharge from hospital.[50] Of patients without significant defect on completion duplex scans, Hansen et al found 98% graft patency after a mean of 12 months of follow up.[49]

Follow-up and Natural History Studies

A large majority of patients (85%) will have a lasting, trouble-free result from renal revascularization. The mortality of renal artery angioplasty and open surgery in the best hands is low at 0.5–1.0%, but the inherent technical failure rate of these procedures is about 5%.[1–2] Late stenosis, aneurysmal dilatation of bypass grafts and graft occlusion will occur in 8–16% patients.[1,51] These complications can occur in the absence of clinical features and so regular follow-up with objective assessment of continued therapeutic success is essential.[1,3,51]

Arteriography can be used for follow-up, but is uncomfortable for the patient and carries a risk of contrast nephrotoxicity. A novel approach using carbon dioxide as a contrast for DSA and can produce reasonable images but there remains the problem of patient discomfort and the occasional complication related to the catheter insertion site.[52]

Duplex ultrasound lends itself well to repeated studies and can visualize aortorenal grafts with a high degree of success.[3,52–53]

This high study completion rate probably relates to knowledge of the site of origin and insertion of the graft. Occlusion and >60% stenosis in main arteries and grafts can be detected with accuracy, but the sensitivity in detection of branch artery restenosis has been found to be low by one group.[53] However, it is not clear how thoroughly the hilar signals were evaluated in this study. The major advantage for duplex studies in follow-up is their noninvasive nature, allowing repeated examinations and providing data that can be compared with previous examinations in the same patient. This allows for a greater understanding of the response of RAS to surgical reconstruction or balloon angioplasty and to monitor the results of revascularization.

The natural history of renal artery stenosis also lends itself to assessment by duplex ultrasound. In an arteriographic study, Schreiber et al demonstrated that almost half of the patients with RAS due to atherosclerosis had progression in the degree of stenosis of the lesion (37/85) over time, and this was associated with a reduction in renal size and deterioration in renal function.[4] Progression to renal artery occlusion occurred in 14 of 85 (16%) patients studied. In the same study, none of the patients with FMD later had renal artery occlusion. In a duplex study from this center, 19 renal arteries with 60–99% stenosis were included in follow-up for 1 year and none progressed to occlusion.[3] However, there was a significant reduction in kidney size and deterioration in renal function during follow-up. If high degrees of stenosis were associated with a poor prognosis for the kidney, this could prove a useful screening test for patients who would benefit from renal revascularisation.

CONCLUSIONS

Duplex ultrasound is a useful and increasingly popular mode of assessment for patients with suspected RVH. In diagnosis of the underlying RAS it performs equally as well as arteriography in the main renal artery. It suffers from lack of sensitivity in the diagnosis of RAS in branch lesions and accessory renal arteries, but as more is learned about renal parenchymal Doppler spectra and signals obtained from the renal hilum this sensitivity could improve. These are the very lesions that are difficult to diagnose by arteriographic methods without resorting to further contrast injection or catheter manipulation. At open surgery, completion duplex ultrasound, compared with a completion arteriogram, is fast and easier and has satisfactory clinical results; it may become the completion study of choice. Important natural history data on the progress of RAS and its response to treatment will accrue with wider application of duplex ultrasound in diagnosis and follow-up. Further experience will allow the difficult problems of renal artery branch stenoses and renal parenchymal disease to be resolved.

Acknowledgments

The authors thank Janette A. Isaacson, R.V.T., and Watson Smith, R.V.T., for obtaining the Doppler waveforms for the illustrations.

REFERENCES

1. Dean RH. Changing concepts in indications for renal artery reconstruction. In: AD Whittemore, ed, *Advances in Vascular Surgery*. Volume 1. St Louis: Mosby; 1993.
2. Greminger P, Steiner A, Schneider E, Kuhlmann U, et al. Cure and improvement of renovascular hypertension after percutaneous transluminal angioplasty of renal artery stenosis. *Nephron* 1989;51: 362–366.
3. Taylor DC, Moneta GL, Strandness DE Jr. Follow-up of renal artery stenosis by duplex ultrasound. *J Vasc Surg* 1989;9:410–415.
4. Schreiber MJ, Pohl MA, Novick AC. The natural history of atherosclerotic and fibrous renal artery disease. *Urol Clin North Am* 1984;11: 383–392.
5. Kaplan NM. Hypertension in the population at large. In: Clinical Hypertension. Williams and Wilkins, Los Angeles, 1986.
6. Gifford Jr RW. Epidemiology and clinical manifestations of renovascular hypertension. In: JC Stanley & CB Ernst (eds), Renovascular Hypertension. W B Saunders, Philadelphia, 1984.
7. Anderson Jr GH, Blakeman N, Streeten DHP. Prediction of renovascular hypertension. Comparison of clinical diagnostic indices. *Am J Hypertens* 1988;1:301–304.
8. Chuang VP, Ernst CB. Angiography for renovascular hypertension. In: HL Neiman & JST Yao (eds), Angiography of Vascular Disease, 151–214. Churchill Livingstone, New York, 1985.
9. Holley KE, Hunt JC, Brown AL, Kincaid OW, Sheps SG. Renal artery stenosis: a clinicopathological study in normotensive and hypertensive patients. *Am J Med* 1964;37:14–22.
10. Drake MD, Ring EJ. Radiologic evaluation of renovascular hypertension. In: RB Rutherford (ed), Vascular Surgery, Volume 2, 1231–1244. W B Saunders, Philadelphia. 1989.
11. Smith HW. Unilateral nephrectomy in hypertensive patients. *J Urol* 1956;76:685–701.
12. Freeman NE, Leeds FH, Elliott WG, Rowland SR. Thromboendarter-

ectomy for hypertension due to renal artery occlusion. *JAMA* 1954; 156:1077–1079.

13. Hamovici H, Zinicola N. Experimental renal artery stenosis: diagnostic significance of arterial haemodynamics. *J Cardiovasc Surg* 1962; 3:259–262.
14. Pickering TG. Renovascular hypertension: medical evaluation and non-surgical treatment. In: JH Laragh, BM Brenner (eds), Hypertension: Pathophysiology, Diagnosis and Management. Raven Press, New York, 1990.
15. Sumner DS. Evaluation of Noninvasive testing procedures: data analysis and interpretation. In: EF Bernstein (ed), Noninvasive Diagnostic Techniques in Vascular Disease. C V Mosby, St Louis, 1985.
16. McKenzie JK. Screening for renal artery stenosis: useful or not? *J Can Med Assoc* 1990;142:845.
17. Simon N, Franklin SS, Bleifer KH, Maxwell MH. Cooperative study of renovascular hypertension: clinical characteristics of renovascular hypertension. *JAMA* 1972;220:1209–1218.
18. Murie JA, Morris PJ. Surgical management of renal hypertension. In: GRD Catto (ed), Management of Renal Hypertension. MTP Press, Lancaster, 1988.
19. Dean RH. Renovascular hypertension. In: WS Moore (ed), Vascular Surgery: A Comprehensive Review; 3rd Edition. W B Saunders Co., Philadelphia, 1991.
20. Svetkey LP, Kadir S, Dunnick NR, Smith SR, et al. Similar prevalence of renovascular hypertension in selected blacks and whites. *Hypertension* 1991;17:678–683.
21. Ying CY, Tifft CP, Gavras H, Chobanian AV. Renal revascularisation in the azotemic hypertensive patient resistant to therapy. *N Engl J Med* 1984;311:1070–1075.
22. Distler A, Spies K-P. Diagnostic procedure in renovascular hypertension. *Clin Nephrol* 1991;36:174–180.
23. Kassirer JP. Atheroembolic renal disease. *N Engl J Med* 1969;280: 812–818.
24. Martin-Paredero V, Dixon SM, Baker JD, Takiff H, Gomes AS, et al. Risk of renal failure after major angiography. *Arch Surg* 1983;118: 1417–1420.
25. Katayama H, Yamaguchi K, Kozuka T, Takashima T, Seez P, et al. Adverse reactions to ionic and non-ionic contrast media. *Radiology* 1990;175:621–628.
26. Pauker SG, Kopelman RI. Screening for renovascular hypertension, a which hunt. *Hypertension* 1989;14:258–260.
27. Kaufman JJ. Renovascular hypertension: the UCLA experience. *J Urol* 1979;121:139–144.
28. Hoffman U, Edwards JM, Carter S, Goldman ML, Harley JD et al. Role of duplex scanning for the detection of atherosclerotic renal artery disease. *Kidney Int* 1991;39:1232–1239.
29. Strandness DE Jr. Duplex scanning in diagnosis of renovascular hypertension. *Surg Clin North Am* 1990;70:109–117.

30. Kohler TR, Zierler RE, Martin RL, Nicholls SC, Bergelin RO et al. Noninvasive diagnosis of renal artery stenosis by ultrasonic duplex scanning. *J Vasc Surg* 1986;4:450–456.
31. Zoller WG, Hermans H, Bogner JR, Hahn D, Middeke M. Duplexsonography in the diagnosis of renovascular hypertension. *Klinische Wochneschrift* 1990;68:830–834.
32. Postma CT, van Aalen J, de Boo T, Rosenbusch G, Thien T. Doppler ultrasound scanning in the detection of renal artery stenosis in hypertensive patients. *Br J Radiol* 1992;65:857–860.
33. Avasthi PS, Voyles WFF, Greene ER. Noninvasive diagnosis of renal artery streosis by echo-Doppler velocimetry. *Kidney Int* 1984;25: 824–829.
34. Norris CS, Pfeiffer JS, Rittgers SE, Barnes RW. Non-invasive evaluation of renal artery stenosis and renovascular resistance. Experimental and clinical studies. *J Vasc Surg* 1984;1:192–201.
35. Miralles M, Santiso A, Gimenez A, Riambau V, Saez A et al. Renal duplex scanning: correlation with angiography and isotopic renography. *Eur J Vasc Surg* 1993;7:188–194.
36. Daigle RJ, Stavros AT, Lee RM. Overestimation of velocity and frequency values by multielement linear array dopplers. *J Vasc Technol* 1990;14:206–213.
37. Taylor DC, Kettler MD, Moneta GL, Kohler TR, Kazmers A, et al. Duplex ultrasound scanning in the diagnosis of renal artery stenosis: a prospective evaluation. *J Vasc Surg* 1988;7:363–369.
38. Kotval PS. Doppler waveform parvus and tardus: a sign of proximal flow obstruction. *J Ultrasound Med* 1989;8:435–440.
39. Patriquin HB, Lafortune M, Jequier J-C, O'Regan S et al. Stenosis of the renal artery: assessment of slowed systole in the downstream circulation with Doppler sonography. *Radiology* 1992;184:479–485.
40. Stavros AT, Parker SH, Yakes WF, Chantelois AE, Burke BJ et al. Segmental stenosis of the renal artery: pattern recognition of tardus and parvus abnormalities with duplex sonography. *Radiology* 1992; 184:487–492.
41. Kliewer MA, Tupler RH, Carroll BA, Paine SS, Kreigshauser JS et al. Renal artery stenosis: analysis of Doppler waveform parameters and tardus-parvus pattern. *Radiology* 1993;189:779–787.
42. Erley CM, Duda SH, Wakat J-P, Sokler M, Reuland P et al. Noninvasive procedures for diagnosis of renovascular hypertension in renal transplant recipients—a prospective analysis. *Transplantation* 1992;54:863–867.
43. Townshend RR, Tomlanovich SJ, Goldstein RB, Filly RA. Combined doppler and morphologic evaluation of renal transplant rejection. *J Ultrasound Med* 1990;9:199–206.
44. Neumyer MM, Gifford RRM, Thiele BL. Identification of early rejection in renal allografts with duplex ultrasonography. *J Vasc Technol* 1988;12:19–25.
45. Fleischer AC, Hinton AA, Glick AD, Johnson HK. Duplex doppler

sonography of renal transplants: correlation with histopathology. *J Ultrasound Med* 1989;8:89–94.

46. Mostbeck GH, Kain R, Mallek R, Derfler K, Walter R et al. Duplex doppler sonography in renal parenchymal disease: histopathologic correlation. *J Ultrasound Med* 1991;10:189–194.
47. Graves FT. The Arterial Anatomy of the Kidney. Williams and Wilkins, Baltimore. 1971.
48. Courbier R, Jausseran JM, Reggi M: Detecting complications of direct arterial surgery. The role of intraoperative arteriography. *Arch Surg* 1977;112:1115–1118.
49. Hansen KJ, O'Neil EA, Reavis SW, Craven TE, Plonk GW et al. Intraoperative duplex sonography during renal artery reconstruction. *J Vasc Surg* 1991;14:364–374.
50. Okuhn SP, Reilly LM, Bennett JB, Hughes L, Goldstone J et al. Intraoperative assessment of renal and visceral artery reconstruction: the role of duplex scanning and spectral analysis. *J Vasc Surg* 1987;5:137–147.
51. Stanley JC, Ernst CB, Fry WJ. Fate of 100 aortorenal vein grafts: characteristics of late graft expansion, aneurysmal dilatation and stenosis. *Surgery* 1973;74:931–944.
52. Harward TRS, Smith S, Hawkins IF, Seeger JM. Follow-up evaluation after renal artery bypass surgery with use of carbon dioxide arteriography and color-flow duplex scanning. *J Vasc Surg* 1993;18: 23–30.
53. Hudspeth DA, Hansen KJ, Reavis SW, Starr SM, Appel RG, Dean RH. Renal duplex sonography after treatment of renovascular disease. *J Vasc Surg* 1993;18:381–390.

5

Diagnosis of Renal Artery Stenosis by Magnetic Resonance Angiography

Abigail K. Hanna, George Holland,
Richard A. Baum, and
Jeffrey P. Carpenter

MAGNETIC RESONANCE ANGIOGRAPHY FOR SCREENING OF THE HYPERTENSIVE PATIENT

Symptomatic renal artery stenosis is a significant and treatable problem. In the United States, as many as forty million persons have hypertension. Although the incidence of renovascular hypertension (RVH) is probably less than 3% within this group,[1,2] repair of renovascular lesions for the treatment of RVH has given durable results in 95% of properly chosen surgical candidates.[3] To achieve such results, the careful screening of potential surgical candidates requires detailed imaging of the renal arteries.

Contrast arteriography has been the standard for renal vascular imaging, but it is impractical as a screening test in patients who are often at high risk for contrast related complications. To address this shortcoming other screening tests have been proposed. Rapid-sequence intravenous pyelography has been extensively used in the past but is associated with a high false-negative rate.[4] Isotope renography is used but has a limited sensitivity. The addition of captopril to the nuclear scan has shown promise in identifying and predicting those patients with renin-dependent hypertension among patients with normal renal function (sensitivity and specificity greater than 90%). However, the utility of renal scintigraphy is limited in patients with renal failure due to increased background activity.[5] Reports of the use of spiral computed tomographic scanning for the detection of renal artery stenosis are beginning to appear, but this technique requires the use of 150 ml of nephrotoxic intravenous contrast.[6] Recent interest has focused on the ability of duplex ultrasound to evaluate the renal artery noninvasively. This technique has been promising in the hands of experienced laboratories, but is operator dependent, time consuming and limited by its inability to image accessory renal arteries.[7]

Advances in magnetic resonance angiography (MRA) hardware and software have established its place in carotid and peripheral vascular disease diagnosis.[8–11] Recently, independent clinical trials have indicated that MRA is also a reliable noninvasive imaging modality for screening patients with suspected RVH.[12–16] MRA offers soft tissue imaging of renal size and parenchymal disease in addition to arteriographic images. Physiologic information related to the velocity and quantity of blood flow can also be obtained and pressure gradients estimated across areas of stenosis.[14] The only contraindications to MRA are those applicable to MR imaging in general: a small percentage of patients (5–10%) are unable to undergo scanning secondary to ferromagnetic implants or claustrophobia.

This chapter will summarize the efficacy of MRA as a screening tool, when compared with contrast angiography. Specific causes of false positives and negatives will be addressed, as well as the utility of MRA in the azotemic patient.

PRINCIPLES OF MAGNETIC RESONANCE ANGIOGRAPHY OF THE RENAL ARTERIES, UNENHANCED TECHNIQUES

Although the physics of MRA are complex, the clinician can grasp a fundamental understanding of the essential differences in the techniques that are available for imaging the renal vasculature. The best images are produced with an understanding of the advantages and limitations of the various MRA techniques available. Three main MRA technique options are available. Time-of-flight (TOF) sequences and phase contrast (PC) sequences are considered "bright blood" techniques because the flowing blood is detected as a signal that is brighter than the surrounding tissue. The third technique, "black blood" MRA, images the flowing blood as black in contrast to the lighter tissue background. All of these sequences can be acquired with either two dimensional (2D) or three dimensional (3D) techniques. Two dimensional acquisition involves the imaging of one cross sectional slice of tissue at a time while 3D techniques image a volume of tissue. Both 2D and 3D techniques can be processed into angiogram-like images that can be rotated 180 degrees around a central longitudinal axis, an advantage over contrast arteriography because one study can provide many views of a vascular lesion. The following is a short description of the principles of these acquisition techniques and their shortcomings. Black blood technique is not useful in imaging the fine detail of the renal vasculature, therefore this section will concentrate on bright blood techniques.

TWO-DIMENSIONAL TIME-OF-FLIGHT

Edelman and associates were the first to describe a 2D TOF scan of renal artery blood flow.[17] An angiogram-like image is obtained by exposing the stationary tissue protons within the imaged body slice to a rapid series of radiofrequency pulses. Since there is insufficient time between pulses for the protons of the stationary tissue to relax, they appear relatively dark. Conversely, the flowing fresh blood appears brighter than the stationary tissue because the newly excited protons of the fresh blood pass quickly through the radiofrequency saturated tissue "slice", emitting a bright signal as they relax (T1 signal). The 2D TOF technique images one 3–5 mm slice of tissue at a time, before the next anatomic slice in the sequence is activated. Because of this, flowing blood has time to relax before it is restimulated with the next radiofrequency pulsation. The strongest signal is given off by rapidly flowing blood in a plane perpendicular to the slice. Sluggish flow, retrograde flow, or flow parallel to the tissue slice will give off little or no signal because it becomes super-saturated with excited protons and has no contrast with the surrounding tissue. The advantage of 2D TOF MRA is that it detects regions of slow flow (distal to a tight stenosis) because it is less susceptible to saturation effects. A disadvantage of 2D TOF MRA is that it has a tendency to overestimate the severity of stenosis. Another problem with 2D TOF MRA is motion artifact. Normal respiratory movements cause loss of the bright signal of flowing blood. Tissues and vessels that are located in the lateral aspects of the body are most affected by respiratory movements. The central vessels such as the aorta and its proximal branch arteries move less and therefore are more accurately imaged. A 2D unenhanced TOF MRA requires a fully cooperative patient who can hold their breath for up to 45 seconds.

THREE-DIMENSIONAL TIME-OF-FLIGHT

Three dimensional TOF MRA relies on the same inflow enhancement theory as the 2D TOF technique but a whole block of tissue is imaged simultaneously. The block of tissue is represented as an image composed of thousands of cubic units called voxels. Voxels are the three dimensional equivalent of pixels. The 3D unenhanced TOF MRA has the capability of achieving higher spatial resolution than the 2D TOF technique. The degree of stenosis is more accurately diagnosed with 3D TOF MRA than with 2D TOF when both are compared to contrast arteriography. Resolution is best when the imaged volume is small. A smaller volume results in smaller voxels which produce narrower effective range of velocity-induced phase shifts. The overall effect is finer spatial resolution by minimizing the resultant cancellation and signal loss caused by adjoining voxel phases that negate each other (phase shifts). A phase shift between voxels is less likely to occur when the flowing blood traverses a tissue volume at its narrowest aspect. Phase shift and loss of signal is more likely to occur the longer the blood dwells within the imaged volume. A limitation of unenhanced 3D TOF MRA is drop out of signal in distal arteries, with loss of contrast between blood and surrounding soft tissues. Although this is a problem in 2D TOF studies, it is more apparent on 3D studies. This phenomenon occurs when the blood traversing the region of excitation travels parallel to the slice, becoming supersaturated like the surrounding tissue. For this reason 3D TOF MRA is less sensitive to slow flow and often unable to detect the artery distal to a tight stenosis. Breath holding is not as critical for 3D TOF MRA, but in unenhanced 2D and 3D TOF techniques, breath holding improves the accuracy significantly.

PHASE-CONTRAST CINEMATIC MAGNETIC RESONANCE ANGIOGRAPHY

In TOF MRA, a slice or volume of tissue is super-saturated with excited protons. The unsaturated blood transiently becomes excited as it passes through the slice, then emits a signal as it quickly relaxes. Phase-contrast MRA differs by employing the principle that moving blood will strongly deflect radiofrequency signals (change phase) relative to stationary tissues. The higher the velocity, the brighter the signal. A tight stenosis and distal artery may not image well due to sluggish flow. As blood flows into the field of study, a sequential time frame acquisition system similar to cinematic film records the blood as it courses through the vasculature. Like TOF techniques, PC MRA can be acquired with 2D or 3D technology and can be formatted into an angiogram-like image that can be viewed through 180 degrees of rotation. This technique has been most efficacious for normal renal arteries, and its accuracy depends on eliminating motion artifact and the presence of uniform flow velocity.[14,16] A major limitation of PC MRA is its extreme sensitivity to a narrow blood velocity range. Any flow that is moving slower or faster than the set velocity sensitivity will not be imaged. Patients with wide pulse pressures will have signal drop out due to pulsation artifact. Another limitation is the poor rate of detection of accessory renal arteries.

MRA AS A NONINVASIVE SCREENING TOOL: COMPARISON TO CONTRAST ANGIOGRAPHY, THE GOLD STANDARD

Practical application of MRA as a noninvasive screening tool for surgical candidates is predicated on the technique having a high sensitivity, high negative predictive value, high specificity, and that it is readily available, cost effective, and easily tolerated by the patient. A routine MRA study takes approximately 60 minutes. The patient is pre-screened for a history of metallic implants, foreign objects and ferromagnetic clips. The average cost of a MRA renal artery study is approximately the same as digital subtraction contrast angiography. In many centers intra-arterial angiography requires a short hospital stay or an overnight hospitalization for monitoring or for intravenous hydration, adding to the overall cost, whereas MRA is performed as an outpatient.

CLINICAL TRIALS, TWO- AND THREE-DIMENSIONAL TIME-OF-FLIGHT MRA

Four independent studies have compared unenhanced TOF MRA as a screening modality for RVH with contrast angiography **(Table 5–1)**. The reported sensitivity of MRA as a screening test ranges from 91 to 100%, the specificity 76 to 94%.

Two clinical trials comparing 2D TOF technique with contrast arteriography were performed by the Beth Israel Hospital group to screen for renal artery stenosis in hypertensive patients. Each study assigned one blinded radiologist to interpret all of the contrast angiograms, and another blinded radiologist to read the MRAs. The earliest study of 25 patients by Kim et al.,[18] correctly determined the number of renal arteries in all patients, detecting all five accessory arteries. With respect to the ability of MRA to detect a 50% or greater luminal narrowing, their study showed 100% sensitivity, and 92% specificity when compared with contrast angiography. Four cases of complete renal artery occlusion were correctly identified. The severity of stenosis was overestimated in 4/55 renal arteries evaluated, yielding a correct interpretation of the degree of stenosis in 88%. Although Kim and col-

Table 5–1. Accuracy of Imaging Methods for Renal Artery Stenoses

Investigator	Year	Sensitivity	Specificity	% Identical	Imaging Method
Kim/Skillman (15)	1990	100%*	92%	88%	2D TOF
Kent/Skillman (8)	1991	100%*	94%	91%	2D TOF
Hertz/Carpenter (5)	1994	91%*	76%	81%	2D TOF + 3D PC
Yucel (12)	1993	100%†	93%	91%	2D TOF + 3D TOF
Debatin (14)	1991	53%*	97%	—	2D TOF vs 2D PC
		84%*	97%	—	
Gedroyc (10)	1994	86%*	94%	—	3D PC

* >50% stenosis detection.
† >70% stenosis detection.

leagues employed breath-hold technique, they observed that only the proximal one third of the renal arterial tree could be reliably imaged using the 2D TOF technology available to them at the time, precluding detection of stenosis in the distal two thirds of the artery.

One year later Kent et al[12] of the same group, presented the results for 37 patients (77 arteries) screened by 2D TOF MRA. Using the same observer protocol, the MRA protocol was varied slightly by evaluating thinner slices (3 mm) in some of the studies, and altering their scan parameters (time/echo time/flip angle). Based on the criterion of detection of a 50% or greater reduction in the luminal diameter, they reported 100% sensitivity and 94% specificity. They accurately predicted the degree of stenosis in 70 of 77 renal arteries (91%). In the group with severe (>75%) stenosis, there were 4 false positives, including one patient with a less than 50% stenosis which was called severe by MRA. All three accessory renal arteries were identified. A distal renal artery stenosis was missed in a patient with fibromuscular dysplasia. Like the previous study, stenoses appeared longer and more critical when compared to contrast angiography. They observed that an artery with a high grade stenosis would appear to be occluded by MRA, but a "reconstituted" distal artery would be present. The authors identified two major limitations: Overestimation of the degree of stenosis and poor imaging of the distal portion of the renal artery.

To avoid the pitfalls of 2D TOF MRA, Yucel et al[16] combined the technique of 3D TOF with 2D TOF MRA. Three dimensional TOF MRA is capable of achieving higher spatial resolution, with slice thickness as small as 0.7 mm. They applied the combined techniques to a cohort of 16 azotemic hypertensive patients with serum creatinine ranging from 1.8 to 5.3 mg/dl. The 3D studies were obtained with normal respirations, while the 2D images required breath holding. Axial, coronal and projection images were reviewed. All renal arteries were identified by MRA. Three of 16 patients had accessory renal arteries, all correctly identified. The degree of stenosis was correctly identified in 32/35 arteries studied (91%). All MRA errors were in the severely stenotic group (stenosis greater than 70%). Two patients with angiographic occlusion and one with moderate stenosis were called severely stenotic by MRA. For severe occlusive disease the sensitivity was 100% and the specificity was 93%. Yucel and colleagues observed that unenhanced 2D and 3D TOF acquisition were complementary. The finer resolution of 3D TOF acquisition gave a more accurate estimate of the degree of stenosis, while the 2D TOF studies displayed greater signal intensity distal to severe stenoses, allowing for detection of slow flow in severely stenotic vessels.

Motivated by such promising preliminary reports, the MRA Study Group at the University of Pennsylvania enlisted 16 patients in a screening trial that combined breath holding 2D TOF MRA with 3D PC MRA to reassess the value of multi-modality MRA in detecting renovascular lesions. The images were interpreted by experienced MR radiologists blinded to the results of contrast angiographic studies and the patients' histories. Although 100% of the proximal stenoses were identified, three of four accessory renal arteries were missed. One distal renal artery lesion was also missed in a patient with fibromuscular dysplasia. Based on the criterion of detection of a 50% or greater reduction in the luminal diameter, the combination of 2D TOF and 3D PC MRA yielded a 91% sensitivity, a 76% specificity and a 94% negative predictive value. A scatter plot diagram graphically depicts the relationship of MRA measurements and contrast arteriographic measurements of percent stenosis **(Fig. 5–1)**. The Pearson correlation coefficient ($r = 0.8$, $P < 0.001$) and the coefficient of determination ($r^2 = 0.64$) imply a significant, but imperfect correlation. In studies using standard MRA techniques, our group agrees with others that visualization of the renal orifice and the proximal renal vessels is far superior to that of the distal vessels. This is due to degradation of the MRA signal by respiratory motion, and over saturation of the blood with radiofrequency pulses, which is more pronounced as one moves laterally from the aorta to the distal artery.[9] To overcome this limitation, a trial of gadolinium enhanced MRA is in progress at the University of Pennsylvania. **Figures 5–2 and 5–3** show the detail that can be achieved by using gadolinium to image the distal renal arteries and post-stenotic segments of renal artery.

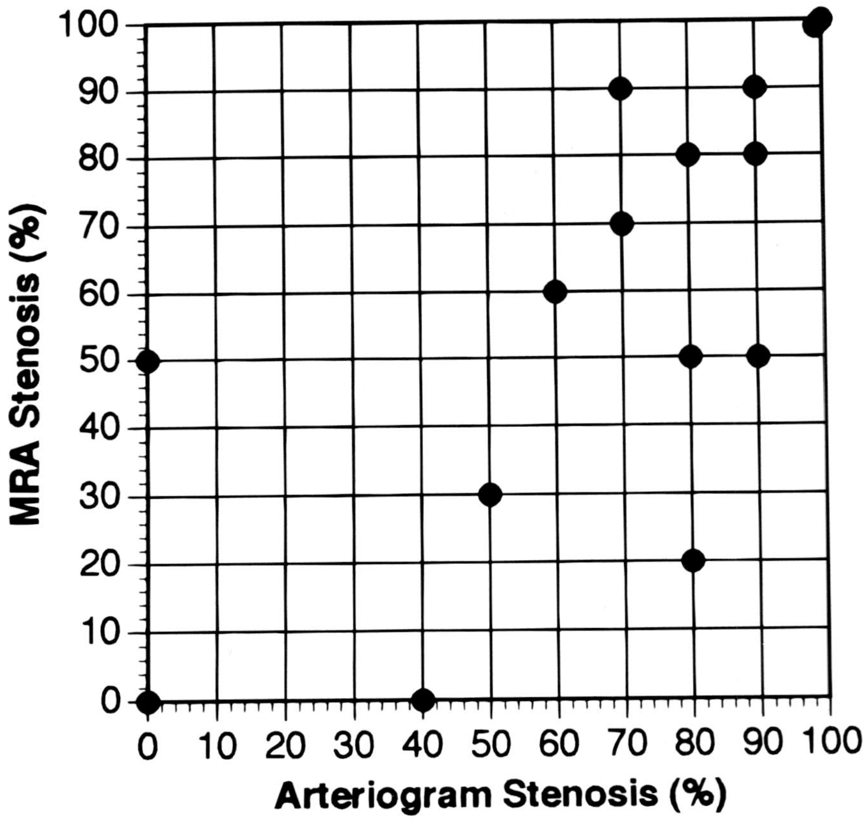

Figure 5–1. Measurement of renal artery stenosis. The relationship between measurements of renal artery stenosis by MRA and contrast arteriography is depicted. The Pearson correlation coefficient (R) equals 0.8 ($P < 0.001$). (Data from 32 arteries are depicted; circles may represent multiple overlapping data points.)[13]

CLINICAL TRIALS, PHASE-CONTRAST MRA

Two independent groups have investigated the utility of phase contrast MRA. Debatin et al[19] initially compared 2D TOF and 3D PC MRA with contrast arteriography. Thirty nine patients underwent 2D TOF study using 7-mm thick slices and 3D PC techniques. The authors reported a sensitivity of 53% for 2D TOF MRA, and 84% for 3D PC MRA. Both modalities had a 97% specificity. The low sensitivity of the 2D TOF technique may have been attributable to very thick slice segments.

Gedroyc and colleagues[14] have evaluated 74 patients with 3D PC MRA and compared it with contrast arteriography. In an evaluation of the first 46 patients of this group, sensitivity was re-

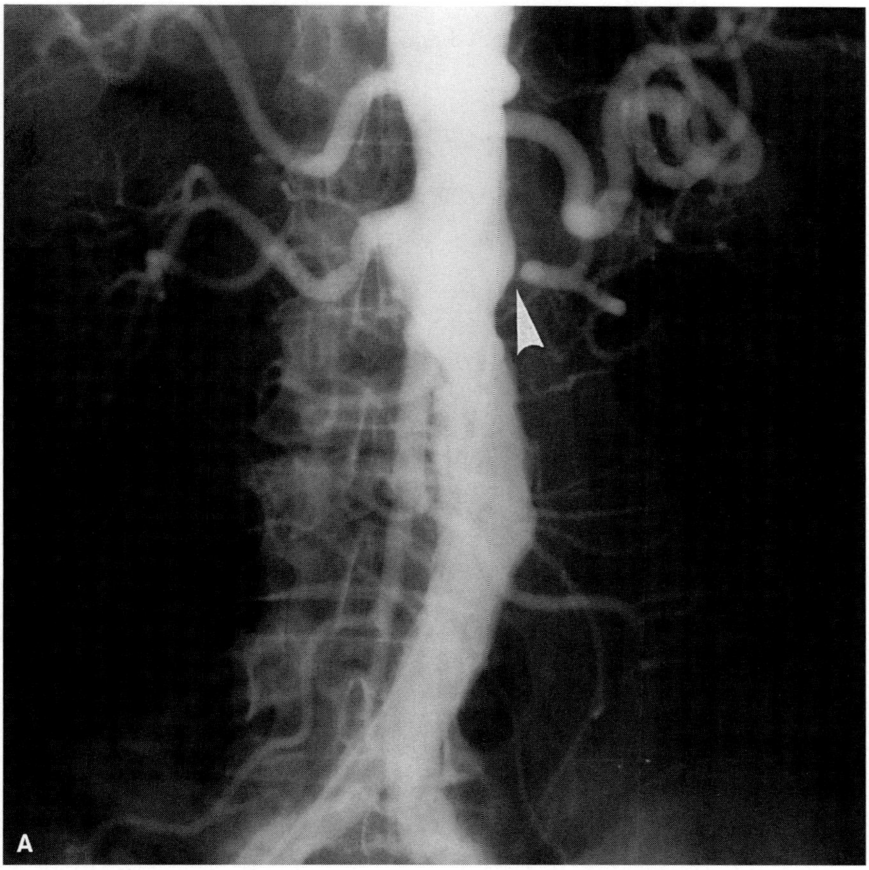

Figure 5–2. Contrast arteriography and MRA of the renal artery. A. Contrast aortogram from a patient with an aortic aneurysm and high grade left renal artery stenosis (arrow). B. Axial image from the MRA in the region of the left renal artery stenosis. The aorta and orifice of the left renal artery with stenotic lesion and post-stenotic dilatation is seen (arrow). C. MRA of the post-surgical appearance of the patient depicted in A and B. An infrarenal aortic bifurcation graft is seen to be patent. A left aorta-renal bypass arising from the left limb of the aortic bifurcation graft is seen to be patent. A normal right renal artery is seen for correlation with the contrast arteriogram depicted in A. D. Compressed axial view along the line drawn through the aortic bifurcation graft in C. This demonstrates the left aorta-renal bypass and anastomosis to the left renal artery (arrow) with patent branch arteries. (Figure continues.)

ported at 84%, and specificity at 90%. More recent data, completing the study, showed sensitivity at 86% and specificity at 94%. Their group has found this modality very useful in the evaluation of renal transplant recipients for narrowing at the line of anastomosis,[20] although 3D PC MRA takes longer than 2D or 3D TOF technique, limiting the anatomical area covered at one sitting.

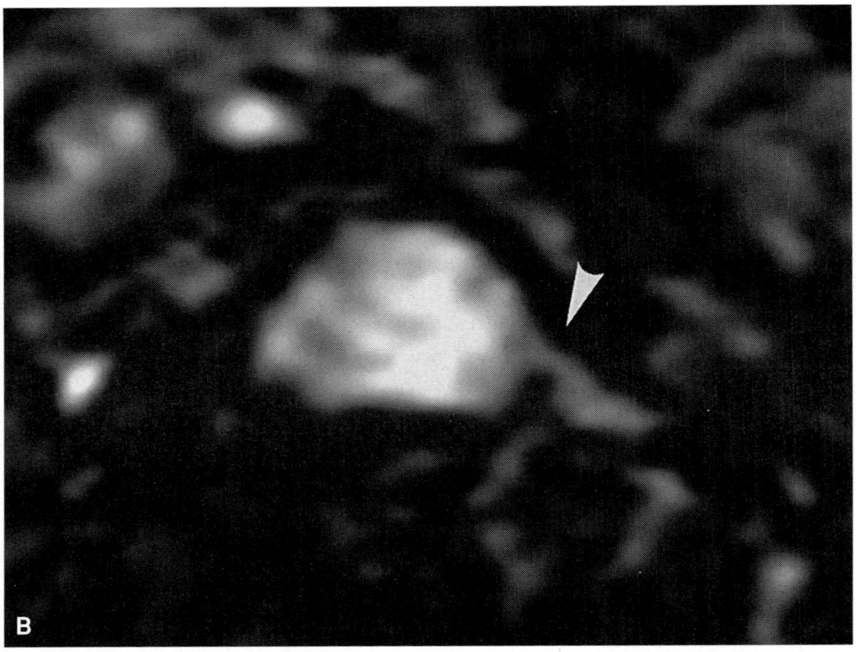

Figure 5–2. *(continued)*

TECHNICAL ADVANCES

Gadolinium-Enhanced MRA

One of the major problems of MRA imaging is loss of signal in the distal vessels. This may be due to a post-stenotic change in the flow velocity, or phase errors due to motion artifact. To overcome problems associated with poor contrast between vessels and background tissue, gadolinium, a non-nephrotoxic rare earth metal, is used in the form of gadopentetate dimeglumine or gadolinium-diethylenetriamine-pentaacetic acid. Gadolinium acts as a paramagnetic reducing agent when present in flowing blood. It decreases the effects of spin saturation, reducing the T1 of blood, permitting intense signals even in the distal vessels.[21] Three dimensional vessel tracking is necessary to follow the first pass of the gadolinium bolus. This is important because a strong venous phase will be seen, and over time the gadolinium will distribute throughout the extracellular space. The technique has been used to evaluate cerebral blood flow and anatomy,[21] coronary artery blood flow,[22] and the study of the intrathoracic great vessels.[23] Ongoing studies of gadolinium enhanced MRA of the renal arter-

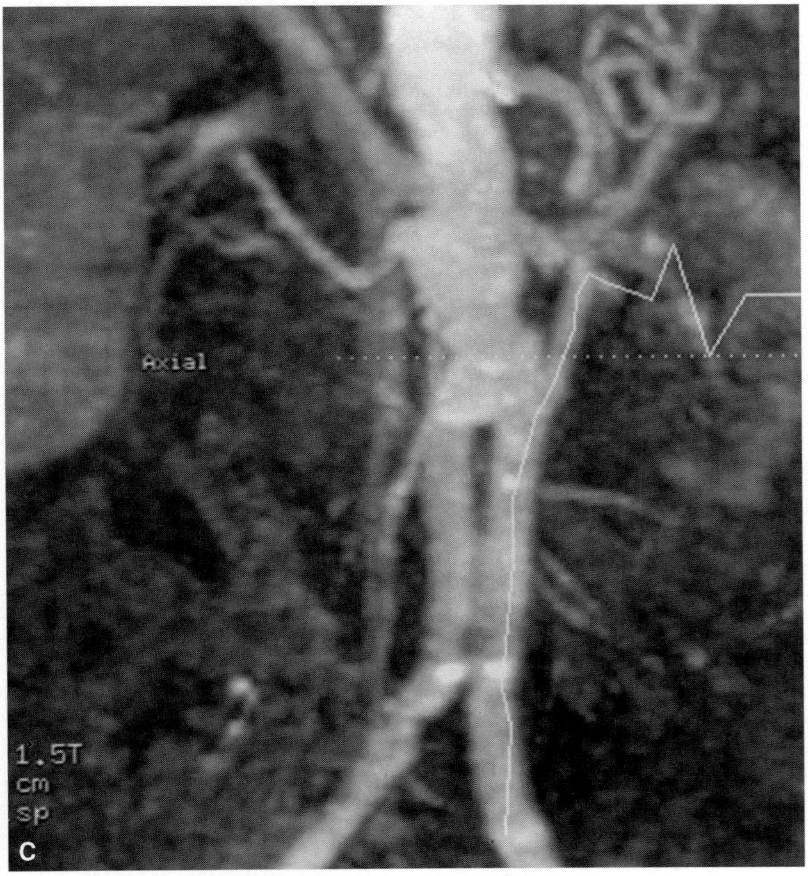

Figure 5–2. *(continued)*

ies, comparing it with 2D and 3D TOF MRA without gadolinium, and conventional contrast arteriography show promising early results at the University of Pennsylvania.

RENAL ARTERY FLOW STUDIES WITH TWO-DIMENSIONAL CINEMATIC PHASE-CONTRAST MRA

Debatin and colleagues[24] using a modified 2D phase-contrast (PC) MRA technique, have accurately measured renal blood flow in 8 normal subjects when compared with para-amino hippurate (PAH) clearance. These authors used a cine technique that records

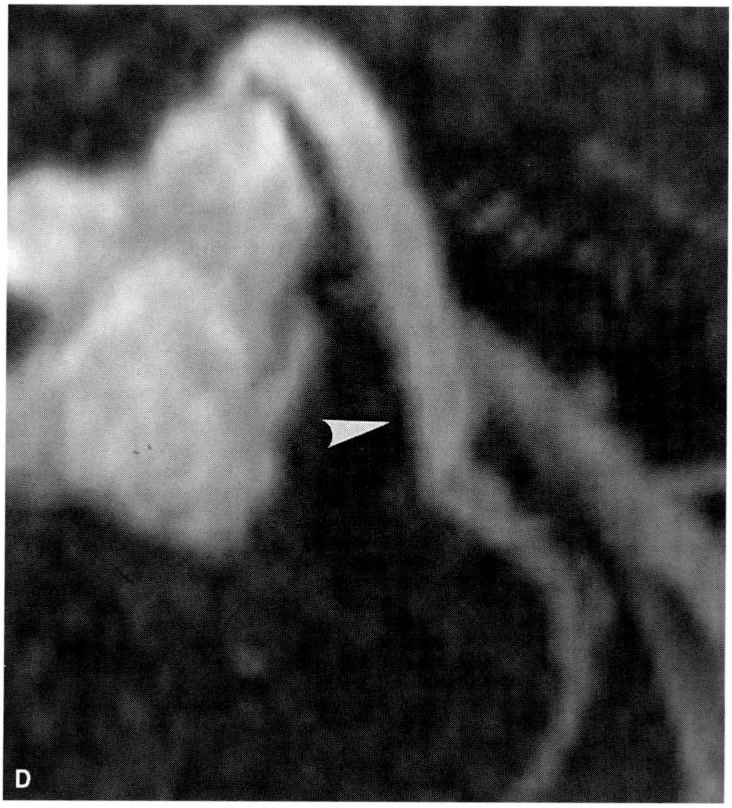

Figure 5–2. *(continued)*

six high spatial-resolution time frames at different moments in the cardiac cycle, over a 37 second breath hold. The frames are stored in their proper flow pattern sequence, that can be played back as a cine-loop dynamic image. The technique combines time resolved imaging with automatic data segmentation (TRIADS) PC. Respiratory motion artifact on the accuracy of the TRIADS PC technique was evaluated in eight patients who underwent TRIADS PC with and without breath holding. The breath holding TRIADS PC MRA had the best correlation with PAH clearance ($r = 0.98$, $P = 0.005$). The patients enrolled in the study group had histories of renal parenchymal disease, membranous glomerulonephritis (5), systemic lupus erythematosus (2), and focal sclerosis (1). All patients had normal renal function. It is not clear whether the patients had normal or diseased renal vasculature, which would greatly alter the ability to visualize the distal renal vessels. Because of this uncertainty, it is not clear whether patients with stenotic lesions will enjoy the same diagnostic accuracy as their counterparts with normal renal function. This technique

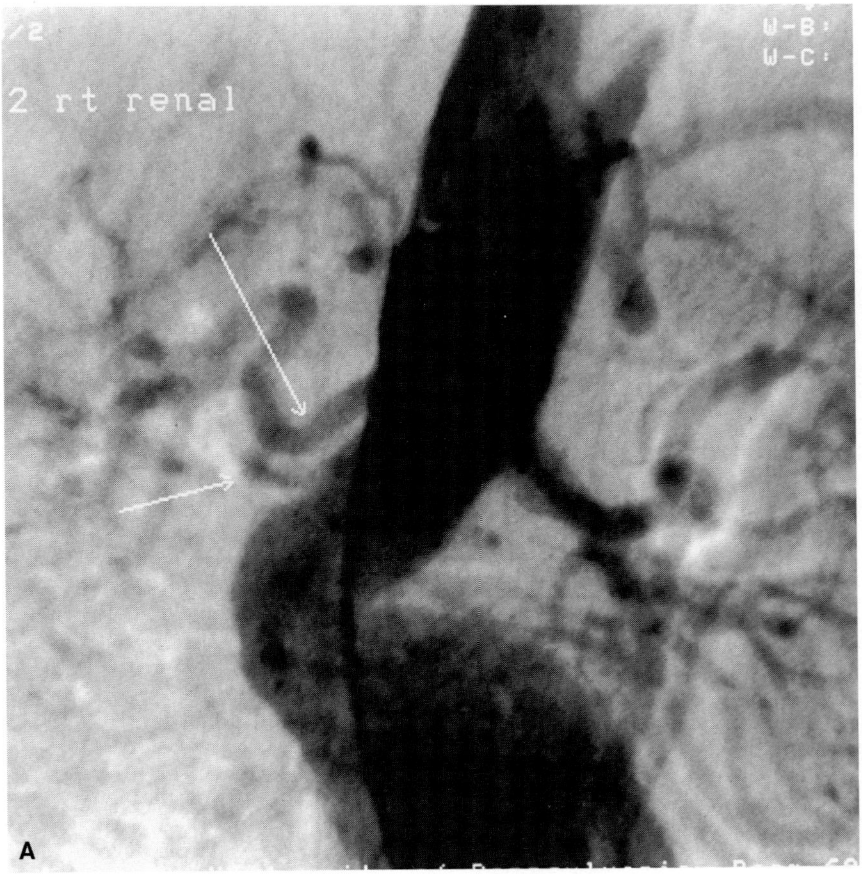

Figure 5–3. Contrast arteriogram and MRA from a patient with an accessory renal artery. A. Contrast arteriogram from this patient with an abdominal aortic aneurysm reveals a double right renal artery and a single left renal artery. B. Gadolinium-enhanced MRA from the same patient which also demonstrates the double right renal artery and single left renal artery. In addition, a retroaortic left renal vein was identified. (Figure continues.)

must be tested on the subgroup of patients with renovascular hypertension. A large study correlating MRI calculated flow data to outcome postintervention will be needed before the technique can be validated.

RECOMMENDATIONS

In centers where MRA has been validated by comparison with standard contrast arteriography it may be employed as the screening test of choice for patients with suspected renovascular disease.

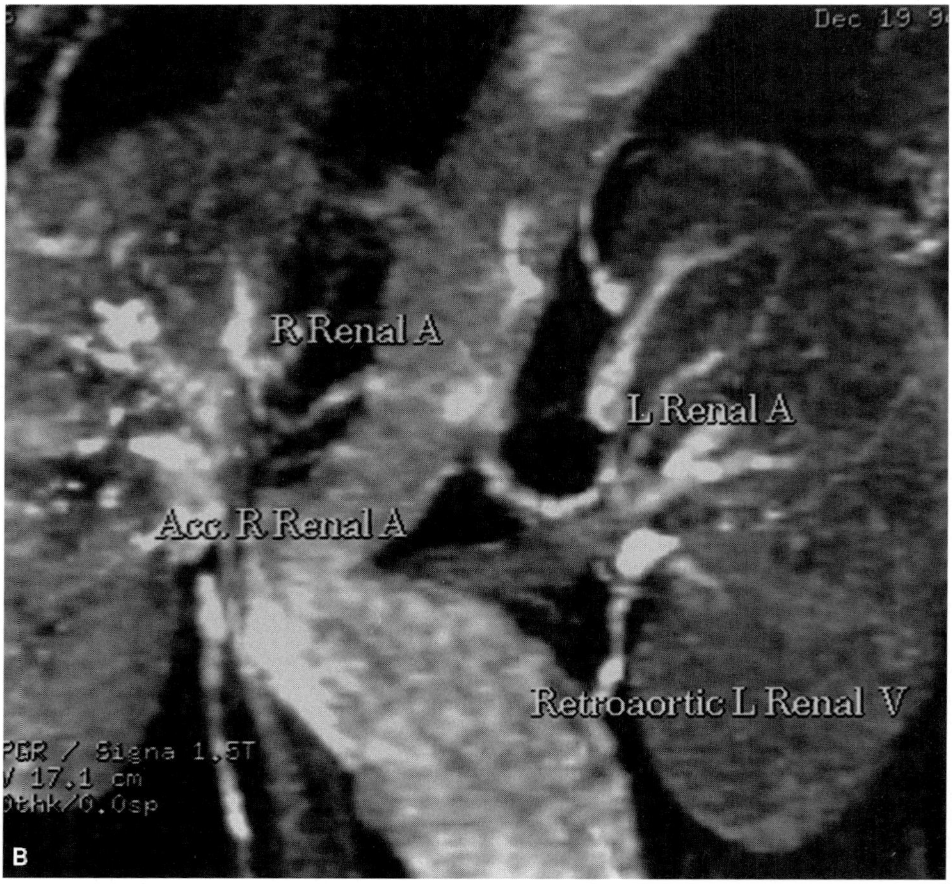

Figure 5–3. *(continued)*

MRA is highly sensitive and has a high negative predictive value in several recent series. It offers the advantage of arteriographic imaging, unlike any other currently employed noninvasive test. The technique can be implemented on a large number of currently installed MR scanners using commercially available software. In the future, due to its outpatient application and low morbidity, MRA will have an increasing role in the diagnosis of renovascular disease.

REFERENCES

1. Dean, RH. Renovascular hypertension: an overview. In: Rutherford, RB, ed. *Vascular Surgery.* 3rd edition. Philadelphia: WB Saunders; 1989, pp. 1211–1218.

Part II

Indications for Renal Artery Revascularization for RENOVASCULAR HYPERTENSION AND RENAL SALVAGE

2. Working group on Renovascular Hypertension. Final Report of the Working Group on Renovascular Hypertension. *Arch Int Med* 1987; 147:820–829.
3. Dean, RH. Changing Concepts in Indications for Renal Artery Reconstruction. In: Whittemore AD, ed. *Advances in Vascular Surgery*. Vol. 1. St. Louis, Mosby-Year Book, Inc.; 1993:171–180.
4. Lawson JD, Boerth RK, Foster JH, et al. Diagnosis and management of renovascular hypertension in children. *Arch Surg* 1977;112: 1307–1311.
5. Meier GH, Sumpio B, Black HR, Gusberg RJ. Captopril renal scintography. An advance in the detection and treatment of renovascular hypertension. *J Vasc Surg* 1990;11:770–777.
6. Galanski M, Prokop M, Chavan A, et al. Renal artery stenosis: spiral CT angiography. *Radiology* 1993;189:185–192.
7. Strandness DE. Duplex scanning in diagnosis of renovascular hypertension. *Surg Clin North Am* 1990;70:109–117.
8. Owen RS, Carpenter JP, Baum RA, et al. Magnetic resonance imaging of angiographically occult runoff vessels in peripheral arterial occlusive disease. *NEJM* 1992;326:1577–1581.
9. Hertz SM, Baum RA, Owen RS, et al. Comparison of magnetic resonance angiography and contrast arteriography in peripheral arterial stenosis. *Am J Surg* 1993;166:1123–1126.
10. Riles TS, Eidelman EM, Litt AW, et al. Comparison of magnetic resonance angiography, conventional angiography, and duplex scanning. *Stroke* 1992;23:341–346.
11. Mittl RL, Broderick M, Carpenter JP, et al. Blinded reader comparison of magnetic resonance angiography and duplex ultrasonography for carotid artery bifurcation stenosis. *Stroke* 1994;25:4–10.
12. Kent CK, Edelman RR, Kim D, Steinman TI, Porter DH, Skillman JJ. Magnetic resonance imaging: A reliable test for the evaluation of proximal atherosclerotic renal artery stenosis. *J Vasc Surg* 1991; 13(2):311–318.
13. Hertz SM, Holland GA, Baum RA, Haskal ZJ, Carpenter JP. Evaluation of renal artery stenosis by magnetic resonance angiography. *Am J Surg* 1994;168:140–143.
14. Gedroyc W. Magnetic resonance angiography of renal arteries. *Urol Clin North Am* 1994;21(2):201–214.
15. Lewin J. Time-of-flight magnetic resonance angiography of the aorta and renal arteries. *Invest Radiol* 1992;27:S84–S89.
16. Yucel KE, Kaufman JA, Prince M, Bazari H, Fang L, Waltman AC. Time-of-flight renal MR angiography; Utility in patients with renal insufficiency. *Mag Res Imaging* 1993;11:925–930.
17. Edelman RR, Wentz KO, Mattle H, et al. Projection arteriography and venography: initial clinical results with MR. *Radiology* 1989; 172:351–357.
18. Kim D, Edelman R, Kent K, Porter DH, Skillman JJ. Abdominal aorta and renal artery stenosis: Evaluation with MR angiography. *Radiology* 1990;174(3):727–731.

19. Debatin JF, Spritzer CE, Grist TM, Beam C, et al. Imaging of the Renal Arteries: Value of MR Angiography. *AJR* 1991;157:981–990.
20. Gedroyc W, Negus R, et al. Magnetic resonance angiography of renal transplants. *Lancet* 1992;339:789–791.
21. Lin W, Haacke M, Smith A, Clampitt M. Gadolinium-enhanced High Resolution MR Angiography with Adaptive Vessel Tracking: Preliminary Results in the Intractanial Circulation. *J Mag Res Imaging* 1992;2(3):277–284.
22. Manning W, Atkinson D, Grossman W, Paulin S, Edelman R. First Pass Nuclear Magnetic Resonance Imaging Studies Using Gadolinium-DTPA in Patients with Coronary Artery Disease. *J Am Coll Cardiol* 1991;18(4):959–965.
23. Revel D, Loubeyre P, Deligenette A, Douek P, Amiel M. Contrast-enhanced Magnetic Resonance Tomography: A New Imaging Technique for Studying Thoracic Great Vessels. *Mag Res Imaging* 1993; 11:1101–1105.
24. Debatin JF, Ting RH, Wegmuller H, et al. Renal artery blood flow: quantitation with phase-contrast MR imaging with and without breath holding. *Radiology* 1994;190:371–378.

6 Renal Revascularization or Nephrectomy for Renovascular Hypertension

Richard H. Dean and Kimberley J. Hansen

The usefulness of the selective use of operation in controlling hypertension secondary to renal artery occlusive disease is widely recognized. The criteria for selection for revascularization versus nephrectomy in the patient with a totally occluded renal artery or a poorly functioning kidney are still controversial. Nevertheless, there is no denying the benefit derived through use of either technique in many patients. Traditionally, study of the sequelae of renovascular occlusive disease has centered on the pathophysiology and management of the resultant renovascular hypertension. More recent reports, however, have emphasized the potential for simultaneous retrieval of excretory function in some patients with combined hypertension and renal insufficiency.[1–3] These observations have renewed awareness of this functional consequence of renal ischemia and have led to the coining of the term *ischemic nephropathy*. By definition, ischemic nephropathy reflects the presence of anatomically severe occlusive disease of the extraparenchymal renal artery in a patient with excretory renal insufficiency.

Hypertension in the patient with renal artery occlusion and a poorly functioning or nonfunctioning kidney can be treated equally well by revascularization or nephrectomy. However, the management of hypertension as well as the retrieval of function by revascularization would be superior if both of these end-results could be predicted and assessed. The practical value of this premise is obvious when one considers that as many as 35 percent of patients with mild contralateral occlusive lesions will progress to hemodynamically severe occlusive lesions within 5 years.[4] When such patients have undergone nephrectomy for renovascular hypertension and their contralateral disease has progressed, global renal function is threatened and operative intervention must then be contemplated for patients who are severely azotemic and have potentially dialysis-dependent renal failure. The atherosclerotic occlusive disease in the remaining kidney may not develop in a manner that will be recognized appropriately or will develop at a site not amenable to surgical correction. On the other hand, a too-aggressive attitude toward revascularization of the poorly functioning or nonfunctioning kidney and attempted recovery of function at the lowest limits of retrievability will sometimes lead to revascularization of a kidney in which no functional response can be achieved. In this instance, primary nephrectomy would be simpler than revascularization and would be equally beneficial in the control of hypertension. Therefore, evaluation of the expected results of revascularizing poorly functioning kidneys and of the value of preoperative predictors of retrieval are important in the management of these patients.

Reports of retrieval of function underscore the potential value of aggressive management.[5,6] We reviewed the effect of revascularization of renal function in 64 patients who had a preoperative creatinine clearance by the affected kidney of less than or equal of 15 ml/min.[7] Results of this study and our subsequent experience have led us to proceed with revascularization whenever the distal vessel is identified and appears normal by arteriography. Similarly, when at least 10% of total renal function is coming from the poorly functioning kidney on isotope renography, we will explore the distal vessel even when it is not visualized by arteriography. In about 40% of such cases, we will find a normal distal vessel and will proceed with revascularization. Nevertheless, if atherosclerotic lesions are present at the level of the branches, we will proceed with nephrectomy.

Although Zinman and Libertino found preoperative renal biopsy to be a useful predictor of functional retrieval in their series of patients,[8] we have not found it worthwhile. Having identified diffuse hyalinization of glomeruli in specimens obtained by open biopsy of selected sections of kidneys with adequate renal function and in kidneys with marked improvement in excretory function, we long ago abandoned the technique as misleading and potentially hazardous.

A number of factors influence the successful revascularization of poorly functioning kidneys. Although studies have not defined limits below which clinically important retrieval of function is impossible, they have identified preoperative variables that may predict a favorable response. Removal of a nonfunctioning kidney does nothing to diminish excretory function. Indeed, subsequent improvement in blood pressure control with the concomitant elimination of high-dose diuretics and other meditations that might adversely affect renal function may lead to improvement in function in the remaining kidney. Nevertheless, long-term follow-up studies of renal function and renal anatomy in patients with renovascular hypertension underscore the frequently progressive nature of the disease in both the ipsilateral and the contralateral kidney.[9,10] For this reason, the aggressive use of revascularization rather than nephrectomy in patients with characteristics favorably predicting retrieval of function should improve the long-term management of these patients. The application of predictors such as urinary hyperconcentration of nonreabsorbable solutes on split renal function studies[7] and the identification of a disease-free distal renal artery on preoperative angiography or intraoperatively should allow a more accurate selection of the appropriate operation and thereby limit the frequency of inappropriate revascularization leading to subsequent nephrectomy.

Finally, renal length has been frequently used as a factor on which the decision has been based for nephrectomy. We evaluated this factor as a predictor of functional retrieval in our previously mentioned group of 64 patients[7] in this group. Preoperative renal length was found to have a statistically significant negative linear relationship ($P = 0.023$; $r = -0.513$) to the extent of change in renal length. Many physicians have adopted a lower limit of renal length below which they suggest that there is no value of revascularization. Although the linear regression analysis only included two kidneys with length less than or equal to 8.0 cm, it suggests that when other parameters predict the presence of retrievable renal function in a kidney with a correctable lesion that short renal length alone is not a valuable negative predictor of response. In contrast, one might expect the greatest percent improvement in length in such kidneys. Nevertheless, the premise that renal length improvement can be equated to improvement in renal function is speculative. The demonstrated interrelationships between preoperative renal length, change in renal length following revascularization, and changes in functional parameters as identified in this study, however, suggest that such a relationship may exist.

Because the question of revascularization versus nephrectomy arises when one has poor vascular anatomy or renal parenchyma a brief discussion of issues surrounding arteriography are appropriate. We have continued to rely on standard "cut film" arteriography in patients with renal insufficiency who have clinical or duplex sonographic evidence of renovascular disease. In our experience, adequate assessment of the renal vasculature and the juxtarenal aorta requires multiple injections when intra-arterial digital subtraction angiography is employed. The use of a single midstream flush aortogram requires no more contrast material than that required for such multiple intra-arterial digital subtraction studies. Additionally, standard arteriography provides information about cortical thickness and renal length, as well as improved clarity for interpretation of the renal artery anatomy.

The fact that arteriography in patients with severe renal insufficiency, especially those with concomitant diabetes mellitus, can aggravate renal failure is widely recognized. Nevertheless, we believe that this risk is justified in such patients who have severe or accelerated hypertension or who have positive findings on renal duplex sonography. In these circumstances, the potential benefit derived from identification and correction of a functionally significant renovascular occlusive lesion exceeds the risk of arteriography.

Finally, we believe nephrectomy is a procedure that should be limited to a subgroup of patients with RVH in whom the kidney responsible for the hypertension has nonreconstructable vessels and negligible or no residual excretory function. In these circumstances of unretrievable renal function, nephrectomy can provide benefit in control of hypertension while not diminishing overall excretory function. In all other circumstances in which there is significant residual excretory renal function, the price of nephrectomy (loss of functioning renal mass) is greater than the potential benefit. Exception to this rule occurs only when hypertension is incontrollable on maximal drug therapy and residual pressures consistently are severely elevated (greater than 120 mm Hg). This extreme conservatism for the role of nephrectomy is based on the knowledge that greater than 35 percent of patients with atherosclerotic lesions will develop contralateral severe lesions during follow-up. Such lesions will place such a patient at risk for clinically severe renal failure and recurrent hypertension. This is of even greater importance in children, in whom 50 percent of those who initially present with a unilateral lesion subsequently will develop contralateral disease.[11]

In summary, we believe nephrectomy should be limited to the subgroup of patients with renovascular hypertension in whom the kidney responsible for the hypertension has non-reconstructible vessels and negligible or no residual excretory function. In these circumstances of irretrievable renal function, nephrectomy can provide benefit in control of hypertension without diminishing overall excretory function using this algorithm, primary nephrectomy alone accounts for only 2.5% of our procedures.

REFERENCES

1. Scobie JE, Maher ER, Hamilton G, et al. Atherosclerotic renovascular disease causing renal impairment—A case for treatment. *Clin Nephrol* 1989;31:119.
2. Bengtsson U, Bergentz S-E, Norback B. Surgical treatment of renal artery stenosis with impending uremia. *Clin Nephrol* 1974;2:222.
3. Novick AC, Pohl MA, Schreiber M, et al. Revascularization for preservation of renal function in patients with atherosclerotic renovascular disease. *J Urol* 1983;129:907.

4. Dean RH, Wilson JP, Burko H, Foster JH. Saphenous vein aortorenal bypass grafts: serial arteriographic study. *Ann Surg* 1974;180: 469–478.
5. Dean RH, Lawson JD, Hollifield JW, et al. Revascularization of the poorly functioning kidney. *Surgery* 1979;85:44.
6. Libertino JA, Zinman L. Revascularization of the poorly functioning and the nonfunctioning kidney. In Novick AC, Straffon RA eds. *Vascular Problems in Urologic Surgery.* Philadelphia: WB Saunders; 1982, pp 173–187.
7. Dean RH, Englund R, Dupont WD, et al. Retrieval of renal function by revascularization. Study of preoperative outcome predictors. *Ann Surg* 1985;202:367.
8. Zinman L, Libertino JA. Revascularization of the chronic totally occluded renal artery with restoration of renal function. *J Urol* 1977; 228:517.
9. Dean RH, Kieffer RW, Smith BM, et al. Renovascular hypertension: Anatomic and renal function changes during drug therapy. *Arch Surg* 1981;116:1408.
10. Dean RH. Renovascular hypertension. *Curr Probl Surg* 1985; 22(2):6.
11. Lawson JD, Boerth RK, Foster JH, et al. Diagnosis and management of renovascular hypertension in children. *Arch Surg* 1977;112:1307.

7

Renal Revascularization for Atherosclerotic Ischemic Renal Disease

Andrew C. Novick

Atherosclerosis is the most common cause of renal artery disease and accounts for 70% of all renal artery lesions. This disease may be limited to the renal artery (15–20% of cases) but is more often a manifestation of diffuse atherosclerosis involving the abdominal aorta, coronary, cerebral, or lower extremity vessels (80–85% of cases). Several epidemiologic studies have shown that atherosclerotic renal artery disease is common in patients with generalized atherosclerosis obliterans, regardless of whether renovascular hypertension is present.[1–5] These data indicate that the anatomic presence of atherosclerotic renal artery disease in older patients is far more common than that of atherosclerotic renovascular hypertension.

INDICATIONS FOR INTERVENTION

The development of chronic renal failure from atherosclerotic renal artery disease, termed ischemic nephropathy, has become an important clinical issue which is separate and distinct from the problem of renovascular hypertension. Studies on the natural history of atherosclerotic renal artery disease have made it possible to identify those patients in whom such disease poses a significant threat to overall renal function.[6,7] This designation applies to patients with high-grade arterial stenosis affecting the entire renal mass, namely where such stenosis is present bilaterally or involves a solitary kidney. In such patients, the risk of complete renal arterial occlusion is significant, and if this occurs, the clinical outcome is a critical decrease in functioning renal mass with resulting renal failure. Intervention to restore normal renal blood flow is indicated in such patients for the purpose of preserving renal function. Such intervention can be achieved with surgical revascularization or percutaneous transluminal angioplasty (PTA).

In considering potential candidates for surgery or PTA to preserve renal function, a determination must be made of the potential for renal salvage. Total occlusion of the renal artery does not necessarily imply irreversible ischemic parenchymal damage, and it is well accepted that with gradual arterial occlusion, the viability of the kidney can occasionally be maintained through the development of collateral arterial supply.[8,9] Helpful clinical clues suggesting renal salvageability in such cases include: 1) angiographic demonstration of retrograde filling of the distal renal arterial tree by collateral vessels on the side of total arterial occlusion, 2) a renal biopsy demonstrating well preserved glomeruli and tubules with minimal arteriolar sclerosis, 3) a kidney size of >9 cm, and 4) function of the involved kidney upon isotope renography or intravenous pyelography. When such criteria are met, restoration of normal renal arterial flow can lead to recovery of renal function.

It is also appropriate to emphasize that revascularization to preserve renal function is generally not worthwhile in patients with severe azotemia (serum creatinine >4.0 mg/dl), because advanced underlying renal parenchymal disease is usually present and obviates improvement in renal function with restored perfusion.[10] Severe nephrosclerosis is the most common form of parenchymal disease; in such cases, however, renal cholesterol embolization may be an additional complicating feature. The single exception to the above admonition regarding preoperative renal function is presented by patients with chronic bilateral total renal arterial occlusion where, fortuitously, the viability of one or both kidneys has been maintained through collateral vascular supply. The degree of preoperative renal functional impairment in such cases is often severe, and the improvement following revascularization may be dramatic.[11,12] Unfortunately, this clinical presentation is rare.

PERCUTANEOUS TRANSLUMINAL ANGIOPLASTY

In patients with atherosclerotic renal artery disease, the success rate of PTA has been excellent and comparable to that of surgical revascularization in patients with non-ostial lesions. These lesions comprise only 15–20% of all atherosclerotic renal artery lesions and PTA has emerged as the treatment of choice. In the more commonly encountered ostial atherosclerotic lesions, the efficacy of PTA is not as well established since most published reports have indicated less satisfactory results in this large clinical subgroup.[13–17] This group also comprises the majority of older patients who require relief of arterial obstruction for treatment of ischemic nephropathy. The major problem with PTA for ostial atherosclerotic lesions has been a high incidence of recurrent stenosis due either to elastic recoil of the dilated artery, neointimal hyperplasia, or recurrent atheromatous disease. At the present time, surgical revascularization is the definitive form of intervention for ostial atherosclerotic renal artery disease.

SURGICAL RENAL REVASCULARIZATION

A variety of surgical revascularization techniques are available for treating patients with significant atherosclerotic renal artery disease. Aortorenal bypass with a free graft of autogenous hypogastric artery or saphenous vein remains a popular method in patients with a non-diseased abdominal aorta.[18,19] Polytetrafluoroethylene aortorenal bypass grafts have been successfully employed by some authors.[20–22] Renal endarterectomy also continues to be utilized to treat atherosclerotic renal artery disease.

In older patients, severe atherosclerosis of the abdominal aorta may render an aortorenal bypass or endarterectomy technically difficult and potentially hazardous to perform. In such cases, alternate surgical approaches have been favored that allow renal revascularization to be safely and effectively accomplished while avoiding clamping of a badly diseased aorta. The most effective alternate bypass techniques have been splenorenal bypass for left renal revascularization[23,24] and hepatorenal bypass for right renal revascularization.[25] The absence of occlusive disease involving the origin of the celiac artery is an important prerequisite for these operations. A recent study indicated the presence of significant celiac artery stenosis in 50% of patients with atherosclerotic renal artery stenosis.[26] This information underscores the importance of obtaining preoperative lateral aortography to evaluate the celiac artery origin in patients who are being considered for hepatorenal or splenorenal bypass.

Use of the supraceliac or lower thoracic aorta for renal revascularization is a new surgical alternative in patients with significant atherosclerosis of the abdominal aorta and its major visceral branches.[27,28] The supraceliac aorta is often relatively disease-free in such patients and can be used for proximal anastomosis of a renal graft. Simultaneous aortic replacement and renal revascularization have been associated with an increased risk of operative mortality,[29,30] and this approach is best reserved for patients with an indication for aortic replacement such as a significant aortic aneurysm or symptomatic aortoiliac occlusive disease.

Reports from several centers indicate that the techniques de-

Table 7–1. Results of Surgical Revascularization for Atherosclerotic Ischemic Nephropathy

Series	No. Pts.	No. (%) Improved*	No. (%) Stable*	No. (%) Deteriorated*
Novick, 1987[31]	161	93 (58%)	50 (31%)	18 (11%)
Hallett, 1987[37]	91	20 (22%)	48 (53%)	23 (25%)
Hansen, 1992[32]	70	34 (49%)	25 (36%)	11 (15%)
Bredenberg, 1992[33]	40	22 (55%)	10 (25%)	8 (20%)
Libertino, 1992[34]	91	45 (49%)	31 (35%)	15 (16%)

* No (%) with improved, stable or deteriorated postoperative renal function.

scribed for renal vascular reconstruction can be safely performed with a high technical success rate.[31–36] Operative mortality rates of 2.1%,[31] 3.1%,[32] 3.4%[33] and 6.1%[34] have been reported following surgical revascularization in patients with atherosclerotic renal artery disease. An increased risk of operative mortality has been observed with bilateral simultaneous renal revascularization,[37] or when renal revascularization is performed in conjunction with another major vascular operation such as aortic replacement.[36] Most studies have indicated a high technical success rate for surgical vascular reconstruction with postoperative thrombosis or stenosis rates of <10%.[31,34,35]

In recent years, surgical revascularization has increasingly been used to preserve renal function in patients with high-grade atherosclerotic arterial occlusive disease affecting both kidneys or a solitary kidney. These are older patients with diffuse atherosclerosis, ostial renal artery lesions, and varying degrees of renal functional impairment. Studies from several centers **(Table 7–1)** have indicated improvement or stabilization of renal function postoperatively in 75 to 89% of patients. Considering the significant risks of progressive occlusive disease and renal failure that have been associated with medical management of such patients, these results demonstrate a favorable influence of revascularization on the natural history of untreated atherosclerotic renal artery disease.

REFERENCES

1. Salmon P, Brown MA. Renal artery stenosis and peripheral vascular disease: Implications for ACE inhibitor therapy. *Lancet* 1990;336: 321.

2. Choudhri AH, Cleland JGF, Rowlands PC, Tran TL, McCarty M, Al-Kutoubi MAO. Unsuspected renal artery stenosis in peripheral vascular disease. *Br Med J* 1990;301:1197–1198.
3. Wilms G, Marchal G, Peene P, Baert AL. The angiographic incidence of renal artery stenosis in the arteriosclerotic population. *Eur J Radiol* 1990;10:195–197.
4. Olin JW, Melia M, Young JR, Graor RA, Risius B. Prevalence of atherosclerotic renal artery stenosis in patients with atherosclerosis elsewhere. *Am J Med* 1990;188:46–51.
5. Harding MB, Smith LR, Himmestein SI, et al. Renal artery stenosis: Prevalence and associated risk factors in patients undergoing routine cardiac catheterization. *J Am Soc Nephrol* 1992;2:1608–16.
6. Schreiber MJ, Pohl MA, Novick AC. The natural history of atherosclerotic and fibrous renal artery disease. *Urol Clin North Am* 1984;11: 383–392.
7. Tollefson DE, Ernst CB. Natural history of atherosclerotic renal artery stenosis associated with aortic disease. *J Vasc Surg* 1991;14: 327–31.
8. Libertino JA, Zinman L, Breslin DJ, et al. Renal artery revascularization: restoration of renal function. *JAMA* 1980;244:1340–1342.
9. Schefft P, Novick AC, Stewart BH, et al. Renal revascularization in patients with total occlusion of the renal artery. *J Urol* 1980;124: 184–186.
10. Mercier C, Piquet P, Alimi Y, Tournigand P, Albrand JJ. Occlusive disease of the renal arteries and chronic renal failure: The limits of reconstructive surgery. *Ann Vasc Surg* 1990;4:166–170.
11. Wasser WG, Krakoff LR, Haimov M, et al. Restoration of renal function after bilateral renal artery occlusion. *Arch Intern Med* 1981;141: 1647–1651.
12. Kaylor W, Novick AC, Ziegelbaum M, Vidt D. Reversal of end-stage renal failure with surgical revascularization in patients with atherosclerotic renal artery occlusion. *J Urol* 1989;141:486–488.
13. Ramsay LE, Waller PC. Blood pressure response to percutaneous transluminal angioplasty for renovascular hypertension. An overview of published series. *Br J Med* 1990;300:569–572.
14. Cicuto KP, McLean GK, Oleaga J, et al. Renal artery stenosis: anatomic classification for percutaneous angioplasty. *AJR* 1981;137: 599–601.
15. Sos TA, Pickering PG, Sniderman KW, et al. Percutaneous transluminal renal angiography in renovascular hypertension due to atheroma or fibrous dysplasia. *N Eng J Med* 1983;309:274–279.
16. Hayes J, Risius B, Novick AC, et al. Experience with percutaneous transluminal angioplasty for renal artery stenosis at the Cleveland Clinic. *J Urol* 1988;139:488–492.
17. Canzanello VJ, Millan VG, Spiegel JE, Ponce SP, Kopelman RI, Madias NE. *Hypertension* 1989;13:163–172.
18. Ernst CB, Stanley JC, Marshall FF, et al. Autogenous saphenous

vein aortorenal autografts: a ten-year experience. *Arch Surg* 1972; 105:855–864.

19. Stoney RJ, Olofsson PA. Aortorenal arterial autografts: The last two decades. *Ann Vasc Surg* 1988;2:169–173.
20. Khauli RB, Novick AC, Coseriu CV. Renal revascularization and polytetrafluoroethylene grafts. *Cleve Clin Q* 1984;51:365–369.
21. Cormier JM, Fichelle JM, Laurian C, Gigou F, Artru B, Ricco JB. Renal artery revascularization with polytetrafluoroethylene bypass graft. *Ann Vasc Surg* 1990;4:471–478.
22. Lagneau P, Michel JB, Charrat JM. Use of polytetrafluoroethylene grafts for renal bypass. *J Vas Surg* 1987;5:738–742.
23. Brewster DC, Darling RC. Splenorenal arterial anastomosis for renovascular hypertension. *Ann Surg* 1979;189:353–358.
24. Khauli R, Novick AC, Ziegelbaum W. Splenorenal bypass in the treatment of renal artery stenosis: Experience with 69 cases. *J Vasc Surg* 1985;2:547–551.
25. Chibaro EA, Libertino JA, Novick AC. Use of hepatic circulation for renal revascularization. *Ann Surg* 1984;199:406–411.
26. Valentine RJ, Martin JD, Myers SI, Rossi MB, Clagett GP. Asymptomatic celiac and superior mesenteric artery stenoses are more prevalent among patients with unsuspected renal artery stenoses. *J Vasc Surg* 1991;14:195–199.
27. Fry RE, Fry WJ. Supraceliac aortorenal bypass with saphenous vein for renovascular hypertension. *Surg Gynecol Obstet* 1989;168: 181–182.
28. Novick AC, Stewart R. Use of the thoracic aorta for renal revascularization. *J Urol* 1990;143:77–79.
29. Shahian DM, Najafi H, Javid H, et al. Simultaneous aortic and renal artery reconstruction. *Arch Surg* 1980;115:1491–1497.
30. Tarazi RY, Hertzer NR, Beven EG, et al. Simultaneous aortic reconstruction and renal revascularization: risk factors and late results in 89 patients. *J Vasc Surg* 1987;5:709–715.
31. Novick AC, Ziegelbaum M, Vidt DG, et al. Trends in surgical revascularization for renal artery disease: ten years' experience. *JAMA* 1987; 257:498–501.
32. Hansen KJ, Starr SM, Sands E, Burkart JM, Plonk GW, Dean RH. Contemporary surgical management of renovascular disease. *J Vasc Surg* 1992;16:319–331.
33. Bredenberg CE, Sampson LN, Ray FS, Cormier RA, Heintz S, Eldrup-Jorgensen PA. Changing patterns in surgery for chronic renal artery occlusive diseases. *J Vasc Surg* 1992;15:1018–1024.
34. Libertino JA, Bosco PJ, Ying CY, Breslin DJ, Woods BO, Tsapatsaris NP, Swinton NW. Renal revascularization to preserve and restore renal function. *J Urol* 1992;147:1485–1487.
35. Van Bockel JH, Van Schilfgaarde R, Felthuis W, Hermans J, Van Brummelen P, Terpstra JL. Surgical treatment of renovascular hypertension caused by arteriosclerosis: Influence of preoperative fac-

tors on blood pressure control early and late after reconstructive surgery. *Surgery* 1987;101:698–705.

36. Lawrie GM, Morris GC, Glaeser DH, DeBakey ME. Renovascular reconstruction: Factors affecting long-term prognosis in 919 patients followed up to 31 years. *Am J Cardiol* 1989;63:1085–1092.
37. Hallett JW, Fowl R, O'Brien PC, Bernatz PE, Pairolero PC, Cherry KJ, Hollier LH. Renovascular operations in patients with chronic renal insufficiency: Do the benefits justify the risks? *J Vasc Surg* 1987;5:622–627.

8

Renal Revascularization Using Percutaneous Balloon Angioplasty for Fibromuscular Dysplasia and Atherosclerotic Disease

Louis Martin

The first renal artery angioplasty was performed by Andreas Gruentzig and reported in *Lancet* in 1974. Now, almost 20 years since this report, the safety and efficacy of renal artery angioplasty are still questioned and its role in the treatment of patients with hypertension and azotemia is not clearly defined. The goals of renal artery angioplasty are cure of renovascular hypertension and improvement or preservation of renal function. It is technically possible to dilate almost all stenoses proximal to the tertiary renal artery branches. The key question is, "Should we?" If every attempted renal angioplasty was technically successful, improved blood pressure control, and had no morbidity, the answer would be "yes." Unfortunately, procedural complications, technical failures and clinical failures are not uncommon. To decide whether to perform renal artery angioplasty, we must know the answers to several important questions: Can renal artery angioplasty be safely performed? Are the results durable? Are the results acceptable compared with medical control and surgical revascularization? Is surgery likely to be complicated by a technical failure? To answer these questions, technical success, morbidity, durability, and clinical success of renal artery angioplasty must be discussed.

TECHNICAL SUCCESS

We will define technical success as safely crossing and dilating the stenosis with no major morbidity, a residual stenosis of less than 50%, and/or a residual pressure gradient of less than 10% of the peak systolic pressure. In experienced hands using currently available angiographic equipment including digital angiography and roadmapping, technical success should be between 85 and 90%. To achieve success this high, the angiographer must also exercise sound judgement in selecting patients for renal revascularization. It is beyond the scope of this chapter to attempt to define the patients on whom angioplasty should *not* be attempted. Suffice it to say that the experienced angiographer should know the limits of his capabilities. The cases that he selects should have a very high chance for technical success and a very low chance of compromising surgical revascularization should failure or complication occur.

All renal artery angioplasties should be done either through long vascular sheaths that extend from the groin to the level of the renal artery or through coaxial guiding catheters through which the guidewire and balloon catheter can be directed across the stenosis **(Figs. 8–1 and 8–2)**. The use of either of these devices enables the angiographer to obtain simultaneous pressure measurements across the stenotic area and to inject contrast media for angiography without having to remove the balloon catheter and/or guidewire from the area which is being treated. Therefore

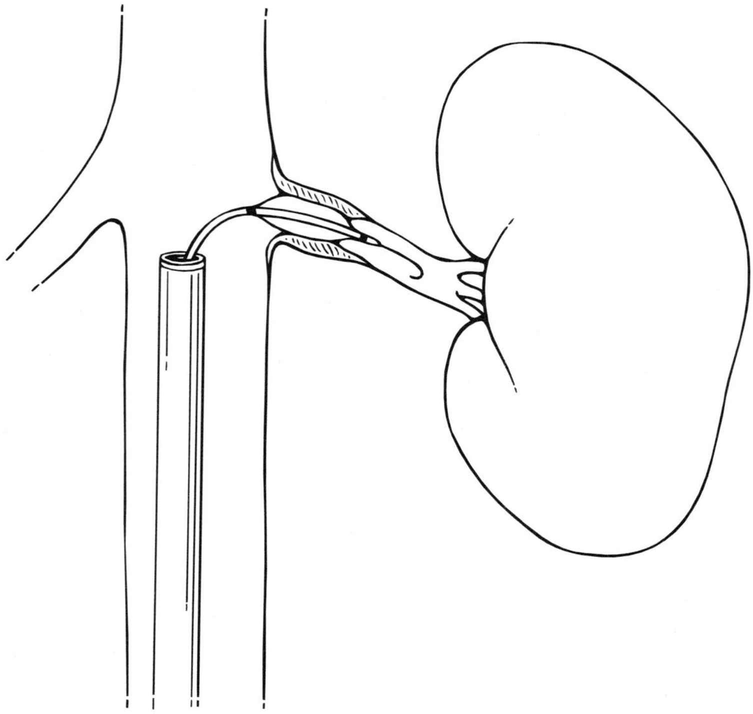

Figure 8–1. Vascular sheath with an opaque tip marker.

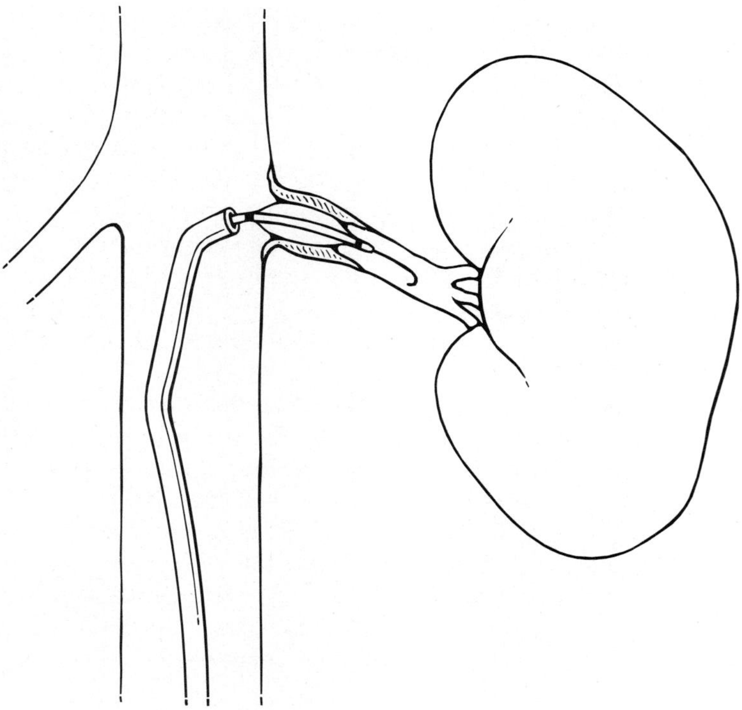

Figure 8–2. Angioplasty balloon introduced through a coaxial renal guiding catheter.

the hemodynamic and anatomic results of the balloon dilatation are known before access across the area of stenosis has been withdrawn **(Fig. 8–3)**. Should it be necessary to redilate with a larger balloon or should a complication requiring treatment occur, this can be determined before removing the balloon catheter or guidewire from the renal artery and can be initiated without the added risk of recrossing the area which has been recently dilated. Equally important is ascertaining the exact position of the balloon before it is inflated in order to ensure the safety of adjacent vascular branches. If necessary, more than one guidewire can be inserted through the same guiding catheter so that an adjacent vascular branch can be protected or treated **(Fig. 8–4)**.

MORBIDITY

Does technical failure compromise surgery? Usually not, but it would be naive to argue that technical failure, should it include intimal dissection or vessel thrombosis, does not compromise surgery. These complications can make required surgical repair

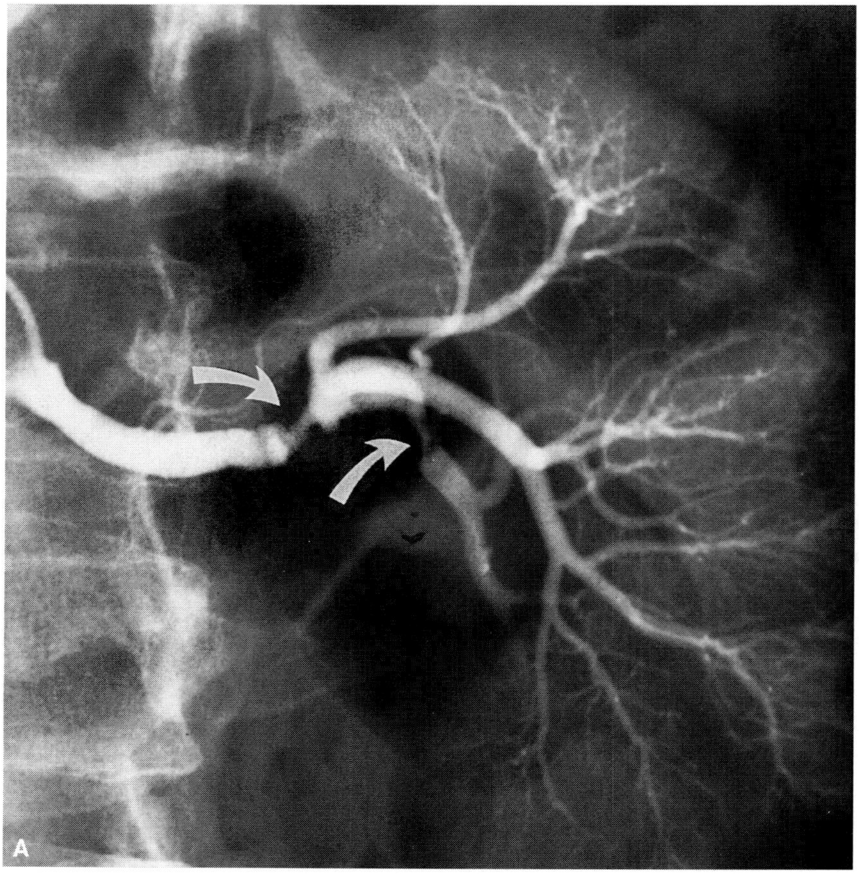

Figure 8–3. A. Selective left renal angiogram showing stenoses of the distal main renal artery and a secondary branch. B. Angiogram performed through a coaxial renal guiding catheter following PTA without withdrawing the guidewire shows successful dilatation of both lesions. (Figure continues.)

emergent and more difficult; in some cases nephrectomy may be necessary. It is important that the angiographer take measures to lessen the risk of compromising future surgery. It is better to accept an uncomplicated technical failure than to persist and cause vascular dissection or thrombosis. In review of almost 1000 patients **(Table 8–1)** including the first 300 patients on whom renal artery angioplasty was performed at Emory University Hospital, trauma to the main renal artery requiring surgical correction occurred in 2.5%, renal artery rupture occurred in 0.7%, and nephrectomy was needed in 0.5%. With increased use of renal guiding catheters, smaller guidewires and balloon catheters, and

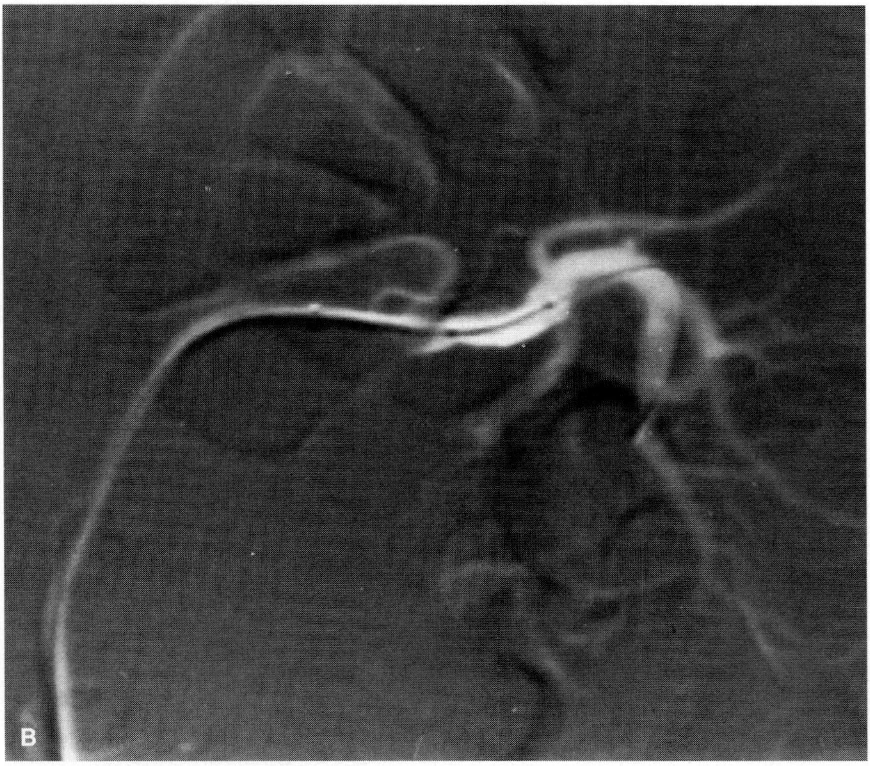

Figure 8–3. *(continued)*

more advanced radiographic equipment, the incidence of these serious complications should lessen. In the last 200 patients on whom angioplasty has been performed at Emory University Hospital, only two have required emergent surgery and none required secondary nephrectomy.

DURABILITY OF RENAL ANGIOPLASTY

In experienced hands, stenosis of the renal artery can be crossed and dilated with low morbidity. Are the results durable or is restenosis sure to occur? **Figure 8–5** demonstrates that long-term patency is possible, but is this case the rule or the exception? Based on 518 patients who underwent follow-up angioplasties, the mean restenosis rate is 30% after PTA of atherosclerotic lesions.[15] Tegtmeyer et al reported 87% ten year cumulative primary patency

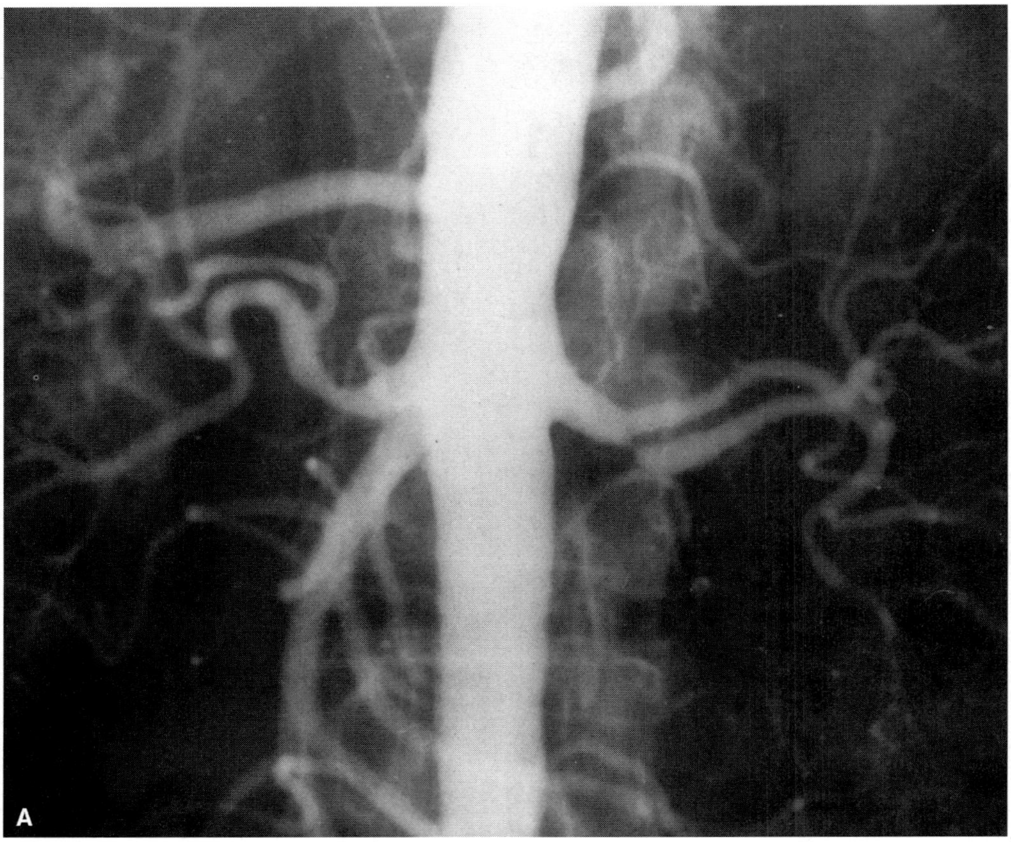

Figure 8–4. A. Aortogram showing stenosis of dorsal renal artery branch. B. Guidewire placed to protect ventral branch should it be damaged while dilating dorsal branch stenosis. C. Aortogram after PTA. (Figure continues.)

based on life table analysis of clinical and angiographic data in 66 patients with fibromuscular dysplasia.[16] Other authors report similarly high primary patency. At Emory University our primary patency is lower: 13 of 66 (20%) patients with FMD required repeat angioplasty to maintain patency. There were no major complications associated with the repeat dilatations nor was secondary surgical revascularization necessary in this group.

Several factors increase the incidence of restenosis. These include ostial location of the lesion, eccentric stenosis, calcification in the vessel wall, and an inadequate initial angioplasty result. Some have suggested that ostial stenoses be treated surgically or by primary stenting. Why are ostial stenoses more difficult to treat effectively? Most interventionalists agree that there are two ana-

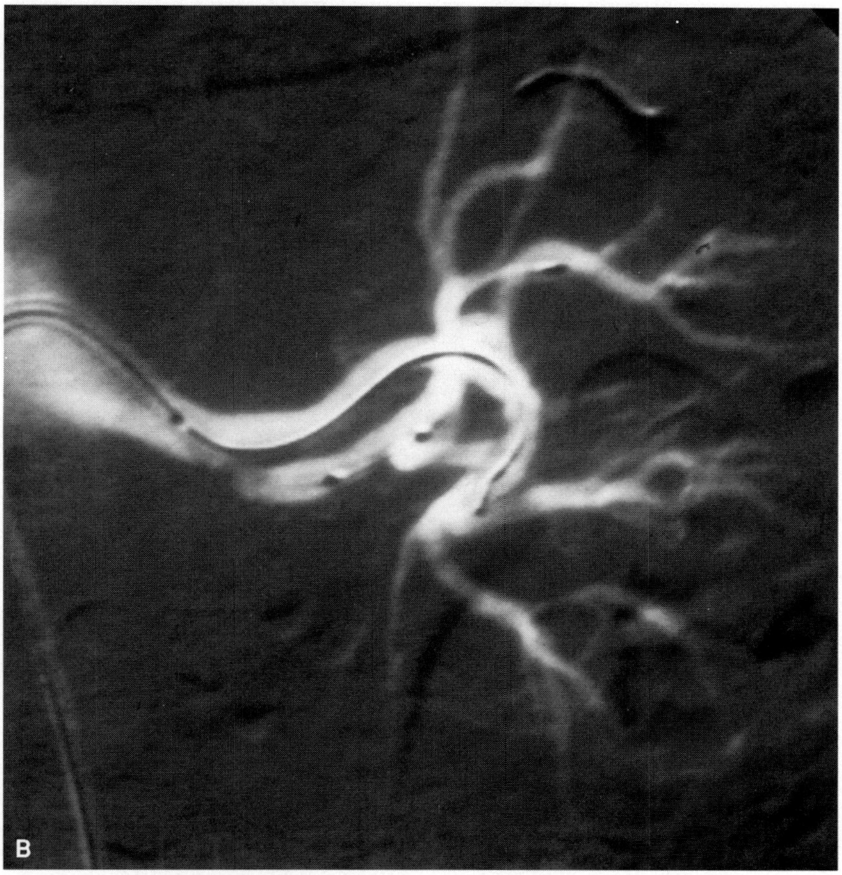

Figure 8–4. *(continued)*

tomic lesions that can narrow the ostium and that these may appear similar angiographically. One involves the lining of the aorta. After displacement during balloon angioplasty, aortic plaque falls like a curtain over the renal artery ostium resulting in technical and clinical failure **(Fig. 8–6)**. The other lesion may appear similar but is secondary to atheromatous plaque involving the most proximal portion of the renal artery. This plaque can be successfully treated by balloon angioplasty **(Fig. 8–7)**. The success of the angiographer in treating ostial stenosis will depend on his ability to distinguish between these two lesions. Unfortunately it is often impossible to tell these lesions apart. In **Figure 8–8,** ostial lesions that appear to be identical were treated similarly by balloon angioplasty. Technical failure on the left required surgical revascularization; treatment on the right was succesful.

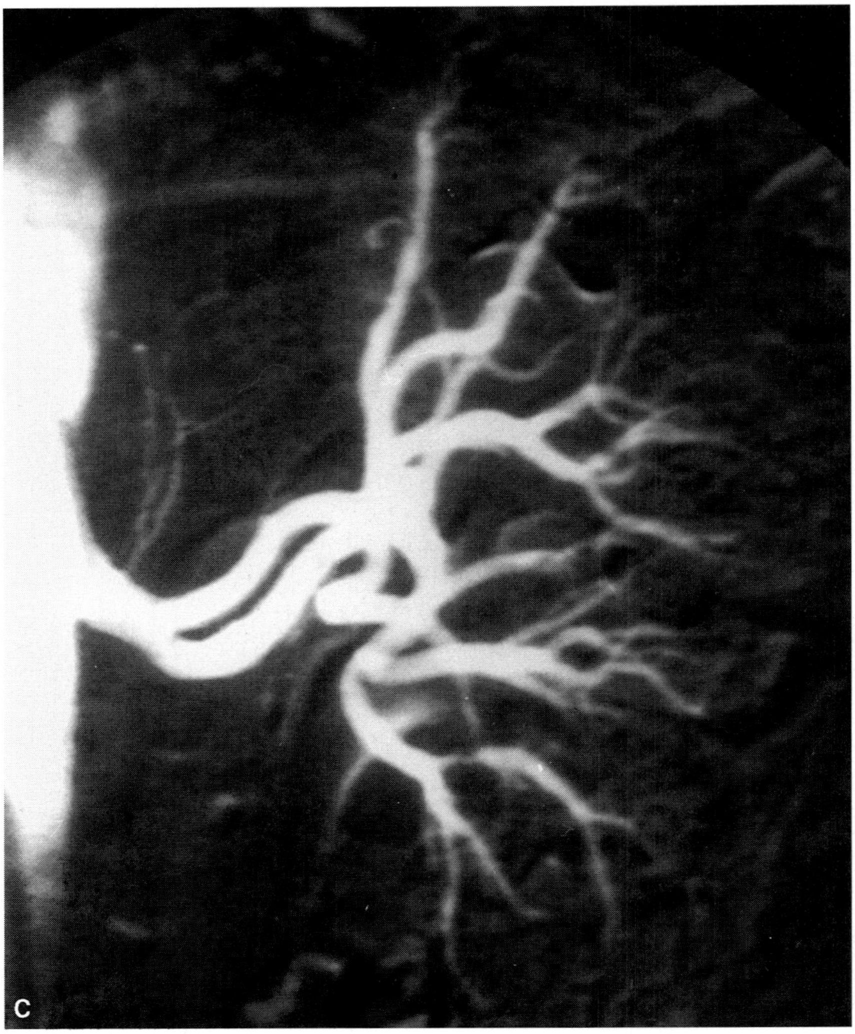

Figure 8–4. *(continued)*

CLINICAL SUCCESS

Certainly with such a high degree of technical success we would expect a very high degree of clinical success to result from renal artery angioplasty. **Tables 8–2 and 8–3** include a review of the published results of renal artery angioplasty for treatment of atherosclerotic and fibromuscular renal artery stenosis reported from major medical centers in the United States and Europe including our own. Disparity exists among the results from these institu-

Table 8–1. Complications Secondary to Renal Artery Angioplasty

Reference Number	1	2	3	4	5	6	7	8	9	Total
Number of patients	300	68	77	70	94	75	89	109	114	996
30-day mortality	1	0	1	1	0	0	0	2	0	5 (0.5%)
Nephrectomy	0	2	0	0	0	0	2	0	0	4 (0.4%)
Trauma to main renal artery										
Injury requiring surgery	5	0	5	1	4	0	4	3	3	25 (2.5%)
Injury not requiring surgery	2	0	5	1	5	0	1	0	15	29 (2.9%)
Rupture	0	0	2	0	2	0	0	1	2	7 (0.7%)
Segmental renal artery occlusion	6	1	0	2	0	0	0	0	11	19 (1.9%)
Renal failure										
Acute	9	1	0	0	1	0	2	0	3	16 (1.6%)
Worsening of chronic	10	0	1	0	0	3	0	6	0	20 (2.0%)
Symptomatic embolization	5	1	1	2	0	0	0	2	0	10 (1.0%)
Puncture site										
Trauma requiring surgery	8	0	0	0	0	0	3	0	4	15 (1.5%)
Other	(4a-c)	(1d)	0	0	(1e)	(1f)	(1g)	(1h)	(2i)	11 (1.1%)

a, perforation of main renal artery by guidewire (no surgery, no sequelae; 1 patient); b, thoracic aortic dissection after SK for opening of totally occluded renal artery (1 patient); c, thrombus in main renal artery lysed by UK successfully (2 patients): d, cardiac arrest (1 patient); e, brachial plexis injury (1 patient); f, small internal dissection; no surgery or sequelae (1 patient); g, transient ideopathic thrombocytopenia and hemolytic anemia (1 patient); h, thrombus main renal artery successfully treated with SK (1 patient); i, perforation of main renal artery by guidewire (no surgery, no sequelae; 2 patients).

tions. Should we expect the 94% benefit reported by Tegtmeyer or the 33% benefit reported by Sos for treatment of atherosclerotic lesions? Can we realistically hope to achieve 100% benefit secondary to angioplasty of fibromuscular renal artery stenoses? Why is there such wide variation in the results of these leading medical centers? The skill of the angiographer may be a factor. Centers in which a select few interventionalists perform a large number of studies tend to have higher rates of technical and clinical success than those with fewer procedures spread over a large number of operators. Of equal importance is how determination of successful outcome is derived. Are technical failures counted as clinical failures? How are restenoses and redilatation dealt with? What is the minimal length of follow-up necessary for inclusion of the patient in the study? How long is the mean follow-up? How is benefit evaluated in the patient who still requires medication to remain normotensive following angioplasty? The answers to these questions will explain some of the differences among the cited angioplasty series; however, the most important factor that influences the results of renal artery angioplasty is patient selection. Selection factors that may adversely affect the results of renal

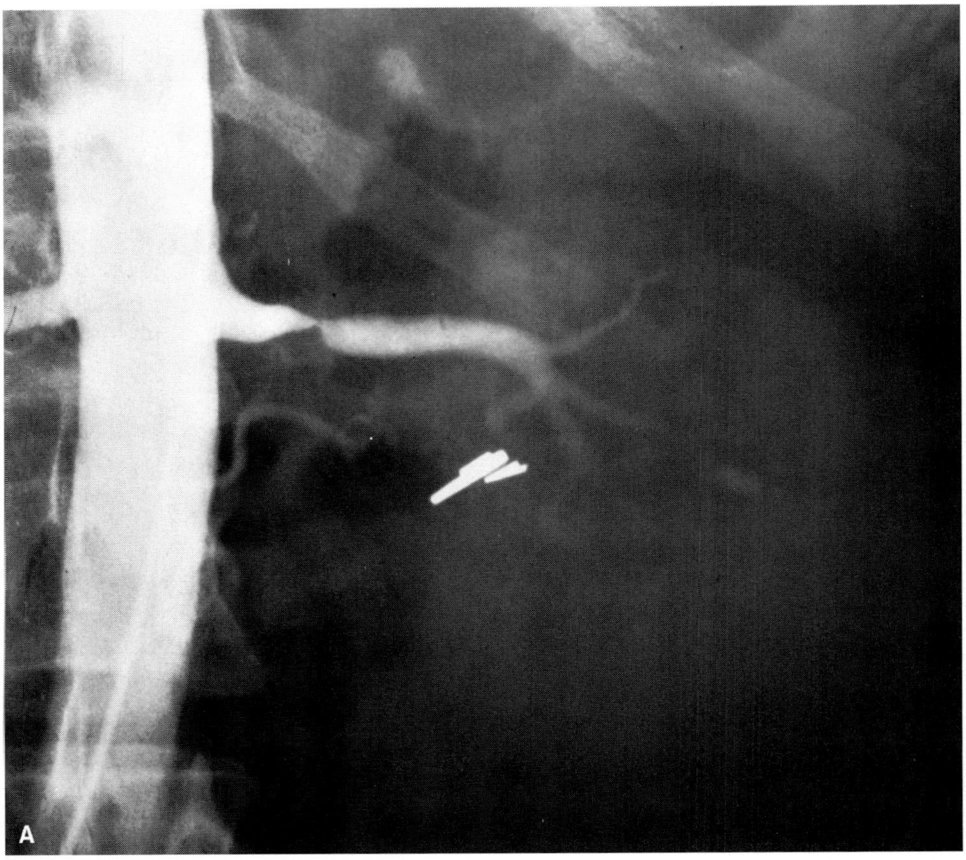

Figure 8–5. A. Aortogram showing left renal artery stenosis. B. Follow-up angiogram 57 months after PTA. (Figure continues.)

artery angioplasty include advanced age, long duration of hypertension, stenoses involving the renal artery ostium or branch vessels, bilateral stenoses, densely calcified arteries, azotemia, loss of renal mass, and arteriolonephrosclerotic changes in the distal renovascular bed. Two other factors that are less obvious are also major determinants in the patient selection process. These are preselection of patients by the referring physicians and patient rejection by the angiographer/interventionalist. Both of these are subtle, extremely difficult to define, and impossible to evaluate when comparing the results of reported series.

Realizing that these are issues that cannot be resolved in this chapter, the clinical success secondary to renal artery angioplasty in 267 consecutive patients treated at Emory University Hospital are reviewed. These results are representative of the patient popu-

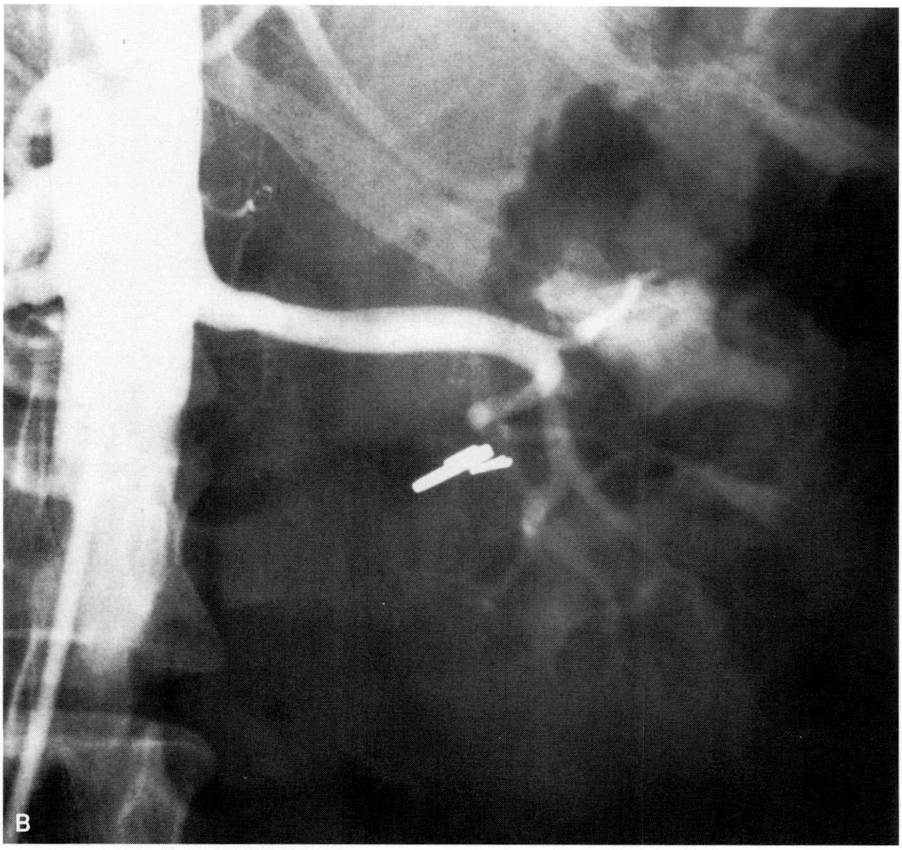

Figure 8–5. *(continued)*

lation treated at tertiary care university centers in the United States. The 267 patients are comprised of 204 patients with atherosclerotic renal artery stenosis, 110 of whom have been treated for ostial stenosis of at least one renal artery and 63 patients with renal artery stenosis secondary to fibromuscular dysplasia. A stenosis was considered significant if there was greater than 50% narrowing of the lumen and/or a greater than 15% peak systolic pressure gradient ($\Delta P \times 100$/aortic peak systolic pressure) was measured across the stenosis. The stenosis was considered ostial if the proximal 4 mm of the renal artery lumen was involved. Follow-up was terminated if surgery was performed to revascularize or remove a kidney that had been treated by angioplasty; otherwise, all patients were included in follow-up for more than 12 months after their last angioplasty. Demographic data is presented in **Table 8–4.** The patients were considered cured if, after

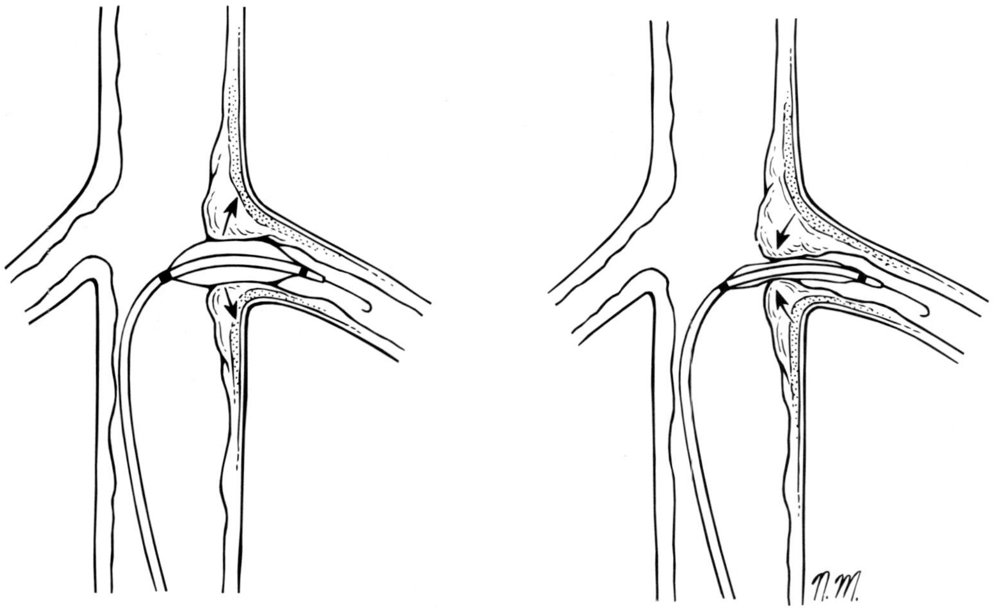

Figure 8–6. On right, aortic plaque falls across renal artery ostium following PTA.

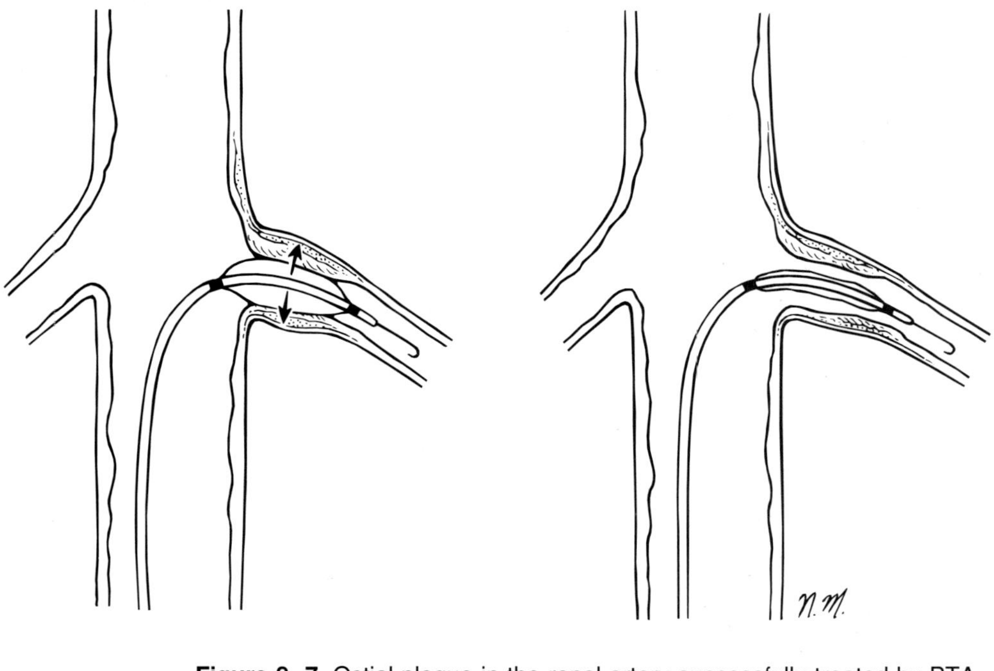

Figure 8–7. Ostial plaque in the renal artery successfully treated by PTA.

Table 8–2. Results of PTRA for Atherosclerotic Renal Artery Stenosis

First Author	No. of Patients	% Benefit	% Cure	% Improved	% Failed
Tegtmeyer	65	94	23	71	6
Schwarten	52	92	44	48	8
Klinge	133	78	10	68	22
Greminger	48	77	23	54	23
Collopinto	51	73	16	57	27
Chiesura-Corona	71	64	17	47	36
Martin	204	63	16	47	37
Baert	141	61	28	33	39
Geyskes	44	52	9	43	48
Miller	46	50	13	37	50
Canzanello	100	43	4	39	57
Grim	25	40	4	36	60
Sos	51	33	15	18	67
Total	1031	64%	17%	47%	36%

the angioplasty, the diastolic blood pressure was less than 90 mm Hg without administration of antihypertensive medication or improved if the diastolic blood pressure was: a) less than 90 mm Hg with the administration of equal or reduced doses of medication or b) greater than 90 but less than 110 mm Hg with at least a 15 mm Hg decrease from the measurements obtained before angioplasty while the patient is receiving a similar or decreased medication regimen. Angioplasty was considered to have failed clinically

Table 8–3. Results of PTRA for Fibromuscular Renal Artery Stenosis

First Author	No. of Patients	% Benefit	% Cure	% Improved	% Failed
Tegtmeyer	27	100	37	63	0
Miller	13	100	85	15	0
Geyskes	21	96	48	48	4
Greminger	34	88	41	47	12
Chiesura-Corona	44	87	64	23	13
Klinge	51	86	35	51	14
Colopinto	11	82	36	46	18
Sos	31	81	52	29	19
Baert	19	79	58	21	21
Martin	63	75	21	54	25
Total	314	85%	43%	42%	15%

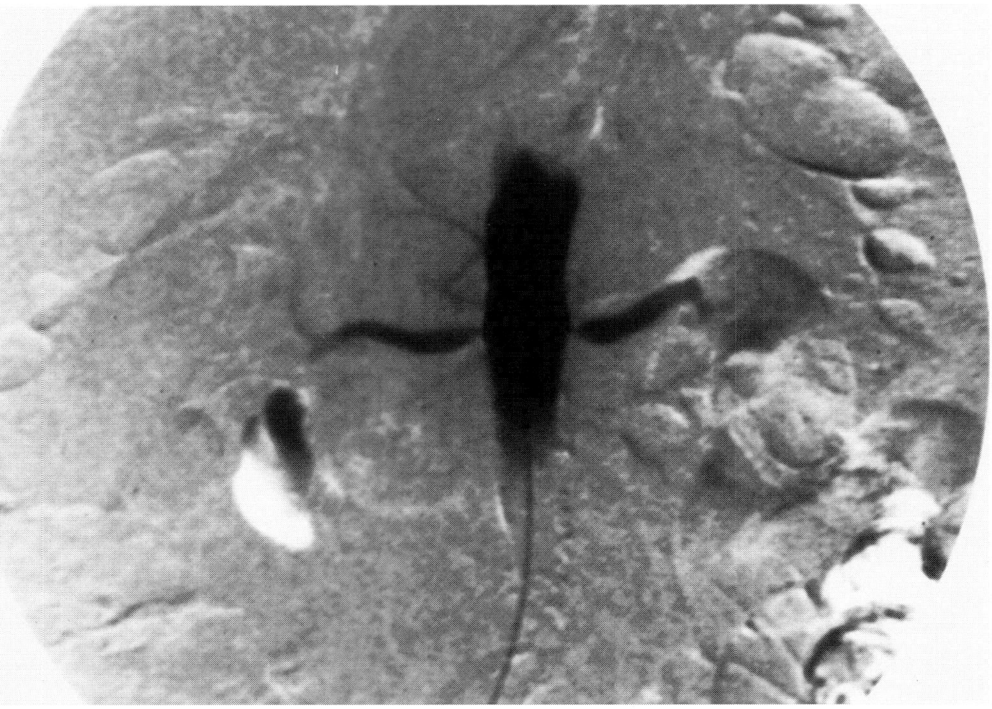

A

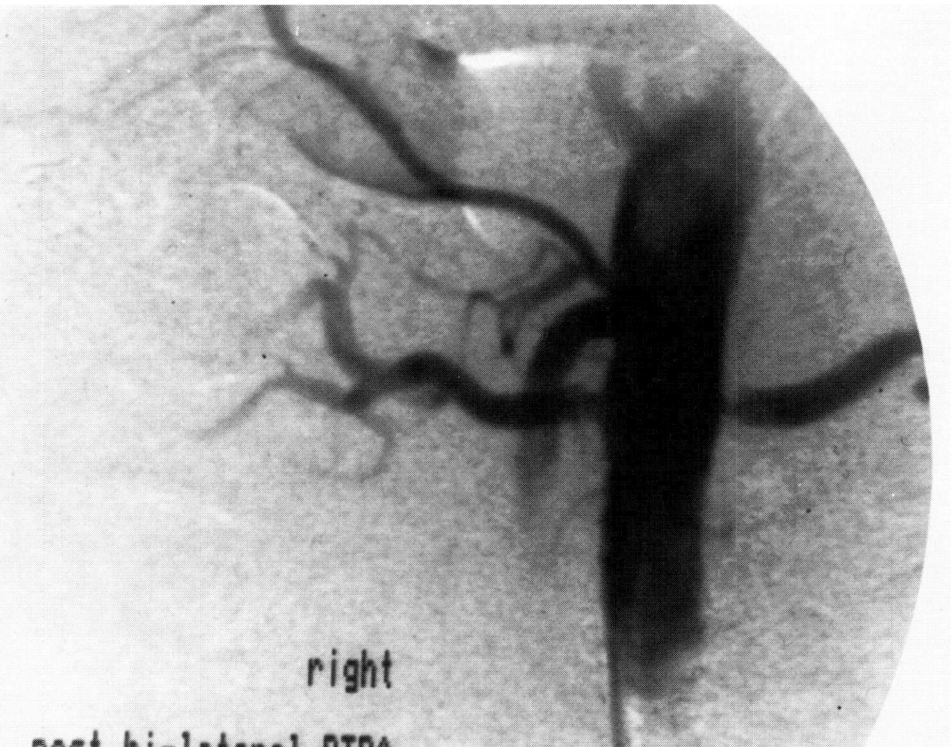

B

Table 8–4. Emory University Study Population (267 Patients)

	AS	FMD
Total patients	204	63
Patients to surgery < 12 months	22	0
Patients to surgery > 12 months	3	0
Patients follow-up > 12 months	181	63
Mean follow-up (months)	38	39
Range follow-up (months)	12–97	12–108
Mean age (years)	60	52
Male/female (percentage)	57/43	8/92
PTRA		
Unilateral	65%	38%
Bilateral	35%	62%
Repeat × 1	26 (13%)	12 (18%)
" × 2	3 (1%)	0
" × 3	0	1 (2%)

if there was no improvement in blood pressure control, if surgery was performed on a vessel following angioplasty, or if the stenosis could not be crossed and dilated. Benefit was determined by adding the number of patients who were cured and improved. Diastolic blood pressure values and number of antihypertensive medications (combination medications are counted as multiple drugs, i.e., the sum of their individual components) recorded before initial treatment and at the latest follow-up were used for evaluation of benefit. Follow-up was measured from the date of the last angioplasty.

Demographic data and results of angioplasty are listed in **Tables 8–4 to 8–8**. No patient was included as a clinical success with less than 1 year follow-up; all patients who required secondary surgical revascularization, whether before or after 12 months of follow-up, were considered clinical failures; and mean follow-up was 38 months for atherosclerotic disease and 39 months for fibromuscular disease. Results of angioplasty of FMD-branch stenoses have been tabulated because of controversy as to whether these lesions should be treated by PTA or surgery.[17,18]

Figure 8–8. A. Aortogram showing bilateral ostial renal artery stenosis. B. Aortogram after bilateral angioplasty shows that treatment was successful on the right but unsuccessful on the left.

Table 8–5. PTRA of 94 Patients with Non-Ostial Atherosclerotic Renal Artery Stenosis

Clinical Result	# (%) Patients	Diastolic-BP pre/post	# Drugs pre/post	% Stenosis pre/post	ΔP-Gradient pre/post
Cured	21 (22)	100/79	1.4/0	70/27	95/9
Improved	43 (46)	106/78	2.3/1.7	70/18	85/7
Failed	30 (32)	103/84	1.5/2.6	74/26	87/17

DISCUSSION

In experienced hands, the results of renal angioplasty are sufficiently good and the morbidity low enough to consider it a viable alternative to surgical revascularization.

Greminger et al retrospectively analyzed the effects of surgery, PTRA, and antihypertensive drugs in 202 patients with renovascular hypertension. Among the three examined groups, patients undergoing operations had the highest pretreatment blood pressure values, youngest age, shortest duration of hypertension, and lowest incidence of bilateral stenoses. They also had normal mean serum creatinine levels. Patients who were treated by angioplasty had slightly impaired renal function, were older, had less severely elevated blood pressures, and a longer history of hypertension than patients on whom operations were performed. Medically treated patients had the oldest mean age, the longest duration of hypertension and the highest incidence of bilateral stenoses. Greminger et al. concluded that certain patient characteristics had influenced the choice of treatment, preventing a direct comparison of these three types of therapy.[19] Although we have not conducted a similar study, the conclusions reached by Greminger et al would be valid in the patients treated at Emory

Table 8–6. PTRA of 110 Patients with Ostial Atherosclerotic Renal Artery Stenosis

Clinical Result	# (%) Patients	Diastolic-BP pre/post	# Drugs pre/post	% Stenosis pre/post	ΔP-Gradient pre/post
Cured	11 (10)	93/79	1.5/0	71/38	95/15
Improved	53 (48)	102/80	2.5/1.9	77/27	90/13
Failed	46 (42)	98/91	1.9/2.4	76/29	97/18

Table 8–7. PTRA of 63 Patients with FMD

Clinical Result	# (%) Patients	Pre-PTA BP	Pre-PTA # Drugs	Post-PTA BP	Post-PTA # Drugs
Cured	13 (21)	182/111	1.7	126/76	0
Improved	34 (54)	179/107	1.8	128/80	1.5
Failed	16 (25)	173/103	1.4	139/90	2.4

University. A prospective randomized trial comparing the three treatment modalities would be necessary to satisfactorily compare their efficacy.

Who then is a candidate for renal artery angioplasty? Because of excellent clinical results and low morbidity, PTRA should be considered the treatment of choice in patients with renin producing stenosis of the renal artery, whether caused by arteriosclerosis or fibromuscular dysplasia. Stenoses in the segmental branches can be dilated as well as those in the main renal artery **(Fig. 8–9)**. Surgical revascularization should be performed: 1) when the stenosis involving the renal artery ostium cannot be successfully treated by percutaneous angioplasty or stenting; 2) when the patient requires replacement of the abdominal aorta; 3) when severe atheromatous plaque lining the abdominal aorta makes the risk of renal, visceral, or peripheral embolization unacceptably high; 4) when PTRA was initially successful but stenosis recurs after one redilation; and 5) when there is no adequate vascular access route to the renal artery.

The major problems confronting PTRA are restenosis after a technically successful angioplasty, and inadequate result in many ostial lesions. Percutaneous atherectomy, laser angioplasty, and placement of an expandable metallic stent, which bridges the area of narrowing and prevents restenosis, are all presently being evaluated in human trials or in the animal laboratory. The acute angles at which the renal arteries arise from the aorta present a

Table 8–8. PTRA of 17 Patients with FMD Branch Stenosis

Clinical Result	# (%) Patients	Pre-PTA BP	Pre-PTA # Drugs	Post-PTA BP	Post-PTA # Drugs
Cured	3 (18)	167/109	1.3	112/72	0
Improved	9 (53)	180/103	2.1	135/85	1.0
Failed	5 (29)	177/107	1.2	137/90	2.2

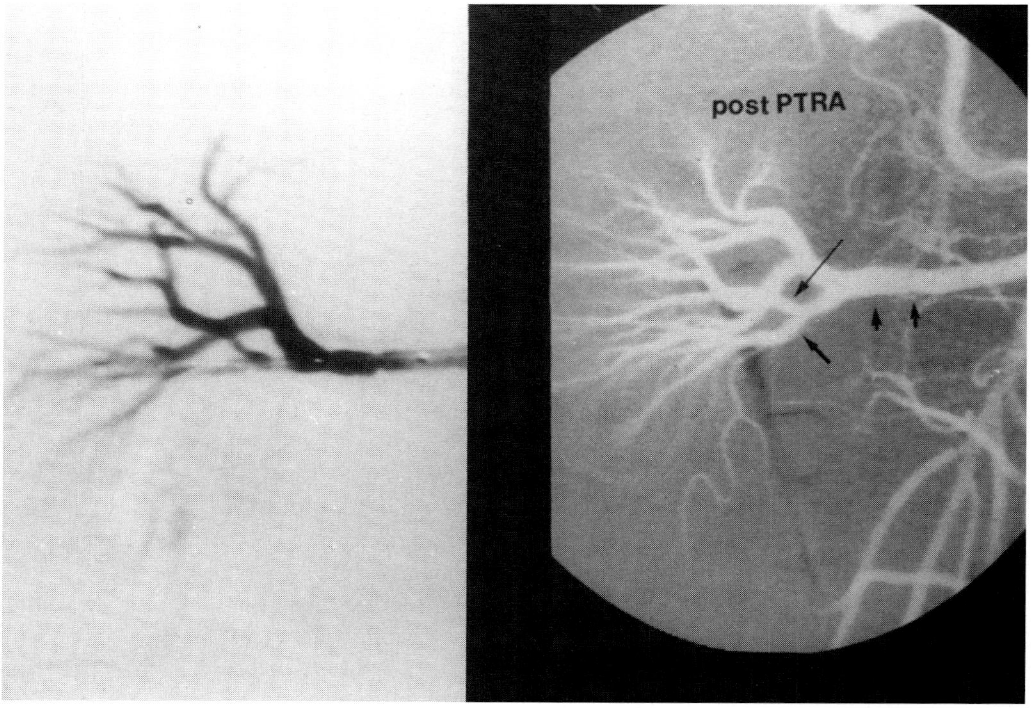

Figure 8–9. Multiple stenoses of inferior branch and distal main renal artery secondary to FMD were successfully treated by PTA.

special problem. Delivery systems are being modified so that these new technologies can be applied to the renal vessels. Removing plaque by laser vaporization or atherectomy may make a high percentage of patients with ostial renal artery stenosis amenable to percutaneous treatment without stenting.

In the future, as in the past, treatment of the patient with renovascular hypertension will remain a team effort. Members of the team include the referring clinician, nephrologist, vascular surgeon, and angiographer-interventionalist. Each member of the team should be thoroughly familiar with all the therapeutic alternatives so that the most appropriate one can be selected.

REFERENCES

1. Martin LG, Casarella WJ, Alspaugh JP, et al. Increased technical success and decreased complications in renal artery angioplasty. The

second and third hundred patients. Presented at Scientific Assembly of the Radiologic Society of North America; Chicago, Illinois; December 2, 1986.

2. Colapinto RF, Stronell RD, Harries-Jones EP, et al. Percutaneous transluminal dilatation of the renal artery: Follow-up studies on renovascular hypertension. *AJR* 1982;139:727–732.
3. Gardiner GA, Meyerovitz MF, Stokes KR, et al. Complications of transluminal angioplasty. *Radiology* 1986;159:201.
4. Geyskes GG, Puylaert CBA, OEI HY, Dorhut Mees EJ. Follow-up study of 70 patients with renal artery stenosis treated by percutaneous transluminal dilatation. *Br Med J* 1983;287:333–336.
5. Lohr E, Weighert HCh, Funke-Volkers R, Strotges MW, Bildstein A. Renal angioplasty: Experiences with 94 patients. *Urol Radiol* 1982; 4:211–214.
6. Schwarten DE. Transluminal angioplasty of renal artery stenosis: 70 experiences. *AJR* 1980;135:969–974.
7. Sos TA, Pickering TG, Sniderman K, et al. Percutaneous transluminal renal angioplasty in renovascular hypertension due to atheroma or fibromuscular dysplasia. *N Engl J Med* 1983;309:274–279.
8. Tegtmeyer CJ, Kellum CD, Ayres C. Percutaneous transluminal angioplasty of the renal artery. *Radiology* 1984;153:77–84.
9. Chiesura-Corona M, Feltrin GP, Miotto D, Savastano S. Complications of renal angioplasty: Incidence and effects on clinical outcome. *J Inter Radiol* 1989;4:75–84.
10. Greminger P, Steiner A, Schneider E, et al. Cure and improvement of renovascular hypertension after percutaneous transluminal angioplasty of renal artery stenosis. *Nephron* 1989;51:362–366.
11. Baert AL, Wilms G, Amery A, Vermylen J, Suy R. Percutaneous transluminal renal angioplasty: Initial results and long-term follow-up in 202 patients. *Cardiovasc Inter Radiol* 1990;13:22–28.
12. Miller GA, Ford KK, Braun SD, et al. Percutaneous transluminal angioplasty vs. surgery for renovascular hypertension. *AJR* 1985; 144:447–450.
13. Canzanello VJ, Millan VG, Spiegel JR, Ponce SP, Kopelman RI, Madias NE. Percutaneous transluminal renal angioplasty in management of atherosclerotic renovascular hypertension: Results in 100 patients. *Hypertension* 1989;13:163–172.
14. Grim CE, Luft FC, Yune HY, Klatte EC, Weinberger MH. Percutaneous transluminal dilatation in the treatment of renal vascular hypertension. *Ann Intern Med* 1981;95:439–442.
15. Martin LG, Rees CR, O'Bryant TO. Percutaneous Angioplasty of the Renal Arteries. In: Strandness DE Jr, van Breda A, eds. *Vascular Diseases: Surgical and Interventional Therapy*. New York: Churchill Livingstone 1994;729.
16. Tegtmeyer CJ, Selby JB, Hartwell GD, et al. Results and complications of angioplasty in fibromuscular disease. *Circulation* 1991; Supp. I, 83:I 155.

17. Dean RH. Reply to letter to the editor. *J Vascular Surg* 1987:821.
18. Novick AC. Management of renovascular disease: A surgical perspective. *Circulation* 1991;83 [Suppl I]:I 167–I 171.
19. Greminger P, Luscher TF, Zuber J, et al. Surgery, transluminal dilatation and medical therapy in the management of renovascular hypertension. *Nephron* 1986;44:suppl 1:36–39.

Indications for and Results of Renal Angioplasty and Stenting

9

Thomas A. Sos and David W. Trost

Despite our comprehensive understanding of renovascular hypertension, diagnostic tests based on the pathophysiology of the disease have been disappointing in their sensitivity and specificity. They are particularly unreliable in the setting of bilateral disease and/or renal dysfunction. The recent results of vascular surgery and renal angioplasty combined with the use of metallic stents have shown dramatic benefits of "revascularization," even in the setting of renal artery occlusion, ostial renal artery stenosis, and renal dysfunction. Timely diagnosis and intervention are imperative; therefore, we recommend the early use of arteriography using digital subtraction angiographic techniques for the definitive diagnosis.

INTRODUCTION

It has been previously estimated that for 1 to 5 percent of patients with hypertension, occlusive renal artery disease is the cause.[1] Recently it has been recognized that ischemic nephropathy can produce renal failure even without accompanying hypertension.[2,3] However, the physiologically based diagnostic and screening tests have been relatively unreliable, especially in the presence of bilateral disease and/or renal dysfunction. The sensitivity and specificity of these tests are of course very dependent on the prevalence of the disease in the patient populations being screened, and on the expertise and interest of the investigators. At tertiary referral centers, in patients for whom there is a strong clinical suspicion, the incidence of renovascular hypertension may be as high as 10 to 30 percent,[4–16] whereas in general populations being screened, it may be lower than 1%.[17–19]

SCREENING, DIAGNOSIS, AND TREATMENT OF PATIENTS WITH SUSPECTED RENOVASCULAR HYPERTENSION (Fig. 9–1)

Clinical Characteristics

The clinical characteristics of renovascular hypertension have been previously described in detail elsewhere.[20] These are summarized in **Table 9–1.**

Ambulatory Screening

Patients with some or all of the clinical characteristics in **Table 9–1** should be suspected of having renovascular hypertension. In this subgroup, the work-up should progress to a peripheral plasma renin assay (PRA) before and after angiotensin converting enzyme inhibition (ACEI) with captopril or a similar drug.[21,22] This is a relatively simple office procedure with a sensitivity and specificity of 74 and 89%, respectively, for the presence of renovascular hypertension. Although some patients with essential hypertension have PRA values of $\geq$ 4 ng/ml per hour, it is very unusual for patients with renovascular hypertension to have PRA values of $\geq$ 3 ng/ml per hour.

Diagnostic Tests

The relative lack of success of the physiologically based tests have resulted in a search for newer diagnostic tests **(Table 9–2)**. These

Table 9–1. Clinical Characteristics of Renovascular Hypertension

Recent onset of hypertension
Relatively difficult to control hypertension
Retinopathy
Continuous systolic/diastolic abdominal bruit
Renal dysfunction
Onset of hypertension after age 55 (etiology most likely atherosclerosis)
Onset of hypertension at relatively young age, particularly in women (etiology most likely fibromuscular dysplasia)
History of smoking
Presence of vascular disease in other organ systems
Recurrent pulmonary edema, even in the absence of severe coronary disease

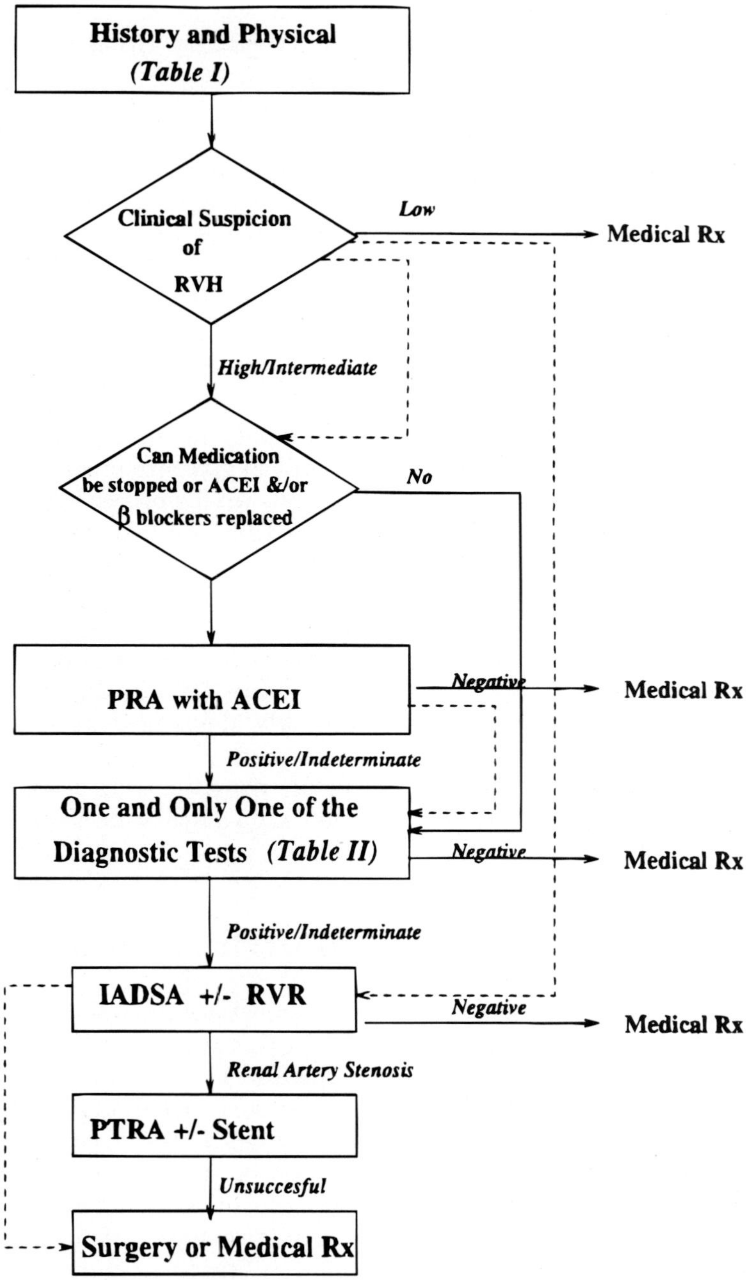

Figure 9–1. Algorithm for the evaluation and treatment of patients with suspected renovascular hypertension.

Table 9–2. Diagnostic Tests for Renovascular Hypertension

Selective renal vein renin sampling and assay with and without ACE inhibition (insensitive and inaccurate in presence of renal dysfunction and/or bilateral disease)
Radionuclide renal scanning with and without ACE inhibition (insensitive and inaccurate in presence of renal dysfunction and/or bilateral disease)
Renal artery duplex sonography
Magnetic resonance angiography
Helical (spiral) computerized tomography (contraindicated in patients with renal dysfunction)

diagnostic tests usually receive an enthusiastic early reception; however, other investigators have difficulty duplicating the results of the original investigators. For these reasons, especially in patients with bilateral disease and renal dysfunction, several of these tests are performed additively only to give either conflicting or inconclusive results. Unless these tests are being performed in the context of a scientific comparative study, we believe that, in the setting of strong clinical suspicion and a positive or equivocal ACEI PRA, any *one* (and only one) of the tests in **Table 9–2** should be performed.

The sensitivity and specificity of hypertensive pyelography is too low to be used as a screening test.[23] Intravenous digital subtraction angiography has been justifiably abandoned in favor of intra-arterial studies.[24–26]

In the appropriate clinical setting, if one of the tests described in **Table 9–2** is positive or equivocal, an arteriogram should be the next step.

Diagnostic Arteriography and Treatment Options

As previously discussed, most of the diagnostic and screening tests are somewhat unreliable, especially in the presence of bilateral renal artery disease or renal dysfunction. For these reasons, a diagnostic arteriogram should be performed sooner rather than later. Arteriography remains the gold standard. In the past, diagnostic arteriography using conventional film screen combinations and contrast boluses of 40 to 50 ml of 76% conventional ionic contrast media has frequently resulted in transient renal failure. With the use of intra-arterial digital subtraction angiography (IADSA), the incidence of this complication has significantly diminished. We currently use 4-French aortic flush catheters and deliver only 15 to 20 ml of 30% ionic contrast media to perform an aortogram to screen for the presence of significant renal artery disease. A single frontal aortogram allows the diagnosis of significant renal artery disease in virtually all patients. Once an atheromatous renal artery lesion has been demonstrated, there is no need (in fact, it is contraindicated) to perform selective catheterization of the involved renal artery for better demonstration of the lesion unless an intervention such as angioplasty or stenting is planned at the same sitting. It is not unusual for the diagnostic selective catheterization itself, if performed by inexperienced operators, to result in a renal artery dissection or occlusion. By contrast, however, in younger patients where the aortogram demonstrates normal main renal arteries, it is imperative to do selective magnification arteriography in several oblique views for detection of branch renal artery disease.[27] This is particularly true in children.

Fifty percent diameter arteriographic stenoses are widely assumed to be physiologically significant based on the assumption that 50% diameter stenoses in two planes result in a 75% cross-sectional area stenosis.[28] In our experience, however, 50% diameter lesions are rarely of physiologic significance. Experimental studies have demonstrated that flow is decreased when the cross-sectional area stenosis reaches 80–90%.[29] Most clinically significant renal artery stenoses compromise 80% of the vessel diameter and are not difficult to recognize as being very severe. When in doubt, the stenosis is usually *not* clinically important. The arteriographic characteristics of physiologically significant renal artery stenoses are detailed in **Table 9–3.**

Selective pharmacoangiography with vasoconstrictive or vasodilator drugs to enhance the accuracy of diagnostic renal arteriography entails additional time and risks, and the information does not justify its use.[30]

IADSA can be performed on outpatients. If the diagnostic arteriogram is negative, the patients can be discharged after 6–8 hours of recovery.

There should be prior agreement between the physicians responsible for the patient's care on how to proceed if a physiologi-

Table 9–3. Characteristics Suggestive of Physiologically Significant Renal Artery Stenosis

Luminal diameter stenosis equal to or exceeding 80%
Presence of collateral circulation
Poststenotic dilatation
Diminished velocity of flow across the stenosis
Diminished ipsilateral renal size mass
Pressure gradient exceeding 20% of peak systolic pressure (unfortunately, the diagnostic catheter itself usually adds significantly to the obstructing lesion, and therefore, pressure measurements are somewhat unreliable.

cally significant renal artery stenosis is demonstrated by arteriography. If angioplasty or stenting is the initial procedure of choice, then a significant lesion should be treated immediately rather than subjecting the patient to the risk of a repeat catheterization. Prior to performing an angioplasty, the surgical options should also be discussed in case the angioplasty or stent fails or produces a complication. If the surgical procedure of choice is a bypass graft from the branches of the celiac axis, then the pressure in the celiac axis itself should be selectively catheterized to determine whether there is a pressure gradient prior to the angioplasty rather than using additional contrast for a lateral aortogram. If the surgeon's preferred operation is an aorto-renal endarterectomy, then stent placement in the ostium should be performed only if it is accepted that this surgical option would probably not be available. A stent should not be deployed near the renal hilum because it may interfere with a subsequent aortorenal bypass graft.

SCREENING, DIAGNOSIS, AND TREATMENT OF PATIENTS WITH SUSPECTED ISCHEMIC NEPHROPATHY (Fig. 9–2)

Clinical Characteristics

In a significant minority of patients with renal failure, renal artery stenosis is the etiology. (1) Patients without clearly documented medical or parenchymal renal disease, particularly those who have other vascular disease; smokers; and those with relatively recent onset and rapid progression of renal dysfunction should be suspected of having renal artery stenosis (Table 9–4). We believe that no patient should be treated by dialysis unless a reversible cause has been looked for and eliminated. It is far less expensive to perform an intra-arterial digital subtraction arteriogram than to dialyze a patient who has reversible renal artery disease. (2) Ischemic nephropathy may or may not be accompanied

Table 9–4. Clinical Characteristics Suggestive of Ischemic Nephropathy

Absence of documented renal parenchymal disease
Presence of vascular disease in other organic systems
History of smoking
Recent onset of renal dysfunction
Rapid progression of renal dysfunction
Presence of hypertension
Unequal kidney size

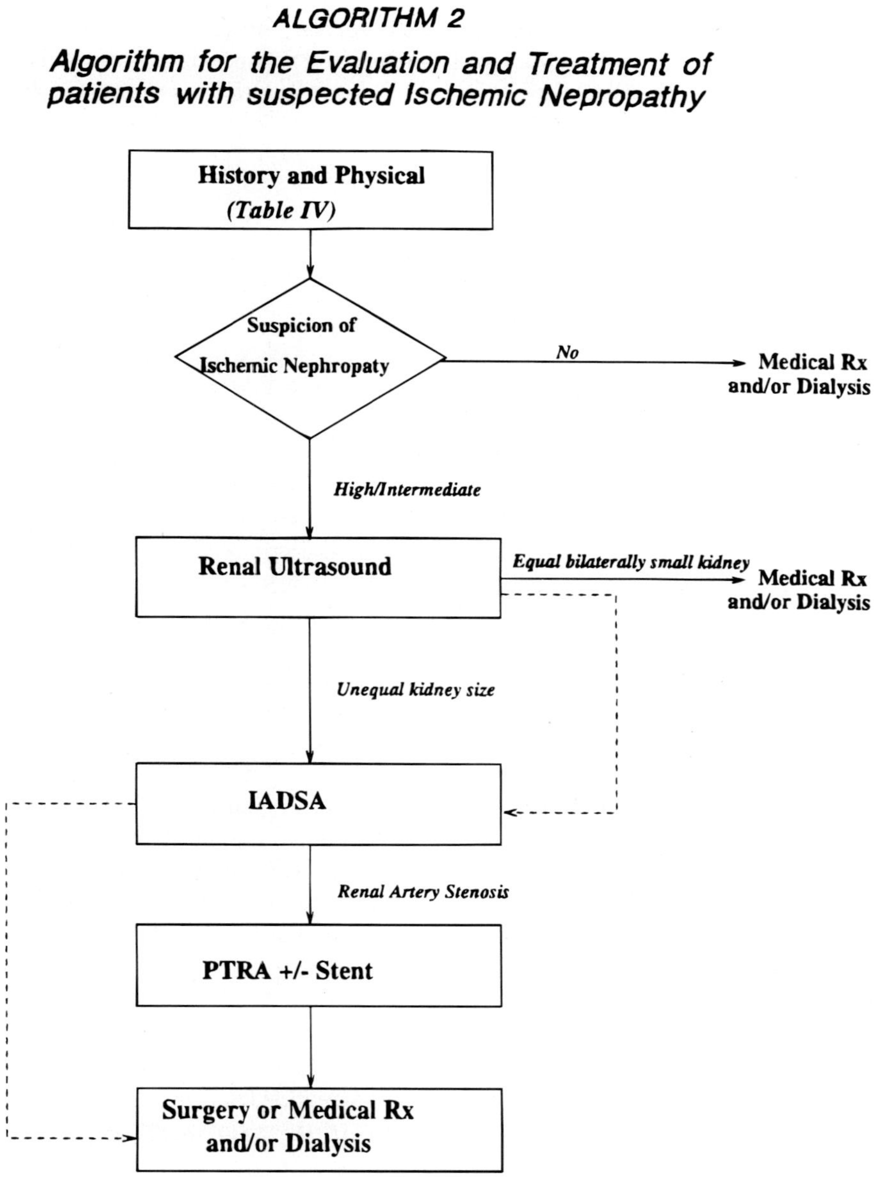

Figure 9–2. Algorithm for the evaluation and treatment of patients with suspected ischemic nephropathy.

by the presence of hypertension. The evaluation of patients with suspected ischemic nephropathy is somewhat simpler than that of renovascular hypertension. Most patients with renal dysfunction due to parenchymal renal disease have a history of a responsible causative systemic illness. These include diabetes mellitus, chronic glomerulonephritis, scleroderma, lupus erythematosis, and other parenchymal and connective tissue disorders. These diseases affect both kidneys equally and produce a symmetrically reduced renal mass.

Diagnostic Tests (Fig. 9–2)

The best way to screen patients for suspected *ischemic nephropathy* is to perform an abdominal sonogram to evaluate renal size and mass. The severity of bilateral renal artery stenosis is usually asymmetrical[31] and results in unequal kidney size. In this patient population, these findings should prompt an IADSA to identify a potentially reversible renal artery lesion.

Physiologically significant renal arterial occlusive disease can produce renovascular hypertension with or without ischemic nephropathy. Although the pathophysiologic basis of renovascular hypertension (renin-angiotensin-aldosterone axis) is now well understood, application of tests based on these physiologic principles has been disappointing. We have outlined the clinical and laboratory work-up necessary in patients suspected of having renovascular hypertension or ischemic nephropathy and strongly urge the early use of IADSA for confirmation of the diagnosis.

The screening, detection, and treatment of renovascular hypertension and ischemic nephropathy must be a multidisciplinary cooperative venture between internist, interventional radiologist, and vascular surgeon. Patients found to have renal artery stenosis can be treated by surgery or by angioplasty and stents immediately following the diagnostic arteriogram.

INTRODUCTION TO PERCUTANEOUS TRANSLUMINAL RENAL ANGIOPLASTY (PTRA)

The concept of percutaneous transluminal angioplasty (PTA) treatment of vascular obstructive disease was first described by Dotter and Judkins in 1964.[32] The initial technique consisted of advancing rigid coaxial teflon dilators over a guide wire sequentially one over the other; this technique was applicable only to relatively straight arteries. Developments in technology culminated in Gruntzig's design of a double lumen balloon dilatation catheter in 1974. This balloon had a flexible small shaft and a cylindrical balloon at its tip, which could be inflated in the stenotic area. Gruntzig reported the first renal balloon angioplasty (PTRA) in 1979.[33]

PATHOPHYSIOLOGY OF ANGIOPLASTY AND BALLOON DILATATION

The mechanical aspects of renal angioplasty are related to the underlying histopathology and pathophysiology of the lesions. It was originally assumed that angioplasty of atherosclerotic stenoses worked by compression and remodeling of the atheromatous material[32,34,35]; later, Wolf and co-workers [36] showed that angioplasty works by controlled trauma. The atheroma is fragmented longitudinally and circumferentially, with the cracks also tearing into the intima and the media. The muscle fibers of the media are stretched and paralyzed, the adventitia is dilated, and the atheromatous material is redistributed radially and laterally into the overdilated adventitia, thus leaving a large patent central lumen that is kept open by the increased flow. This explanation holds true for lesions within the renal artery. Ostial lesions behave differently.

In order to understand the reason why angioplasty of the renal ostium does not work well, the ostial lesion must be defined. Ostial renal artery stenoses consist of two entities: (1) Aortic plaque encroaching on the renal artery orifice, and (2) disease of the renal artery origin. These two can be difficult or impossible to discriminate by arteriography. Frequently, the disease is a combination of the two types.[37]

In ostial stenoses, the sheet of atheroma surrounding the renal artery ostium is acted upon in a longitudinal rather than a radial fashion by the dilating balloon. Soon after deflation of the balloon, the atheroma recoils, and the stenosis recurs.

It is likely that the mechanism of action of angioplasty in fibromuscular dysplasia (FMD) is similar to that in atheroma in that overdilatation of local stenotic segments leads to healing in the dilated state. Most patients with the medial form of fibromuscular dysplasia respond to a low pressure inflation of the balloons. In intimal fibroplasia,[38,39] Takayasu's arteritis,[38] and neurofibromatosis,[40] initial response is disappointing despite repeated inflations at high pressures. The initial dilatation ruptures the large intimal fibrous cushions and dilates the vessel wall, but spasm and the large bulk of tissue continue to produce a residual stenosis. With increased pressure and flow in the vessel, however, delayed continued expansion of the lumen to normal size has been observed. In these lesions, aggressive repeated overdilatation can result in vessel rupture. For this reason, in these patients we do not persist in trying to eliminate the "waist" of the angioplasty balloon. Infants and young children with the midaortic syndrome[41,42] have shown very poor response to angioplasty, and aggressive dilatation can produce severe complications, including rupture of the artery in these small vessels.

Technique of Angioplasty

If a lesion is considered significant and/or pressure gradient measurement is desired, the artery must be selectively catheterized. Even selective catheterization can be risky, but certainly crossing stenotic renal arteries can be risky, and should not be attempted unless an angioplasty is planned.

The vast majority of renal interventions can be performed easily and safely from a femoral approach; however, a minority of cases require an axillary approach.

Because the renal vessels usually have a caudally directed origin, "recurve" catheters are desirable. "Recurve" catheters have another benefit: because the catheter is pulled down into the artery rather than pushed across it, the operator can exert more axial force to cross lesions. One of the most popular "recurve" designs for renal angiography and intervention has been the Simmons series of catheters and their Chuang visceral modification.

At The New York Hospital, we generally use the Omni series of catheters (AngioDynamics, Glens Falls, NY) as our primary catheter.

An extremely floppy soft-tip guide wire such as a "Bentson" (Cook, Inc, Bloomington, Indiana) or a TAD II (Mallincrodt, Inc, St. Louis, Mo), with the guide wire extending several centimeters out the end of the catheter tip, is the least traumatic way to cross stenoses. Most lesions can be crossed if care is taken to line up the catheter tip with the axis of the stenosis while gently advancing the guide wire. Once the guide wire is across the stenosis, the catheter can be pulled down through or pushed across the lesion. The soft wire is removed, and arterial pressure distal to the stenosis is obtained. If there is any question that the catheter is subintimal, then a careful test injection can be performed. Most stenoses and some short occlusions, especially proximal lesions, can be traversed using this method. If initial attempts at crossing the lesion are unsuccessful, reevaluate the angle of the axis of the stenotic vessel and the eccentricity and irregularity of the plaque, and reposition or use a different catheter. The catheter position can be adjusted to alter the course of the guide wire, and respiratory motion can also be used.

In exchange of the diagnostic for the balloon catheter, a guide wire that has a very soft, atraumatic tip and a rapid transition to a stiff shaft is useful. This type of wire can be safely advanced into the segmental branches and provides the needed shaft stiffness to facilitate advancing a balloon across the stenosis. The TAD II wire has a very stiff 0.035-inch shaft tapering to a very floppy 0.018-inch tip. The rigid shaft of the TAD II wire can be shaped to closely match the natural curve of the renal artery and its origin from the aorta, facilitating passage of the balloon catheter. Prior to the placement of the wire, nitroglycerin 100–200 mcg should be injected directly into the renal artery to prevent spasm of the vessel during guide wire passage and balloon dilatation.

Balloon Sizing

As a general rule, in the proximal main renal artery we use 2-cm long 8-mm balloons for large men, 7 mm for small men and large women, and 6 mm for small women. We have never used a balloon smaller than 6 mm in the proximal main renal artery of an adult. The lesion should be overdilated by 15–20% compared with the size of the normal artery.[43,44] The standard way to chose the correct balloon is to directly measure the "normal" vessel on a standard cut film arteriogram that has an inherent 20% magnification factor. In order for this technique to be accurate and reproducible, the film changer distance must be constant, and the patient must be as close to the film changer as possible. Even with careful technique, the exact magnification factor is quite variable. With the advent of good digital subtraction angiographic equipment, many of the interventional procedures and even the diagnostic angiography are being performed without cut film. The newer digital equipment can provide accurate measurement of the vessel lumen by basing the measurements on the catheter shaft size or other reference sources, which eliminates magnification error. A balloon 10–20% larger than the measured vessel should be selected. If in doubt use the smaller size balloon initially and redilate with a larger balloon if needed. Patients normally experience mild-to-moderate back or flank pain during the inflation that should resolve quickly following deflation, usually within a minute. If the patient experiences severe pain, inflation should not be continued and the balloon immediately deflated. If the pain rapidly resolves, it is probably safe to reinflate, possibly with a smaller balloon. If the pain continues or increases, it may be a sign of severe injury to the renal artery, such as rupture or occlusion. If a severe injury is suspected, an angiogram should be performed without losing guide wire position across the lesion.

Renal Artery Stenting

Renal stents are currently under evaluation. They are best used for ostial stenoses that have restenosed following PTRA and for ostial lesions that respond poorly to initial angioplasty. Placing renal stents is associated with a new set of considerations. Although angioplasty does not usually affect subsequent surgical renal artery revascularization, stenting can. Stents prevent the performance of an aortic endarterectomy, a procedure not widely used. A proximally placed stent will not usually have an effect on most bypass procedures, unless the stent extends too far toward the branching of the artery. Positioning the stent in the stenosis is of utmost importance. It is essential that the artery origin is imaged in the proper oblique so that the origin is exactly in profile. Only in that position can the stent be accurately positioned at the renal origin. The goal is to place the stent so that it extends slightly into the aortic lumen approximately 1–2 mm to ensure that it covers the ostium adequately.

Complications and Their Prevention

Complications are reported to occur in 5–10% of patients.[45] The most frequent major complications in PTRA are initiated by thrombosis and spasm of the renal artery. The manipulation of guide wires in arteries with spasm and/or thrombosis increases the risks of dissection, occlusion, or perforation. Adjunctive medications can prevent or diminish the incidence and severity of complications.

Spasm

The normal response of the vessel wall to trauma (even to the controlled trauma of angioplasty) is to release serotonin and thromboxane, especially if clot and atheromatous material are present. The renal artery responds to these substances by spasm and thrombosis.

Calcium channel blockers such as oral nifedipine are useful in preventing spasm, as is liberal use of intra-arterial nitroglycerin (NTG). The NTG is administered as 100- to 300- microgram intra-arterial boluses. Intra-arterial papaverine (15–30 mg) intra-arterially and verapamil hydrochloride 2.5 mg intra-arterially have also been used.[46]

Acute Occlusion

Acute occlusion is usually caused by dissection and/or thrombosis, although rarely severe spasm can simulate total occlusion. For nonocclusive dissection, the balloon can be gently inflated for 2 minutes in an attempt to “tack” it down. Stents can also be used to treat dissections of the main renal artery, but should be used only if their position will not interfere with subsequent surgical repair or when surgery is not an option.

Thrombosis can occur during PTRA from thrombus formation

on the catheter and guide wire and from low flow states resulting from spasm, balloon inflation, catheter occlusion of the stenosis, and dissection. The risk of thrombus formation can be reduced by preprocedural administration of antiplatelet agents (aspirin [ASA] 300 mg), intraprocedural heparin, and spasmolytics. Should the procedure last more than 1 hour, heparin should be continued as boluses or a continuous infusion. Inexpensive activated clotting time (ACT) measuring units are helpful in determining if an adequate level of anticoagulation is present. An ACT value between 250 and 300 seconds is adequate. If a thrombus forms, the thrombosed vessels can be frequently opened with urokinase (Abbott Laboratories, Abbott Park, Ill).[46] The pulse spray method may be preferred if the occlusion is total, because it will restore at least partial flow faster than a continuous infusion.[47] For a nonocclusive thrombus, a continuous infusion is usually adequate.

Perforation, Rupture

The difference between arterial perforation and rupture is important. Frank rupture with retroperitoneal extravasation of contrast requires surgical repair. Perforation by only a guide wire is almost always self sealing. Perforations that do not stop bleeding can be embolized.

Following rupture a latex occlusion balloon or an angioplasty balloon can be gently inflated across the tear to tamponade the bleeding. Iced saline can be infused through the catheter to help preserve the kidney while the operating room is being set up. If this does not control the hemorrhage, a large occlusion balloon can be inflated across the renal origin, effectively cross-clamping the aorta at that level.

Every patient should be closely monitored following renal intervention. If the patient has persistent or increasing back or flank pain, arterial rupture or impending rupture as well as total occlusion must be considered. Even if the completion angiogram shows no extravasation, a CT scan is a more sensitive test to look for extravasation around the renal artery and kidney.

EMBOLIZATION

Macroembolization

When performing any intravascular procedure there is always the chance of causing embolization of plaque, thrombus, and/or cholesterol, usually to the lower extremities. The risk of embolization can be minimized by limiting the number of catheter exchanges, and using soft tipped catheters and guide wires. Macroembolization of atherosclerotic plaque or thrombus can usually be treated with surgical embolectomy and/or bypass. If the emboli are thought to be fresh thrombi, then thrombolysis may be attempted.

Microcholesterol Crystal Embolization

Symptomatic distal embolization of dislodged large plaque is rare. However, as more and more patients with uncomplicated focal atheromatous disease have renal angioplasty performed in smaller institutions, the patients referred to larger tertiary care centers have more complex disease. In this patient group, all complications are more frequent. Microcholesterol crystal embolization (CCE), a complication that occurs in approximately 1% of patients, is almost limited to this group.[48] CCE can be the result of simple diagnostic angiography alone; however, it is more frequently seen if multiple catheter manipulations are performed in a diseased aorta. Microemboli can lodge in the kidneys, bowel, or extremities and can produce permanent renal failure, severe ischemia, or organ necrosis. Unfortunately, these events can be severe and even fatal.

There is no specific treatment for CCE. Some authors believe it is safe to anticoagulate these patients,[49] whereas others feel that since anticoagulation is speculated to be a causative agent, it may make the patient worse.[50] Partial function can be regained with time.

PTRA in patients with diffusely atheromatous abdominal aortas should be performed with the least amount of manipulation. The use of a long sheath introduced to just below the renal arteries facilitates transmission of torque and may help prevent microembolization.

RENAL FAILURE

Contrast-Induced

The risk factors for renal failure following administration of iodinated contrast material are well known. They include preexisting renal insufficiency, dehydration, diabetes mellitus, hyperuricemia, and multiple myeloma. Patients with diabetes and renal disease, particularly if the serum creatinine is greater than 3.5 mg/dl,[51,52] are at high risk. Renal dysfunction is usually temporary, but permanent renal dysfunction is a small but real risk. The risks of contrast-induced renal failure can be reduced by liberal patient hydration, if tolerated. Reducing the total contrast load reduces the incidence of contrast-induced renal failure in patients with preexisting renal disease. Administration of Lasix and mannitol has been widely used to prevent contrast-induced renal failure, but the benefit of these infusions has not been clinically proved.[53] The use of low osmolality contrast media has not proved to prevent contrast-induced renal failure. CO_2 with IADSA may be the optimal contrast agents in these patients.

POSTPROCEDURE CARE

Immediately post procedure, patients are hydrated as much as they can tolerate. The heparin given during the procedure is not reversed. Additional doses of heparin are not used immediately following PTRA or stent placement. Blood pressure, fluid intake and output, as well as the serum creatinine are monitored closely. Deterioration of the patient's renal status may warrant reangiography, further intervention, or surgical bypass. We recommend that our angioplasty and stent patients take an antiplatelet agent, usually ASA po 80–300 mg qod, post procedure indefinitely. We do not routinely give systemic anticoagulation, except to patients with known hypercoagulable states.

RESULTS OF PTRA

The overall technical success is approximately 90–95%.[54–57] Technical success is higher in the FMD and unilateral nonostial atheroma categories. Technical success in occlusions is obtainable about 50% of the time.[58] Overall hypertensive benefit after PTRA is about 70–90%; atheroma, 65–95%; FMD, 85–100%[54–57] **(Table 9–5)**. In unilateral nonostial atheromatous stenosis, benefit is approximately 70%[54–57,59,60] **(Table 9–6)**. Ostial benefit is only 25%. Bilateral atheroma benefit is only 46%.[57] Ostial lesions respond poorly because angioplasty must be performed with the balloon parallel to the direction of the vessel to be effective.[61] These are the lesions best suited to stenting. Patients in whom renins lateralize can expect a higher therapeutic benefit rate than those in whom renins do not lateralize.[55] With respect to the following categories, various groups have reported their benefit rate results: Arteritis, 86%[62]; azotemia, 43%[63]; renal allografts, 76%[64]; and pediatrics, 100%.[27] **Figure 9–3** shows a renal artery stenosis due to fibromuscular dysplasia that was treated with angioplasty.

Table 9–5. Immediate and Long-Term Clinical Results of Renal Angioplasty in Fibromuscular Dysplasia

Author (Ref. No.)	No. of Patients	Successfully Dilated (%)	Cured (%)	Improved (%)	Follow-Up (mo) Mean (Range)
Sos[54]	31	27 (87)	16 (59)	9 (33)	16 (4–40)
Tegtmeyer[56]	27	27 (100)	10 (37)	17 (63)	NA (2–51)
Geyskes[59]	21	21 (100)	10 (48)	10 (48)	NA (12–48)
Martin[63]	20	20 (100)	5 (25)	12 (60)	16 (3–36)
Martin[73]	11	8 (73)	5 (63)	1 (13)	13 (NA)
Grim[60]	10	9 (90)	5 (56)	4 (44)	10 (1–14)
TOTAL	120	112 (93)	51 (46)	53 (47)	

Key: NA = Not Available.

RESTENOSIS

Recurrences within the first couple of weeks to few months are probably due to inadequate and incomplete dilatations that stretch the elastic vessel but fail to rupture the plaque and inadequately overdilate the adventitia. In recurrences at or after 6 months, the pathophysiology is more complicated. The initial controlled trauma of angioplasty results in platelet deposition and activation at the dilatation site, followed by fibrocellular prolifera-

Table 9–6. Immediate and Long-Term Clinical Results of Renal Angioplasty in Unilateral Nonostial Atheroma

Author (Ref. No.)	No. of Patients	Successfully Dilated (%)	Cured (%)	Improved (%)	Follow-Up (mo) Mean (Range)
Tegtmeyer[56]*,†	13	11 (84)	3 (27)	8 (73)	NA (1–60)
Schwarten[74]	54	49 (91)	23 (47)	25 (51)	NA (1–18)
Geyskes[59]*	44	44 (100)	4 (9)	19 (43)	NA (12–48)
Martin[63]†	38	38 (100)	10 (25)	19 (47)	19 (3–36)
Sos[54]	20	15 (75)	4 (27)	9 (60)	16 (4–40)
Martin[73]	15	13 (87)	2 (15)	4 (31)	13 (NA)
Grim[60]	15	15 (100)	1 (7)	7 (47)	10 (3–24)
TOTAL	199	185 (93)	47 (24)	91 (46)	

* Includes some patients with bilateral disease
† Includes some patients with ostial stenoses
Key: NA = Not Available.

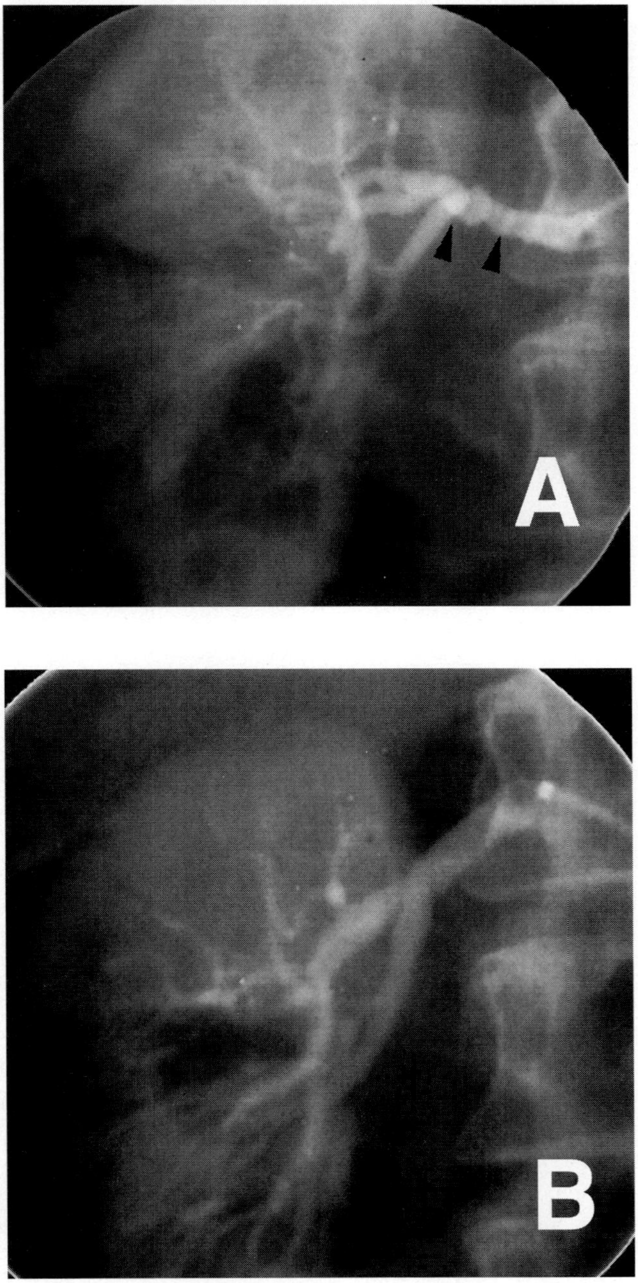

Figure 9–3. Forty-nine-year-old female patient with hypertension. A. Classic beaded appearance of the medial form of fibromuscular dysplasia is seen in the right renal artery. (Arrowheads) B. Appearance of the artery immediately post balloon angioplasty. C. Eight-year follow-up arteriogram shows normal appearance of renal artery. The patient is normotensive.

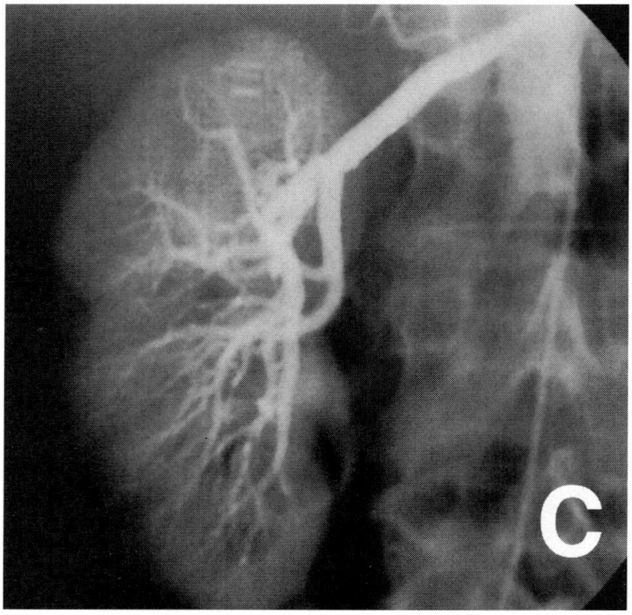

Figure 9–3. *(continued)*

tion. Smoking and hyperlipidemia also contribute to the frequency and severity of restenosis.[64,65]

In most PTRA series, recurrence rate is reported as 15–20%. Unfortunately, most authors combine atheromatous and fibromuscular recurrences, and since recurrence in fibromuscular disease is rare, the combined recurrence rate is significantly lower than the recurrence rate would be for atheromatous disease alone. Additionally, most authorities base recurrence data on clinical follow-up or angiographic examination of only those patients clinically suspected of restenosis. There are very few studies and very few patients in whom routine nonselected follow-up angiography has been performed. These studies indicate that, although some patients with clinical suspicion of recurrence indeed have recurrent stenoses, in other cases the dilated renal artery is normal, whereas the contralateral previously normal artery had developed a stenosis. In other instances, there can be angiographic recurrence without clinical manifestation of hypertension.[66] For these reasons, only recurrence data based on nonselected angiographic follow-up is statistically valid.

We attempted to restudy by angiography 36 patients with unilateral nonostial atheromatous disease. At an approximately 30-month (mean) follow-up, half of these patients were restudied, and the restenosis rate was 17%.

RENAL ARTERY STENTING

Although stents are approved for several locations in the vascular system by the United States FDA, there are none approved for use in the renal arteries. Stents placed in this location are currently under evaluation, and several large multicenter trials have been completed or are under way in the United States, Europe, and Australia. Renal artery stents are probably best used for ostial stenoses, restenoses following PTRA, complications of PTRA, and for other lesions that responded poorly to conventional angioplasty. From the published data, it appears clear that stenting of ostial stenoses has a higher initial success rate[67] and a greatly improved intermediate term patency rate over balloon angioplasty alone. This information probably justifies primary placement of stents for ostial disease regardless of the appearance of the angioplasty.

Technical Considerations

Placing renal stents is associated with a set of considerations not normally encountered by the interventionist who only performs conventional balloon angioplasty. Although angioplasty does not usually affect subsequent surgical renal artery revascularization, stenting can. Stents in the ostial location prevent the performance of aortorenal endarterectomy, a procedure that waxes and wanes in popularity but is recently becoming popular again. A proximally placed stent will not usually have an effect on most bypass procedures, unless the stent extends near the branching of the artery. Placement of stents further out in the renal artery will severely limit the options for subsequent surgical reconstruction.

RESULTS

Stents

Early reports of stenting of the renal arteries are now being published. Rees presented the results of a multicenter trial of the Palmaz-Schatz stent at the 1994 meeting of the Cardiovascular and Interventional Radiological Society of Europe.[68] Three hundred and four stents were placed in 296 arteries in 263 patients. Technical success was 95%. Eighty percent of the lesions were ostial. Ninety-eight percent of lesions were atherosclerotic. At 6-month follow-up, 64% of patients had improvement or cure of hypertension. In 123 patients with renal insufficiency (creatinine > 1.5 mg/dl), there was improvement in 34%, stability in 39%, and deterioration in 27%. Angiographic follow-up at 6 months was performed in 150 patients. Angiographic restenosis (diameter < 50%) occurred in 32.7%. Restenosis was lower in men (23%, $p < .05$); for stents dilated to > 6 mm (26%, $p < .05$); and lowest for men with stents dilated to > 6 mm (10.5%).

At The New York Hospital, we have placed 25 Palmaz stents in 23 arteries of 21 patients.[69] Twenty-two of these were used for atheromatous ostial stenoses. All patients were hypertensive; 11 had serum creatinine ≥ 1.5 mg/dl, and 8 had serum creatinine ≥ 2.0 mg/dl. Thirty percent of the patients were functionally or anatomically uninephric. Ninety-five percent of procedures were technically successful. Repeat angiography was performed in half of the patients at a mean of 7.5 months. Thirty-six percent of the patients had 50% or greater luminal diameter restenosis; however, in only one patient was this accompanied by deterioration of renal function and worsening of hypertension. Mean clinical follow-up was 11.2 months, with a range of 1–21 months; 10 patients were followed up for a minimum of 15 months. Seventy-one percent of patients had cure or improvement of hypertension. All patients with serum creatinine ≤ 1.5 mg/dl were stable at last clinical follow-up. Of eight patients with serum creatinine ≥ 2.0 mg/dl, three were improved, three were stable, and two deteriorated (one of whom had microcholesterol embolization).

In 1994, Hennequin, Joffre, and Rousseau et al.[70] reported the long-term follow-up of 25 Wallstents (Schnieder USA, Inc, Minneapolis, Minn) placed in 21 patients for restenosis after previous balloon angioplasty ($n = 13$) or inadequate immediate postangioplasty response ($n = 8$). Indications for angioplasty were: hypertension in all patients and renal preservation in seven. The stenoses were atheromatous in 15 patients and involved the ostium in seven. Initial stent placement was successful in 91% (19/21) patients. In two patients, the initial stent did not cover the lesion, and an additional stent was placed at 2 and 3 months, respectively. At follow-up angiography (range, 12-60 months; mean, 29 ± 14.22 months), four patients (20%) had stent restenosis. Of these, three had undergone treatment for restenosis after angioplasty, and three had ostial lesions. Cumulative primary patency rate was 95%, 85%, and 77% at seven, nine, and fifteen months, respectively. The cumulative secondary patency was 92% at 15 months. Hypertension was improved in all cases and felt to be cured in three. Renal function was improved in one patient, worse in one patient, and unchanged in the remainder of patients. There were three complications. Thrombosis of a small branch vessel ($n = 1$), renal hilar hemorrhage ($n = 1$), and progressive renal dysfunction thought to be secondary to cholesterol embolization ($n = 1$).

Also in 1994, Raynaud et al.[71] reported their experience with the Wallstent. Twenty-five stents were deployed in 18 renal arter-

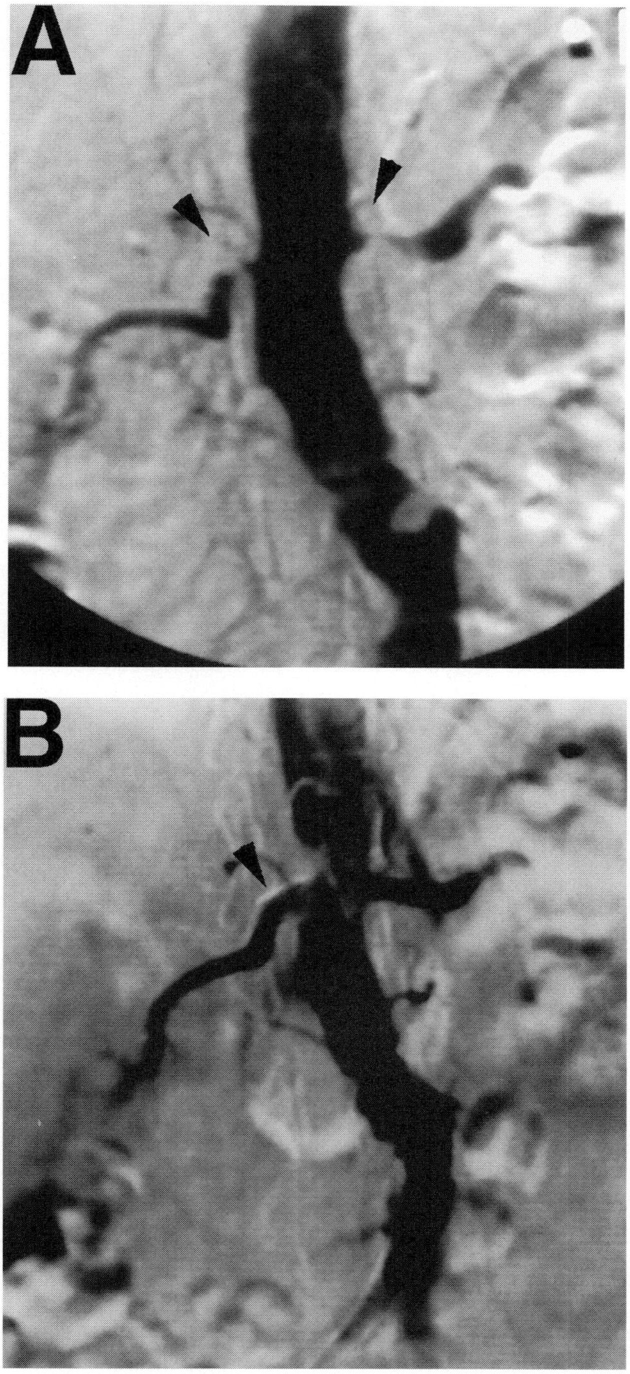

Figure 9–4. Sixty-seven-year-old woman with recurrent flash pulmonary edema and renal insufficiency; serum creatinine 4.0 mg/dl. A. Severe ostial stenosis of the right renal artery. Severe proximal stenosis of the left renal artery. B. Post stent placement; the right renal arterial lumen is normal. Left

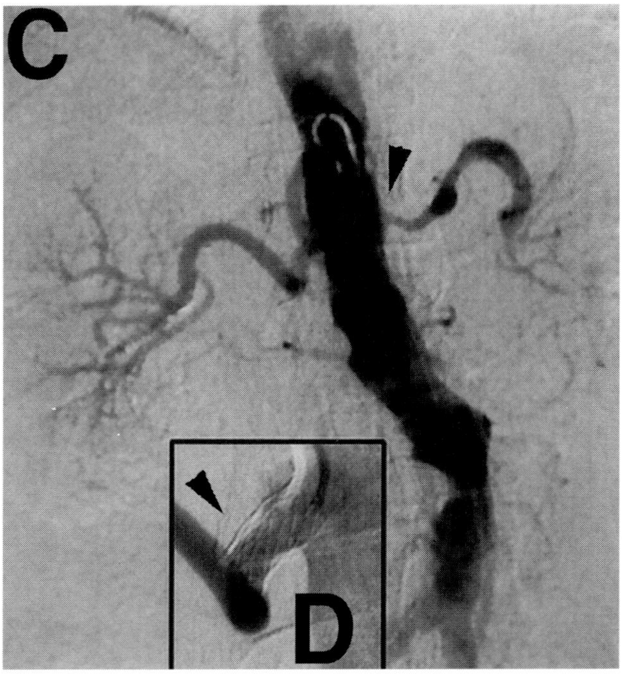

Figure 9–4. *(continued)*
renal arterial lumen is normal post angioplasty. C. At 1-year follow-up, the proximal left renal artery is moderately stenotic (arrowhead). Right renal stent is widely patent. D. Inset, stent with only minimal neointimal hyperplasia (Arrowhead).

ies in 18 patients. Fifteen were atheromatous lesions, four of which were ostial. Thirteen were placed for PTRA failures, and the others were placed for post PTRA dissections. Five patients required a second stent because the initial stent was malpositioned. There were two stent-related complications: one acute thrombosis 15 days post placement and an early restenosis or thrombosis. Hypertension at 6 months was cured in one patient, improved in eight, and unchanged in eight. Sixteen of eighteen patients had follow-up angiograms at a mean of 11 months. One patient had a restenosis greater than 50%, and one patient suffered occlusion.

In 1992 Kuhn et al.[72] reported their use of the Strecker flexible balloon-expandable tantalum stent for treatment of renal artery stenosis. Indications were inadequate immediate postangioplasty response (n = 16), and obstructing intimal flaps following transaortic endarterectomy (n = 2). Seventeen patients were hypertensive, and one was normotensive. In two of the patients, renal artery stenosis had developed after kidney transplantation.

Stent placement was technically successful, and patency was preserved in 14 patients. Midterm results (mean, 12–13 months) for 11 patients showed restenoses (> 50%) in two patients, and improvement of hypertension in eight patients. The initial result and 1-year follow-up of a renal stent placed for ostial disease is shown in **Figure 9–4.**

The current literature is encouraging with regard to the immediate and intermediate results of the use of stents in the renal arteries; however, longer follow-up is needed to really prove the durability of stents in comparison to surgical reconstruction. The available stent designs are working well, but there is still room for improvement in the stents themselves and the delivery systems. Many researchers are currently working on improvements to the current designs and exploring radically new concepts such as covered, biodegradable and chemically impregnated stents.

Although there has never been a randomized prospective study to compare medical therapy, surgery, and angioplasty with stents, many physicians intuitively feel that revascularization and salvage of the ischemic kidney is preferable to long-term systemic antihypertensive therapy. If this assumption is accepted, then it is reasonable to perform angioplasty or stent deployment initially, since these procedures rarely interfere with a subsequent open surgical revascularization.

REFERENCES

1. Gifford R. Evaluation of the hypertensive patient with emphasis on detecting curable causes. *Millbank Mem Fund Q* 1969;47:170.
2. Mailloux LU. Predictors of survival in patients undergoing dialysis. *Am J Med* 1988;84:855.
3. Dean RH, Tribble RW, Hansen KJ, O'Neil E, Craven TE, Redding JF 2nd. Evaluation of renal insufficiency in ischemic nephropathy. *Ann Surg* 1991;213:446.
4. Horvath JS, Waugh RC, Tiller DJ, Duggin GG. The detection of renovascular hypertension: a study of 490 patients by renal angiography. *Q J Med* 1982;51:139.
5. Foster JH, Dean RH, Pinkerton JA, Rhamy RK. Ten years experience with the surgical management of renovascular hypertension. *Ann Surg* 1973;177:755.
6. Anderson GH, Blakemam N, Streeten DH. Prediction of renovascular hypertension. Comparison of clinical diagnostic indices. *Am J Hypertens* 1988;1:301.
7. Nicholson JP, Alderman MH, Pickering TG, Teichman SL, Sos TA, Laragh JH. Cigarette smoking and renovascular hypertension. *Lancet* 1983;2:765.
8. Svetkey LP, Kadir S, Runnick NR, Smith SR, Dunham CB, Lambert

M, et al. Similar prevalence of renovascular hypertension in selected blacks and whites. *Hypertension* 1991;1:678.

9. Simon N, Franklin SS, Bleifer KH, Maxwell MH. Clinical characteristics of renovascular hypertension. *JAMA* 1972;220:1209.
10. Tilman DM, Malatino LS, Cumming AM, et al. Enalarpil in hypertension with renal artery stenosis: long term follow-up and effects on renal function. *J Hypertens* 1984;2(suppl 2):93.
11. Reams GP, Bauer JH, Gaddy P. Use of the converting enzyme inhibitor enalapril in renovascular hypertension. Effect on blood pressure, renal function, and the renin- angiotensin-aldosterone system. *Hypertension* 1986;8:290.
12. Case DB, Atlas SA, Merion RM, Laragh JH. Long-term efficacy of captopril in renovascular and essential hypertension. *Am J Cardiol* 1982;49:1440.
13. Aldigier JC, Plouin PF, Guyenne TT, Thibonnier M, Corvol P, Menard J. Comparison of the hormonal renal effects of captopril in severe essential and renovascular hypertension. *Am J Cardiol* 1982;49: 1447.
14. Davis BA, Crook JE, Vestal RE, Oates JA. Prevalence of renovascular hypertension in patients with grade III or IV hypertensive retinopathy. *N Engl J Med* 1979;301:1273.
15. Hricik DE, Browning PJ, Kopelman R, Goorno WE, Madias NE, Dzau VJ. Captopril-induced functional renal insufficiency in patients with bilateral renal-artery stenoses or renal- artery stenosis in a solitary kidney. *N Engl J Med* 1983;308:373.
16. Jackson B, Matthews PG, Mcgrath BP, Johnston CI. Angiotensin converting enzyme inhibition in renovascular hypertension: frequency of reversible renal failure. *Lancet* 1984;1:225.
17. Lewin A, Blaufox MD, Castle H, Entwisle G, Langford H. Apparent prevalence of curable hypertension in the hypertension detection and follow-up program. *Arch Intern Med* 1985;145:424.
18. Berglund G, Anderson O, Wilhelmsen L. Prevalence of primary and secondary hypertension: studies in a random population sample. *Br Med J* 1976;2:554.
19. Tucker RM, Labarthe DR. Frequency of surgical treatment for hypertension in adults at the Mayo Clinic from 1973 through 1975. *Mayo Clin Proc* 1977;52:549.
20. Mann SJ, Pickering TG. Detection of renovascular hypertension: state of the art 1992. *Ann Intern Med* 1992;117:845.
21. Case DB, Laragh JH. Reactive hyperreninemia in renovascular hypertension after angiotensin blockade with saralasin or converting enzyme inhibitor. *Ann Intern Med* 1979;91:153.
22. Muller FB, et al. The captopril test for identifying renovascular disease in hypertensive patients. *Am J Med* 1986;80:633.
23. Thornbury JR, Stanley JL, Fryback DG. Limited use of hypertensive excretory urography. *Urol Radiol* 1982;3:209.
24. Dunnick NR, et al. Intravenous digital subtraction renal angiogra-

phy: Use in screening for renovascular hypertension. *Radiology* 1989; 171:219.
25. Illescas FF, Braun SD, Cohan RH, Sussman SK, Saeed M, Dunnick NR. Fibromuscular dysplasia of renal arteries: Comparison of intravenous digital subtraction angiography with conventional angiography. *J Can Assoc Radiol* 1988;39:167.
26. Wilms GE, Baert AL, Staessen JA, Amery AK. Renal artery stenosis: Evaluation with intravenous digital subtraction angiography. *Radiology* 1986;160:713.
27. Sos TA, Saddekni S. Pediatric renovascular hypertension: the role of renal angioplasty. *Dialogues Ped Urol* 1985;8(12):7.
28. Gensini GG. *Coronary Arteriography*. Mount Kisco, New York: Futura Publishing, 1975.
29. May AG, DeBerg LV, DeWeese JA, Rob CG. Critical arterial stenosis. *Surgery* 1963;54:250.
30. Bookstein JJ, Walter JF, Stanley JC, Fry WJ. Pharmacoangiographic manipulation of renal collateral blood flow. *Circulation* 1976;54(2): 328.
31. Pickering TG, Sos TA, James GD, Vaughan ED Jr, Sealey JE, Laragh JH. Comparison of renal vein renin activity in hypertensive patients with stenosis of one or both renal arteries. *J Hypertens* 1985;3(suppl 3):291.
32. Dotter CT, Judkins MP. Transluminal treatment of arteriosclerotic obstruction: description of a new technique and a preliminary report of its applications. *Circulation* 1964;30:654.
33. Gruntzig A, Hopff H. Perkutane rekanalisation chronischer arterieller verschlusse mit einem neuen dilatations katheter. Modifikation der Dotter-Technik. *Deutsch Med Wochenschr* 1974;99:2502.
34. Block PC, Myler R, Sterzer S. Morphology after transluminal angioplasty in human beings. *N Engl J Med* 1981;305:382.
35. Castaneda-Zuniga WR, Formanek A, Tadavarthy M, et al. The mechanism of balloon angioplasty. *Radiology* 1980;135(3): 565.
36. Wolf GL, LeVeen RF, Ring EJ. Potential mechanism of angioplasty. *Cardiovasc Intervent Radiol* 1984;7:11.
37. Cicuto KP, McLean GK, Oleaga JA, et al. Renal artery stenosis: anatomic classification for percutaneous transluminal angioplasty. *AJR* 1981;137:599.
38. Srur MF, Sos TA, Saddekni S, et al. Intimal fibromuscular dysplasia and Takayasu arteritis: delayed response to percutaneous transluminal renal angioplasty. *Radiology* 1985;157:657.
39. Archibald GR, Beckmann CF, Libertino JA. Focal renal artery stenosis caused by fibromuscular dysplasia: treatment by percutaneous transluminal angioplasty. *AJR* 1988;151:593.
40. Gardiner GA Jr, Freedman AM, Shlansky-Goldberg R. Percutaneous transluminal angioplasty: delayed response in neurofibromatosis. *Radiology* 1988;169:79.
41. Stanley JC. Renovascular hypertension: The surgical point of view.

In: Schilfgaarde RV, et al, eds. *Clinical Aspects of Renovascular Hypertension*. Boston: Martinus Nijoff, 1983;259.
42. Berkmen YM. The midaortic syndrome: diagnosis and treatment. (letter). *Radiology* 1989;170:571.44.
43. Katzen BT, Chang J, Knox WG. Percutaneous transluminal angioplasty with the Gruntzig balloon catheter: a review of 70 cases. *Arch Surg* 1970;114:1389.
44. Hessel SJ, Adams DF, Abrams HL. Complications of angiography. *Radiology* 1981;138:273.
45. Tegtmeyer CJ, Sos TA. Techniques of renal angioplasty. *Radiology*. 1986;161:577.
46. Sos TA. Renal artery occlusions and stenosis: Thrombolysis in conjunction with angioplasty. Presented at Sixth Biennial Oakwood Hospital Winter Imaging Conference. Steamboat Springs, Colo, 1991.
47. Kandarpa K, Drinker PA, Singer SJ, Cararamore D. Forceful pulsatile local infusion of enzyme accelerates thrombolysis: In vivo evaluation of a new delivery system. *Radiology* 1988;168:739.
48. Flory CM. Arterial occlusions produced by emboli from eroded aortic atheromatous plaques. *Am J Pathol* 1945; 21:549.
49. Fuks DF, Griguoli RE, Borracci RA, Sala C. Cholesterol embolization following coronary angioplasty. *Rev Port Cardiol* 1992;11:1089.
50. Hollier LH, Kazimer FJ, Ochsner J, et al. "Shaggy" aorta syndrome with atheromatous embolization to visceral vessels. *Ann Vasc Surg* 1991;5:439.
51. Cohan RH, Dunnick NR. Intravascular contrast media: Adverse reactions. *AJR* 1987;149:665.
52. Parfrey PS, Griffiths SM, Barrett BJ, et al. Contrast material induced renal failure in patients with diabetes mellitus, renal insufficiency, or both: A prospective controlled study. *N Engl J Med* 1989;320:143.
53. Cruz C, Hricak H, Samhouri F, et al. Contrast media for angiography: effect on renal function. *Radiology* 1986; 158:109.
54. Sos TA, Pickering TG, Sniderman KW, et al. Percutaneous transluminal renal angioplasty in renovascular hypertension due to atheroma or fibromuscular dysplasia. *N Engl J Med* 1983;309:274.
55. Schwarten DE. Transluminal angioplasty of renal artery stenosis: 70 experiences. *AJR* 1980;135:969.
56. Tegtmeyer CJ, Kellum CD, Ayers C. Percutaneous transluminal angioplasty of the renal artery. *Radiology* 1984;153:77.
57. Martin LG, Price RB, Casarella WJ, et al. Percutaneous angioplasty in the clinical management of renovascular hypertension: initial and long term results. *Radiology* 1985;155:629.
58. Sniderman KW, Sos TA. Percutaneous transluminal recanalization and dilatation of totally occluded renal arteries. *Radiol* 1982;142: 607.
59. Geyskes GG, Puylaert CBA, Dei HY, et al. Follow-up study of 70 patients with renal artery stenosis treated by percutaneous transluminal dilatation. *Br Med J* 1983;287: 333.
60. Grim CE, Luft FC, Yune HY. Percutaneous transluminal dilatation

in the treatment of renal vascular hypertension. *Ann Intern Med* 1981;95:439.

61. Freiman DB. Transluminal angioplasty of the renal arteries. *Urol Clin North Am* 1985;12(4):737.
62. Dong ZJ, Li S, Lu X. Percutaneous transluminal angioplasty for renovascular hypertension in arteritis: experience in China. *Radiology* 1987;162:477.
63. Martin LG, Casarella WJ, Gaylord GM. Azotemia caused by renal artery stenosis: treatment by percutaneous angioplasty. *AJR* 1988; 150:839.
64. Kent KM. Restenosis after percutaneous transluminal coronary angioplasty. *Am J Cardiol* 1988;61(14):67G.
65. Wolinsky H. Insights into coronary angioplasty-induced restenosis from examination of atherogenesis. *Am J Cardiol* 1987;60(3):65B.
66. Schwarten DE. Percutaneous transluminal angioplasty of the renal arteries: intravenous digital subtraction angiography for follow-up. *Radiology* 1984;150:369.
67. Dorros G, Prince C, Mathiak L. Stenting of a renal artery stenosis achieves better relief of the obstructive lesion than balloon angioplasty. *Catheterization Cardiovascular Diagnosis 1993;29:191.*
68. Rees CR, Niblett R, Snead D. United States multicenter study of Palmaz-Schatz stents in the renal arteries. CIRSE Annual Meeting and Postgraduate Course of the Cardiovascular and Interventional Radiological Society of Europe. Crete, June 1994.
69. Trost DW, Sos TA. Palmaz stents for the treatment of ostial renal artery stenosis. Abstract presented at 19th Annual Scientific Meeting of SCVIR. San Diego, Calif, 1994.
70. Hennequin LM, Joffre FG, Rousseau HP, et al. Renal artery stent placement: long term results with the Wallstent endoprosthesis. *Radiology* 1994;191(3):713.
71. Raynaud AC, Beyssen BM, Turmel-Rodrigues LE, et al. Renal artery stent placement: immediate and midterm technical and clinical results. *JVIR* 1994;5:849.
72. Kuhn FP, Malms J, Kutkuhn B, et al. The current indications, two-year results and the possibilities for percutaneous stent recovery. *Rofo Fortschr Geb Rontgenstr Neuen Bildgeb Verfahr* 1992;157(1): 65.

10

Renal Revascularization for the Chronically Occluded Renal Artery

John W. Hallett

MANAGEMENT OF THE CHRONICALLY OCCLUDED RENAL ARTERY

Chronic renal artery occlusion is a well-known cause of hypertension. Since the most common etiology is atherosclerosis, occlusion follows a long period of progressive stenosis in most patients. Consequently the involved kidney tends to shrink over time. When occlusion finally occurs and is identified, a surgeon may be consulted to address a dilemma: Can a functional kidney be saved by revascularization or will nephrectomy be necessary to alleviate the hypertension? This chapter addresses this dilemma.

The Clinical Setting

The typical clinical setting of a chronic renal artery occlusion involves a long history of hypertension that may worsen suddenly when a high-grade stenosis progresses to occlusion. The occlusion often precipitates an episode of malignant hypertension, rising serum creatinine and pulmonary edema.[2,5,9] The typical patient is 55–70 years of age and is predominantly male (M:F = 3:1). Diffuse atherosclerosis **(Fig. 10–1)** is present in 85% with the remaining 15% affected by fibromuscular disease, chronic dissection, abdominal aortic coarctation, or neurofibromatosis. Extrarenal atherosclerosis involves the aortoiliac region in 75% of such patients, the coronary arteries in 40%, and the cerebrovasculature in 10%. In a 10-year experience with 625 patients undergoing operation for renovascular disease, we identified 150 (25%) with a chronic renal artery occlusion.

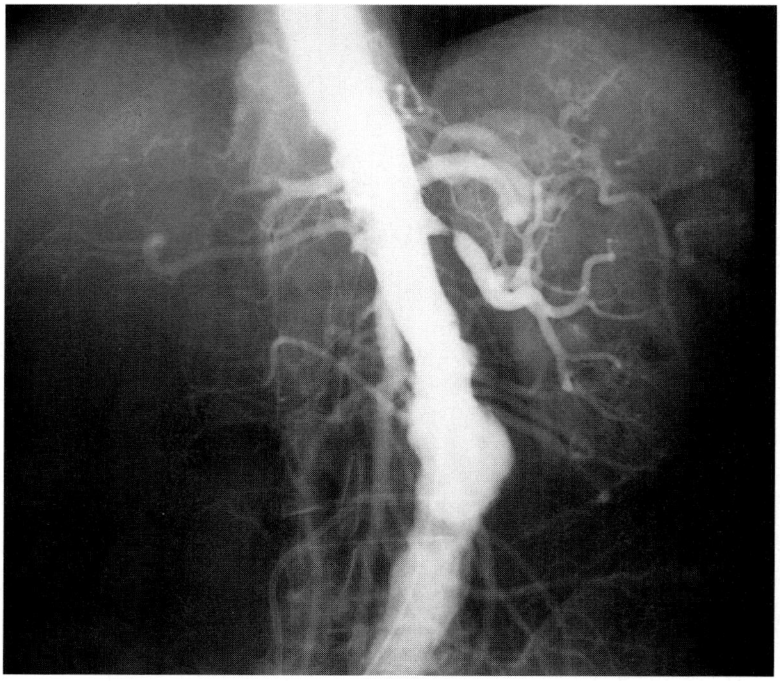

Figure 10–1. Typical patient with a chronically occluded renal artery (right in this case) also has a contralateral high-grade stenosis and infrarenal aortic disease.

Diagnostic Characteristics

Serum creatinine is usually elevated in patients with a chronic renal artery occlusion.[1–12] The mean value approaches 2.0 mg/dl indicating that the contralateral renal artery and kidney are also diseased. The kidney with the renal artery occlusion is generally smaller than the contralateral kidney (a mean length of 11.5 cm versus 13.5 cm). Colorflow Duplex ultrasonography may identify no flow in the proximal occluded renal artery with some collateral refilling in the hilum of the kidney. Renal scan typically shows markedly reduced size and function of the involved kidney. Generally the kidney with the occlusion has less than 25% of the total renal function. If the involved kidney shows minimal uptake on the renal scan and the renal size is less than 8 cm, it is unlikely that a salvageable kidney is present. **(Fig. 10–2)**

The definitive test for ascertaining salvageability of a kidney with chronic renal occlusion is a standard arteriogram with delayed views. **(Fig. 10–3)** Although the distal renal artery and nephrogram may not be seen on early films, delayed images may

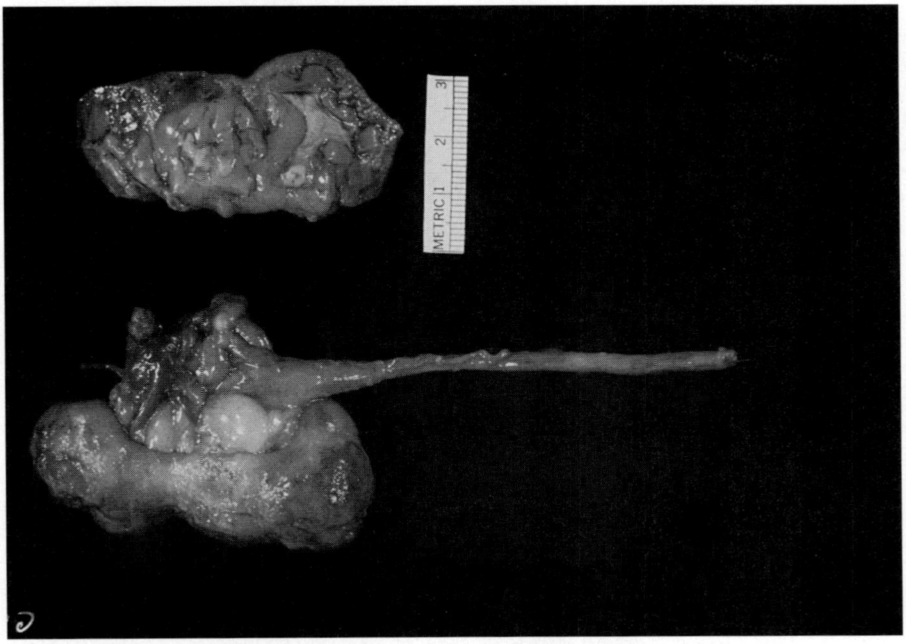

Figure 10–2. About two-thirds of patients with a chronically occluded renal artery will have an atrophic (<8 cm) pressor kidney needing nephrectomy.

reveal opacification of the distal renal artery. A nephrogram may also show on the delayed views. In our experience, failure to see the distal main renal artery or nephrogram on delayed films is a poor prognostic sign for saving the involved kidney, especially if it is less than 8 cm in length. Sampling renal vein renins from the kidney with the occlusion can be helpful. If the kidney does not appear salvageable and the renal vein renins are elevated (greater than 1.5 times the contralateral kidney), a nephrectomy may help to alleviate the hypertension.

Options for Revascularization

Some type of surgical procedure is the treatment of choice for most patients with a chronic renal artery occlusion.[1–12] Although percutaneous transluminal angioplasty may successfully recanalize an occluded renal artery, the durability of this option is limited. There is also the real risk of embolization of clot and atheroma into the renal parenchyma with angioplasty of a chronic occlusion. A nephrectomy will be necessary in many patients with a shrunken pressor kidney. In our experience with 150 chronic renal ar-

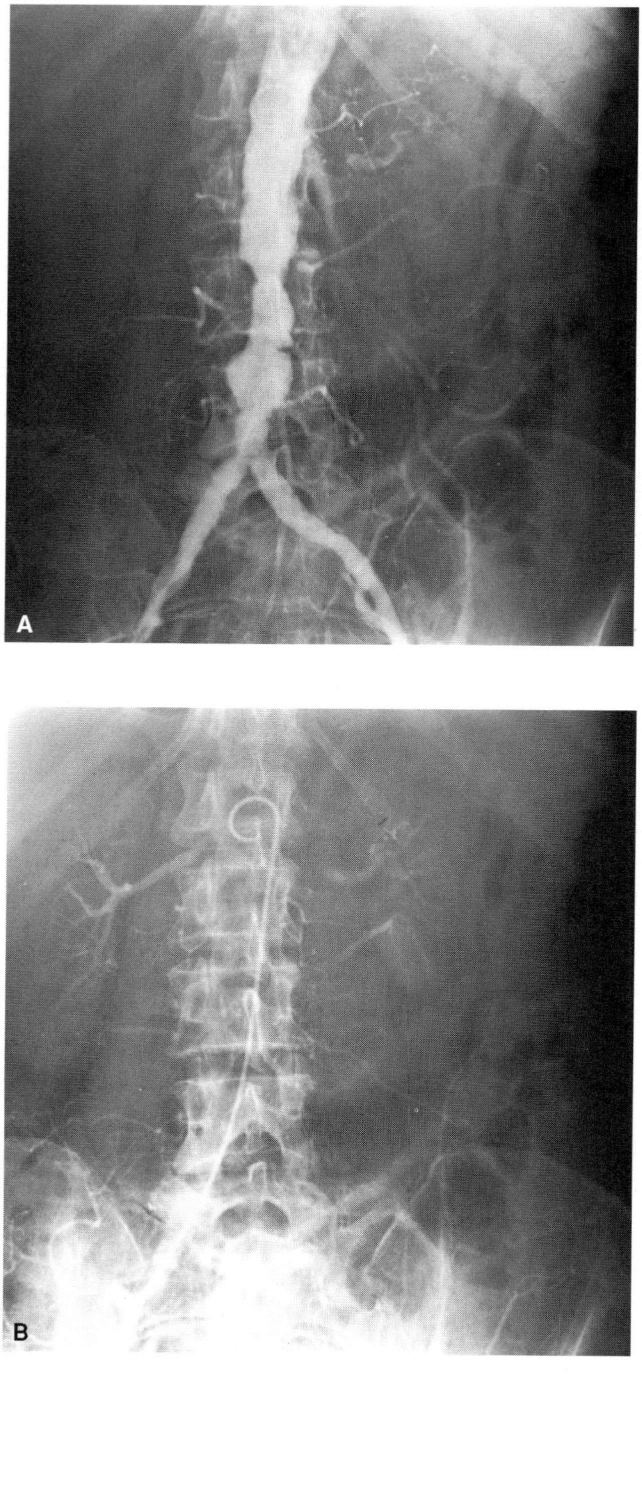

Figure 10–3. The two most important favorable prognostic signs for revascularization of a chronically occluded renal artery are: (1) distal refilling of the main renal artery and (2) a good nephrogram. This patient presented with recent onset of renal failure needing hemodialysis and bilateral renal artery occlusions. A. Early aortogram showing bilateral renal artery occlusion. B. Late refilling of renal arteries.

tery occlusions, 50 patients had kidneys suitable for revascularization while the other 100 had atrophic (<7–8 cm) kidneys that were removed, often at the time of revascularization for a contralateral high-grade renal artery stenosis.

The surgical approach can be considered in three anatomic settings.

1. Renal Artery Occlusion Suitable for Revascularization and a Normal Contralateral Renal Artery (Fig. 10–4) This situation is ideal for a bypass graft. If the celiac axis is normal, a hepatorenal bypass is a good option for a right renal artery lesion while a splenorenal arterial anastomosis is an alternative for the left kidney. These options depend, of course, on excluding significant celiac axis disease on a lateral aortic view which should be requested with the initial renal arteriogram. Other choices include a supraceliac aortorenal bypass, an infrarenal aortorenal bypass or

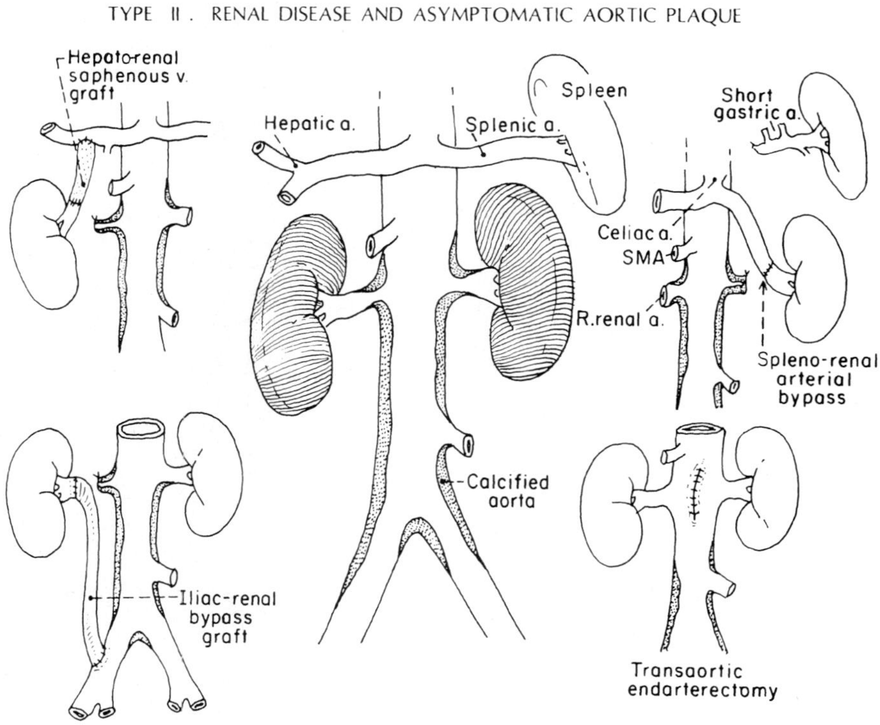

Figure 10–4. Surgical options for unilateral renal revascularization in the presence of asymptomatic but troublesome aortic occlusive or early aneurysmal disease.

an iliorenal bypass. Except for an aortorenal bypass, all of these options avoid cross-clamping the aorta. This is an important consideration in elderly patients with calcified aortic atheroma and significant cardiac comorbidity.

2. Bilateral Severe Renal Artery Occlusive Disease (Fig. 10–5) This anatomic challenge is common in patients with advanced aortorenal atherosclerosis. In fact, nearly 50% of patients with a renal artery occlusion require contralateral renal artery revascularization. Aortic disease (occlusive or aneurysmal) is frequently present as well. The morbidity and mortality for concomitant bilateral renal revascularization and aortic replacement can be significant. Most mortality reports range between 7 and 10% although these rates have dropped recently to 3–5% in centers with larger volumes of renovascular cases.

Transaortic bilateral renal endarterectomy has become our procedure of choice for bilateral proximal renal artery atheroma. This technique can disobliterate a chronic renal artery occlusion. The

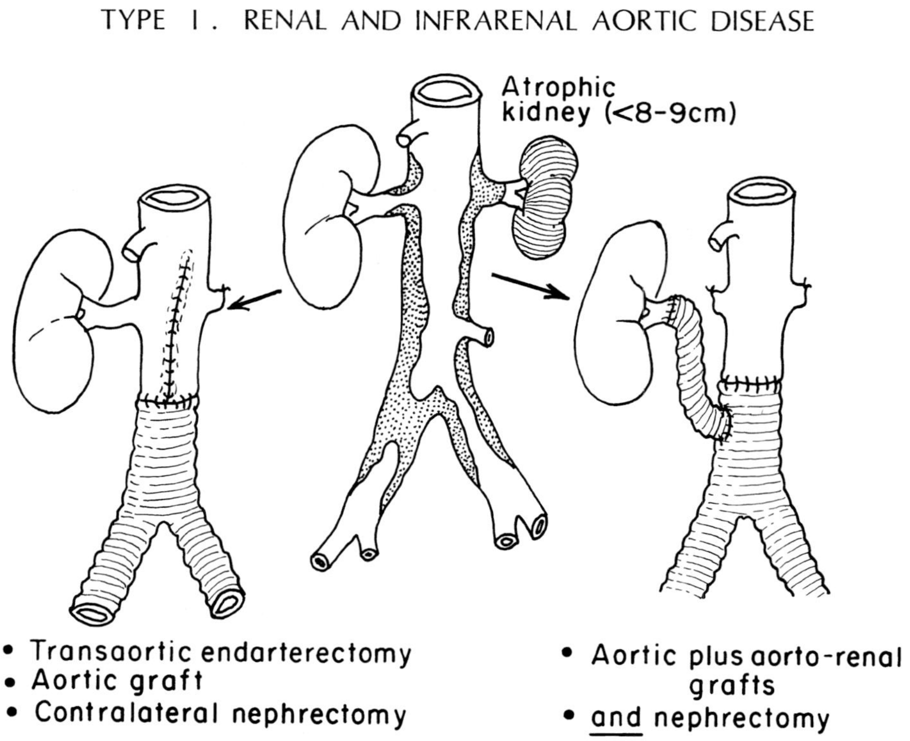

Figure 10–5. Surgical options for bilateral renal artery disease and significant aortic disease needing concomitant reconstruction.

primary advantages of endarterectomy are anatomic restoration of flow and its speed. Renal ischemic time averages 20–30 minutes. The key to its success with an occlusion is extensive mobilization of the involved renal artery so that the plaque can be adequately inverted into the aorta and removed with a satisfactory endpoint. We use intraoperative colorflow duplex ultrasonography to ascertain that the endarterectomy has been technically successful. Problems requiring correction are detected in 10% of patients.

Bypass grafting is our choice when the occlusive plaque extends beyond the proximal one half of the renal artery. The choice of graft material depends on the distal renal size. If the artery is greater than 5 mm in diameter, we use a 6 mm polyester graft. Smaller renal arteries are treated with reversed saphenous vein grafts. These prosthetic or vein grafts are generally attached to the Dacron aortic graft that is placed for aortic disease.

3. Renal Artery Occlusion With a Nonsalvageable Kidney
Nephrectomy is indicated in this situation. In many cases, however, the contralateral kidney has a high-grade renal artery stenosis that needs correction. Consequently, a simple nephrectomy via a flank incision is not adequate therapy. In these cases, we select the best option for the contralateral renal revascularization and perform a nephrectomy at the same operation. In our experience, this simultaneous approach provides the best relief of hypertension and preservation of renal function.

Surgical Results

Several surgical series have provided encouraging results for saving a kidney with a chronic renal artery occlusion. Our previously reported experience with 50 such patients is typical of expected outcome.[10] Several findings of this past study deserve emphasis.

The early perioperative results depend on the extent of aortorenal disease and other medical comorbidity. Bypass grafting was used in seven out of ten patients. Saphenous vein was selected in the vast majority of cases (80–90%). The remaining three out of ten had endarterectomy or reimplantation of the renal artery. Simultaneous contralateral renal revascularization was necessary in nearly one half of patients. Thirty-day mortality was 6%, but all these deaths occurred in patients undergoing concomitant major aortic or other visceral reconstruction. The primary cause of death was myocardial infarction.

Early control of hypertension and preservation of renal function was achieved in the vast majority. At discharge 98% of patients had a lower diastolic blood pressure. Fifty percent were no longer on any antihypertensive medication. The type of operative procedure did not correlate with the blood pressure response. Only one

(2%) renal revascularization occluded in the early postoperative period. In the 74% of patients with a normal preoperative serum creatinine, only 5% required early dialysis. In contrast, 25% of those patients with a creatinine greater than 2 mg/dl needed early dialysis.

Late results were also good. Eighty five percent of patients maintained satisfactory control of hypertension. Ten percent eventually required nephrectomy of the affected kidney. Seven percent of those remaining alive progressed to chronic dialysis. The most common cause of late death remained myocardial infarction and stroke.

SUMMARY

The decision to perform revascularization or nephrectomy in the setting of a chronic renal artery occlusion is influenced by several factors. Most important are the condition of the distal renal artery and the size of the kidney. If the preoperative arteriogram demonstrates a normal renal artery beyond the obstruction, revascularization should be attempted, especially when the kidney is at least 8 cm in length. If contralateral severe stenosis exists, it should be repaired simultaneously to achieve the best control of hypertension and preservation of renal function. If the distal renal artery is not identified angiographically and the kidney is large or functional on renal scan, surgical exploration should be done. Nephrectomy is appropriate when the occluded renal artery is associated with an atrophic (<7 cm) pressor kidney and the opposite kidney can be revascularized. Surgical management of the chronically occluded renal artery provides significant early and late control of severe renovascular hypertension and averts chronic renal failure in the majority of patients. These results are achieved despite diffuse atherosclerosis and considerable medical comorbidity in most patients.

Acknowledgments

The author thanks Renee Brandt for editorial assistance.

REFERENCES

1. Alexander RH, Brient BW. Revascularization of kidneys with totally occluded renal arteries. *South Med J* 1982;75:1087–92.
2. Dean RM, Tribble RW, Hansen KJ, O'Neil E, Craven TE, Redding

JF. 2d. Evolution of renal insufficiency in ischemic nephropathy. *Ann Surg* 1991;213:446–455.

3. Dean RH, Lawson JD, Hollifield JW, Shack RB, Polterauer P, Rhamy RK. Revascularization of the poorly functioning kidney. *Surgery* 1979;85:44–52.
4. Hansen KJ, Starr SM, Sands RE, Burkart JM, Plonk GW Jr, Dean RH. Contemporary surgical management of renovascular disease. *J Vasc Surg* 1992;16:319–330.
5. Hallett JW Jr, Fowl R, O'Brien PC, Bernatz PE, Pairolero PC, Cherry KJ, Hollier LH. Renovascular operations in patients with chronic renal insufficiency: do the benefits justify the risks? *J Vasc Surg* 1987;5:622–7.
6. Lawrie GM, Morris Jr GC, DeBakey ME. Long-term results of treatment of the totally occluded renal artery in forty patients with renovascular hypertension. *Surgery* 1980;88:753–9.
7. Magilligan Jr DJ, DeWeese JA, May AG, Rob CG. The occluded renal artery. *Surgery* 1975;78:730–8.
8. May J, Sheil AGR, Horvath J, Tiller DJ, Johnson JR. Reversal of renal failure and control of hypertension in patients with occlusion of the renal artery. *Surg Gynecol Obstet* 1976;143:411–3.
9. Messina LM, Zelenock GB, Yao KA, Stanley JC. Renal revascularization for recurrent pulmonary edema in patients with poorly controlled hypertension and renal insufficiency: a distinct subgroup of patients with arteriosclerotic renal artery occlusive disease. *J Vasc Surg* 1992;15:73–80.
10. Vogt PA, Pairolero PC, Hollier LH, Fowl RJ, Cherry KJ Jr, Bernatz PE. The occluded renal artery: Durability of revascularization. *J Vasc Surg* 1985;2:125–132.
11. Whitehouse Jr WM, Kazmers A, Zelenock GB, Erlandson EE, Cronenwett JL, Lindenauer SM, Stanley JC. Chronic total renal artery occlusion: Effects of treatment on secondary hypertension and renal function. *Surgery* 1981;89:753–63.
12. Zinman L, Libertino JA. Revascularization of the chronic totally occluded renal artery with restoration of renal function. *J Urol* 1977; 118:517–21.

11

Renal Revascularization for the Acutely Occluded Renal Artery

Kenneth Ouriel

Acute renal artery occlusion occurring as a result of thrombosis or embolism is an infrequently encountered entity, with a paucity of literature on which to form clinical decisions. Elective renal revascularization is an accepted therapeutic modality in patients with renovascular hypertension or renal insufficiency as a result of *chronic* renal artery stenotic disease. By contrast, the precise role of intervention in patients who experience acute occlusion is less well defined. There exist four choices in the management of acute renal artery occlusion; observation, thrombolytic therapy, operative revascularization, and nephrectomy. Although objective data documenting the clinical results of these modalities do not exist, each play an important role in specific clinical settings.

A variety of etiologic mechanisms associated with acute renal artery occlusion exists. Renal artery embolism develops when embolic material is deposited in the renal arterial vasculature, resulting in sudden and frequently irreversible parenchymal ischemia. Renal artery thrombosis occurs in the setting of preexisting atherosclerotic stenotic disease or fibromuscular dysplasia, but renal artery dissection and traumatic etiologies are also encountered. Acute renal artery occlusion is associated with a characteristic spectrum of signs and symptoms, yet diagnosis is frequently delayed because of the relative rarity of the disorder and the failure to consider it as a possibility. The primary sequelae of acute renal occlusion are renal insufficiency and hyperreninemic hypertension, but systemic azotemia is rare in the absence of bilateral renal involvement. The exception to this rule occurs with unilateral renal artery disease and chronic renovascular hypertension; contralateral parenchymal damage and renal failure develop from the long term microangiopathic effects of systemic hypertension.

When sudden renal artery occlusion occurs, the timing and the magnitude of the ischemic insult are dependent on the adequacy of preexisting collateral circulation. Thus, renal artery embolism is frequently associated with irreversible ischemia by the time the diagnosis has been made.[1] In contrast to patients with embolic occlusion, patients with thrombosis usually maintain renal viability indefinitely, since the slow progression of a stenotic lesion provides ample time for the development of protective collateral circulation when the main renal artery occludes.

PATHOPHYSIOLOGY

Acute renal artery occlusion occurs as a result of embolism or thrombosis. Embolism to a solitary kidney or simultaneously to both kidneys comprise a surprisingly high proportion of the cases reported in the literature, probably because of the difficulty in diagnosing unilateral embolism in the presence of a normally functioning contralateral kidney. Similarily, acute thrombosis of one renal artery may go unnoticed until the contralateral vessel occludes, resulting in anuria. Thrombosis may develop following the slow progression of an atherosclerotic or fibrodysplastic stenosis or suddenly after traumatic disruption. Rarely, spontaneous dissection of the renal artery occurs, usually in the setting of underlying atherosclerotic or fibrodysplastic disease. Renal artery emboli are almost always of cardiac origin and may be associated with atrial arrhythmias, valvular disease, or acute myocardial infarction **(Table 11–1)**. Thrombotic occlusion is most commonly associated with calcific atherosclerotic lesions at the renal ostia. These plaques are usually in continuity with dense, circumferen-

Table 11–1. Etiology and Location of Renal Artery Emboli in Combined Series in the Literature

		Frequency
Etiology[1,5]		
	Atrial fibrillation	53%
	Valvular vegetation	12%
	Acute myocardial infarction	23%
	Aortic aneurysm	7%
	Other	5%
Kidney[3,7]		
	Right	55%
	Left	45%
	Solitary (Left or Right)	26%
	Bilateral	10%

tial aortic atherosclerotic disease, a feature which attains significance when contemplating balloon dilatation or aortorenal bypass. Alternatively, renal artery thrombosis may occur in the setting of fibrodysplasia. Fibrodysplastic lesions may occur along the length of the body of the renal artery and have been grouped into four histologic varieties; intimal fibroplasia, medial hyperplasia, medial fibroplasia, and perimedial dysplasia. Thrombosis after traumatic injuries may occur following complete disruption, encountered with or without an arteriovenous fistula. Isolated intimal disruption occurs as a result of traction injuries from blunt trauma to the abdomen. Of the two types of traumatic renal artery occlusion, the primary therapeutic aim is the arrest of hemorrhage in the former and the preservation of renal function in the latter.

Whereas thrombosis of a renal arterial atherosclerotic or fibrodysplastic lesion results in both renovascular hypertension and chronic renal insufficiency, renal embolism is less frequently associated with hypertension. The explanation of this observation may relate to sudden infarction of the renin producing juxtaglomerular cells in the latter entity. When sudden onset of hypertension does develop, one may assume that the collateral flow around the embolus is sufficient to maintain viability of at least the endocrine cells of the organ.

The mechanisms described by Goldblatt explain the pathophysiology associated with the development and maintenance of renovascular hypertension. The renin-angiotensin-aldosterone system is the critical hormonal pathway responsible for the preservation of the normotensive state. Hypertension may develop as a result of overfilling of the arterial system, arteriolar vasoconstriction, or by a combination of these factors. Lowered renal perfusion pressure produces a compensatory increase in unilateral renin secretion, increased angiotensin-II formation, and elevated blood pressure secondary to vasoconstriction and hyperaldosteronemic-induced volume overload. A normal contralateral kidney can partially compensate for the hyperreninemic state by increasing salt excretion. This compensatory response does not occur in the presence of an abnormal or absent contralateral kidney or in the presence of contralateral renal artery disease. Thus, the two forms of Goldblatt hypertension provide experimental corollaries to renovascular hypertension with unilateral versus bilateral renal arterial disease. In the two-kidney, one-clip Goldblatt model a single renal artery is clamped and the opposite kidney is left undisturbed. Unilateral renal artery disease corresponds to this form of Goldblatt hypertension. In the one-kidney, one-clip model, one renal artery is clamped and the contralateral kidney is removed. The clinical corollary of this model is observed in patients with bilateral renal artery disease, where one kidney is completely infarcted and the other is ischemic.

Renin levels are elevated indefinitely in the two-kidney model and the administration of angiotensin inhibitors results in decreases in blood pressure both initially and in the established phase. By contrast, renin levels are only transiently increased in the one-kidney model. Increased renin secretion is soon suppressed by volume expansion from sodium and water retention, and the established phase of hypertension is maintained by volume expansion and not by renin-mediated vasoconstriction. Predictably, angiotensin blockade is ineffective in treating the hypertensive state in the established phase of the one-kidney model or its clinical corollaries.

Morris and colleagues emphasized the importance of subfiltration arterial pressure on the development of irreversible renal ischemic injury.[2] Deterioration of renal function did not develop in canine kidneys subjected to suprarenal aortic occlusion and mean perfusion pressures of 24 mm Hg for up to 2 hours. By contrast, those kidneys with negligible renal perfusion pressures suffered irretrievable damage within 60 minutes of onset. These laboratory studies suggest that renal salvage is unlikely in patients with complete renal artery obstruction and the absence of preexistent collateral arterial channels. Most series of renal arterial occlusions document poor rates of salvage in embolic disease and satisfactory rates of salvage in thrombotic disease.[3] Moreover, the timing of renal revascularization is poorly correlated with successful restoration of function. These observations are likely explained by the adequacy of collateral circulation in renal artery thrombosis and the absence of significant collaterals in most embolized kidneys. Not all renal emboli, however, are totally obstructing and occasional patients may have flow around the embolus or adequate preexisting collateral circulation to maintain perfusion at a level insufficient to provide renal excretory function but yet adequate to preserve viability. Thus, an accurate and timely diagnosis of embolic renal artery occlusion remains the only means of effecting renal salvage and reducing the risk of subsequent embolic episodes.

DIAGNOSIS

Patients with acute renal artery occlusion most often present with flank, back, or abdominal pain **(Table 11–2)**. Nausea and vomiting may occur, and patients may note gross hematuria. A low-grade fever is common, as is new onset hypertension. On examination, patients typically manifest flank tenderness to deep palpation. Laboratory findings consist of leukocytosis, and elevation in the lactate dehydrogenase level is common. The presence of erythrocytes, leukocytes, and protein is almost uniform on urinalysis. The differentiation of embolic versus thrombotic etiologies can some-

Table 11–2. Clinical and Laboratory Presentation in Acute Renal Artery Occlusion[3,5,8]

Parameter	Frequency (%)
Pain	
Abdominal	41
Chest	24
Flank	77
Back	12
Fever (>38°C)	69
Hypertension (>170/100)	85
Creatinine elevation (>2.0 mg/dl)	46
Leukocytosis (>12,000/mm^3)	94
Urinalysis	
Protein	93
Leukocytes (>10/hpf)	59
Erythrocytes (>10/hpf)	71
LDH elevation (>2x normal)	88

times be made on clinical grounds alone, with a history of hypertension in most patients with thrombotic occlusion and cardiac disease in patients with embolic processes **(Table 11–3)**.

When performed, an intravenous pyelogram will document absent function in complete renal artery obstruction and poor function when the obstruction is partial. Renal nuclear medicine studies mirror these findings, but renal arteriography is necessary and diagnostic in all cases where revascularization is contemplated. The differentiation between renal embolism and renal artery thrombosis is sometimes difficult on arteriography. A meniscus may be seen in cases of embolism, while a smooth, tapering lesion is common in thrombotic occlusion. An aorta relatively free of atherosclerotic change is most unusual in cases of atherosclerotic renal artery thrombosis and suggests a diagnosis of embolic occlu-

Table 11–3. Clinical Characteristics of Patients with Embolic (n = 13) and Thrombotic (n = 16) Renal Artery Occlusion[3]

	Embolic	Thrombotic
Previous history of hypertension	23%	69%
Cardiac arrhythmia	62%	2
Valvular heart disease	46%	0
Previous embolic event	69%	0

sion. The presence of abundant collateral channels feeding the distal renal artery implies a preexistent hemodynamically significant renal artery stenosis and a thrombotic rather than embolic etiology. Disease entities that mimic renal arterial occlusion include aortic dissection and pyelonephritis. These entities can usually be excluded on the basis of an accurate history and physical examination and arteriographic study.

The initial diagnostic modality when renal ischemia is suspected is isotope renography. Unlike arteriography or intravenous pyelography, the isotope studies do not produce additional damage to an already compromised kidney and arteriography may be avoided in cases where renal insufficiency is not a result of arterial compromise. Renal arteriography, however, should follow immediately if the renal scan documents an abnormality in perfusion.

THERAPY

The prompt diagnosis of acute renal artery occlusion is essential to the preservation of functional renal parenchyma.[4] Involvement of a solitary kidney or both kidneys simultaneously comprise a surprisingly high proportion of the cases reported in the literature, probably because of the difficulty in diagnosing unilateral occlusion in the presence of a normally functioning contralateral kidney. Acute thrombosis of one renal artery may go unnoticed until the contralateral vessel occludes, resulting in anuria. Systemic anticoagulation is important to preclude propagation of the clot and to prevent embolism to other organs.[5]

There are three options for managing acute renal artery occlusion; revascularization, nephrectomy, and observation alone. Observation predictably results in loss of most if not all functional renal parenchyma and carries the risks of subsequent necrotic abscess formation and long term hypertension. Therefore, expectant management should be reserved for those patients least likely to tolerate any invasive intervention. Nephrectomy is a reasonable alternative in patients without sufficient viable renal parenchyma to warrant revascularization. The therapeutic dilemma, however, is predicting which kidneys will yield measurable excretory function following successful restoration of arterial flow.

Regardless of the etiologic mechanism, therapeutic decisions must be predicated on a determination of renal viability and the potential for salvage of functional parenchyma. The renal perfusion scan and late phase of an aortogram have both been found to be predictive of renal viability.[3] Any degree of perfusion or the visualization of a nephrogram are indicative of adequate residual perfusion and an attempt at revascularization is appropriate. In the absence of either criterion, renal salvage is sufficiently unlikely that attempts at revascularization are warranted only when the loss of the involved kidney would render the patient dialysis dependent.[1,5] Observation is indicated in the absence of prospects for salvage of significant renal mass, but the presence of concurrent factors such as persistent hypertension, pain, or infection mandate early nephrectomy.

Two general methods of restoring renal arterial perfusion exist: catheter-directed thrombolytic therapy, and immediate operative revascularization. Thrombolytic therapy may restore arterial flow more rapidly than can be achieved with operation, but the speed of clot lysis is unpredictable and may take many hours in some cases. Operative revascularization is more predictable in its ability to restore renal arterial perfusion, but this advantage must be weighed against the risks associated with a major surgical intervention in this medically compromised patient group.

A number of anecdotal reports of renal arterial thrombolysis have appeared in the literature, but the merits of this procedure remain to be defined.[6] The infusion catheter must be positioned within the substance of the thrombus if successful dissolution of the thromboembolic material is to be achieved. This factor is probably the most important determinant of successful thrombolysis. The choice of plasminogen activator is less consequential; streptokinase, urokinase, and recombinant tissue plasminogen activator are each acceptable agents. Although the complete dissolution of arterial thromboembolism may require many hours, initial reperfusion through a partially recanalized clot can be achieved within a much shorter period of time. Successful renal artery thrombolysis may be definitive in patients with embolic occlusion, but subsequent balloon angioplasty or operative bypass is required to correct the underlying stenotic lesion in patients with renal artery thrombosis.

A variety of operative techniques suitable for renal arterial exposure exists. Either an anterior or retroperitoneal approach may be undertaken. Using an anterior transperitoneal approach, both renal arteries may be exposed after reflecting the right or left colon medially. Alternatively, the left renal artery may be identified through a lessor sac exposure and the right renal artery after performing a generous Kocher maneuver. A third technique involves retraction of the transverse colon cephalad and following the infrarenal aorta proximally to the renal orifices. The renal vein is usually identified first, and the artery is encountered with mobilization and gentle retraction of the vein.

Balloon catheter thromboembolectomy is necessary in all embolic cases and in those thrombotic cases where the clot has propagated distally. The renal artery is exposed over a sufficient length and balloon catheters are passed proximally and distally in an attempt to clear all thromboembolic debris. Intraoperative arteriography, angioscopy, or Duplex ultrasound may be beneficial to assure the complete removal of thrombus; backflow is almost always scant and its absence should not dissuade attempts at revascularization. Diuretics and mannitol may be useful after revascularization, as may be dopamine in doses of 3 to 5 μg/kg/min. A period of acute tubular necrosis should be expected, but renal excretory function usually returns slowly over a period of several weeks.

Whereas thromboembolectomy alone is sufficient therapy in cases of renal embolization to a previously normal renal artery, the treatment of thrombotic occlusion must address the underlying stenotic lesion. Bypass with saphenous vein, prosthetic conduits, or hypogastric artery (in pediatric patients) all provide acceptable choices. The choice of inflow is very important when performing a renal bypass in the setting of thrombotic occlusion, and the status of the abdominal aorta is critical in this regard. We have utilized hepatorenal, splenorenal, or iliorenal bypass grafts in patients with atherosclerotic disease to minimize the complications associated with clamping a markedly diseased abdominal aorta. Such extensive aortic disease is unusual in patients with fibrodysplastic lesions, and aortorenal bypass is most appropriate in this subgroup.

RESULTS

Failure to revascularize an acutely ischemic kidney is associated with a high rate of complications in the form of chronic hypertension and renal infarction with abscess formation **(Table 11–4)**. These observations suggest that expectant management should be reserved for only the most medically compromised patients.

A review of reported series suggests that renal infarction has already occurred by the time the diagnosis is entertained in cases where the embolus completely occluded the main renal artery.[1,3] Operative or thrombolytic is most successful in cases with partial

Table 11–4. Results of Observation in Patients with Acute Renal Artery Occlusion[3]

	Improved Renal Function	Subsequent Hypertension	Subsequent Necrotic Abscess
Embolism (n = 8)	1 (13%)	4 (50%)	3 (38%)
Thrombosis (n = 8)	0	5 (63%)	1 (13%)
Traumatic (n = 3)	0	0	1 (33%)

renal artery occlusion or in the rare instance of embolization to a kidney with ample preexistent collateral channels. These patients can be identified by the presence of a nephrogram on the late phase of an arteriogram or when the renal perfusion scan reveals persistence of renal blood flow; otherwise, revascularization is inappropriate and therapeutic strategies are directed at the prevention of recurrent embolization with prompt institution of systemic anticoagulation.

Operative intervention was reported to be successful in over 50 percent of cases in the early series[7] However, these studies included *partially* occluding emboli, emboli to branch renal vessels, and patients with poorly documented embolic events that may have represented renal artery thrombosis in some cases. Unfortunately, most patients who experience complete embolic obstruction of a main renal artery do not have sufficient preexistent collateral arterial bloodflow to maintain viability until revascularization can be effected. Literature reports comprising patients with completely occluding main renal artery emboli document an extremely poor rate of salvage. We were unable to save any of 13 embolized kidneys, despite successful restoration of arterial flow in three-fourths of the patients who underwent operative revascularization **(Table 11–5)**.[3]

The operative results in patients with thrombotic occlusion of a preexisting stenotic lesion are strikingly improved over those achieved in patients with emboli. We documented improvement in renal function in five of eight patients presenting with acute thrombotic renal artery occlusion, with relief of hypertension in six (75%) of the cases. The timing of revascularization did not appear critical, although a slow decline in the mass of viable renal tissue can be predicted to occur as the interval between occlusion and revascularization lengthens.

By contrast, the results with revascularization of kidneys rendered ischemic as the result of traumatic renal artery occlusion were dismal. None of three organs were salvaged in our original series[3] and we have been unsuccessful in three additional cases. The absence of collateral circulation renders these kidneys severely ischemic following total obstruction of flow through the ar-

Table 11–5. Results of Operative Intervention in 16 Patients with Acute Renal Artery Occlusion[3]

	Salvage of Function	Nonsalvage
Embolism (n = 5)	0	100%
Thrombosis (n = 8)	63%	37%
Traumatic (n = 3)	0	100%

tery. Infarction is likely to develop within sixty to ninety minutes following injury, thwarting any attempt at salvage.

SUMMARY

The diagnosis of acute renal artery occlusion is frequently elusive, primarily as a result of the rarity of the condition and the failure to promptly recognize the associated signs and symptoms. The options for renal revascularization include thrombolytic therapy, embolectomy, and arterial bypass grafting. Timing is not crucial in cases of thrombotic occlusion, since the preexistence of collateral circulation maintains renal viability despite compromised arterial flow. By contrast, the rapid institution of appropriate intervention is critical in cases of embolic occlusion. Despite valiant efforts at revascularization, renal salvage is rare in patients with totally occluding renal artery emboli. Primary nephrectomy is appropriate in these cases, as well as in cases of thrombotic occlusion with minimal residual renal viability.

REFERENCES

1. Schoenbaum S, Goldman MA, Siegelman SS. Renal arterial embolization. *Angiology* 1971;22:332–343.
2. Morris G.C. Jr, Heider CF, Moyer JH. The protective effect of subfiltration arterial pressure in the kidney. *Surg Forum* 1956;6:623–627.
3. Ouriel K, Andrus CH, Ricotta JJ, DeWeese JA, Green RM. Acute renal artery occlusion: When is revascularization justified? *J Vasc Surg* 1987;5:348–355.
4. Moyer JH, Heider C, Morris GC Jr, Handley C. Renal failure. I. The effect of complete renal artery occlusion for variable periods of time as compared to exposure to sub-filtration arterial pressures below 30 mm Hg for similar periods. *Ann Surg* 1957;145:41–58.
5. Lessman RK, Johnson SF, Coburn JW, Kaufman JJ. Renal artery embolism. Clinical features and long-term follow-up of 17 cases. *Ann Intern Med* 1978;89:477–482.
6. Campieri C, Raimondi C, Ratone F, et al.. Normalization of renal function and blood pressure after dissolution with intra-arterial fibrinolytics of a massive renal artery embolism to a solitary functioning kidney. *Nephron* 1989;51:399–401.
7. Lacombe M. Surgical versus medical treatment of renal artery embolism. *J Cardiovasc Surg* 1977;18:281–290.
8. Winzelberg GG, Hull JD, Agar JWM, Rose BD, Pletka PG. Elevation of serum lactate dehydrogenase levels in renal infarction. *JAMA* 1979; 242:268–269.

12

Renal Revascularization for Recurrent Pulmonary Edema and Renovascular Hypertension

James C. Stanley and Louis M. Messina

Recurrent pulmonary edema, poorly controlled hypertension, and renal insufficiency were first reported as a trimarker of advanced arteriosclerotic renovascular disease by Pickering and colleagues in 1988,[1] and subsequently by Messina and his associates in 1992.[2] Bilateral disease was an important component of this entity and was present in 36 of the 37 patients reported by the two former groups.

Treatment of this subgroup of renovascular hypertensives is difficult.[1–4] Intensive medical therapy, especially with utilization of angiotensin converting enzyme (ACE) inhibitors, may provide control of the hypertensive state, but often is achieved at the expense of further reductions in renal perfusion, a worsening of renal insufficiency, and subsequent volume retention. Volume overload is the preeminent cause of these patient's symptoms. Recurrent pulmonary edema in this form of renovascular hypertension mandates that these patients be treated aggressively.

UNIVERSITY OF MICHIGAN CLINICAL EXPERIENCE

Renal revascularization for recurrent pulmonary edema and poorly controlled renovascular hypertension has been performed in 23 patients, 10 men and 13 women, at the University of Michigan Hospital from over an 8 year time period.[3] The patients ranged in age from 52 to 80 years, with mean ages of the men and women being 68 and 60 years, respectively. Their preoperative blood pressures averaged 200/104 mm Hg. Hypertensive encephalopathy affected three patients in this series. Numbered preoperative antihypertensive medications averaged 3.9 per patient.

Significant renal insufficiency was commonplace, with the preoperative serum creatinine averaging 3.6 mg/dl in this group. Preoperative dialysis was necessary in three patients.

Severe acute pulmonary edema requiring hospitalization affected all 23 patients, including three who required intubation and mechanical ventilation for respiratory failure immediately prior to operation. Left ventricular hypertrophy (LVH) affected 70% of these individuals, yet 52% exhibited normal biventricular function by echocardiography or MUGA studies. Thus poor myocardial compliance appeared more important than primary myocardial contractile failure in this clinical setting. Interestingly, recurrent pulmonary edema and renal insufficiency was not encountered among more than 160 patients with renovascular hypertension due to arterial fibrodysplasia treated at the University of Michigan. Fixed structural changes within the circulatory tree and reduced vasoadaptive mechanisms are more likely to affect older patients with arteriosclerosis than younger patients with fibrodysplastic renal artery disease. This may account for the absence of fibrodysplastic patients in the presently reported subset of renovascular hypertensives.

Advanced arteriosclerosis was common in the Michigan series, with bilateral aortic spillover renal artery disease affecting 96% of these individuals, including 57% with occlusion of one or both renal arteries. Coronary artery disease was common, with 35% having experienced earlier myocardial infarctions and 17% having undergone prior coronary artery bypass. Cerebrovascular accidents affected 35% of these patients, and 70% had evidence of lower extremity occlusive disease.

Intensive antihypertensive drug treatment to improve renal function and lessen the risks for pulmonary edema was pursued initially in all patients, but failed in every instance. Subsequent treatment was highly individualized, including revascularization of 33 kidneys by the performance of: aortorenal bypass-10, aortorenal endarterectomy-6, iliorenal bypass-12, splenorenal bypass-1, hepatorenal bypass-1, renal artery-aortic reimplantation-2, and transluminal renal angioplasty-1. A contralateral nephrectomy was performed in ten patients (43%) for irreparable ischemic renal damage. Concomitant aortic reconstruction for aneurysmal or occlusive disease was undertaken in 22% of this series. In no case was the aortic procedure undertaken simply to provide a better conduit from which to originate a graft for the renal revascularization.

Specific aspects of renal revascularization in this subgroup of renovascular hypertensives deserve comment. Conventional aortorenal bypass using reversed saphenous vein was a common procedure in this series. When treating patients who had undergone earlier aortic reconstructions, grafts to the kidney usually originating from the limb of the previous aortofemoral or aortoiliac

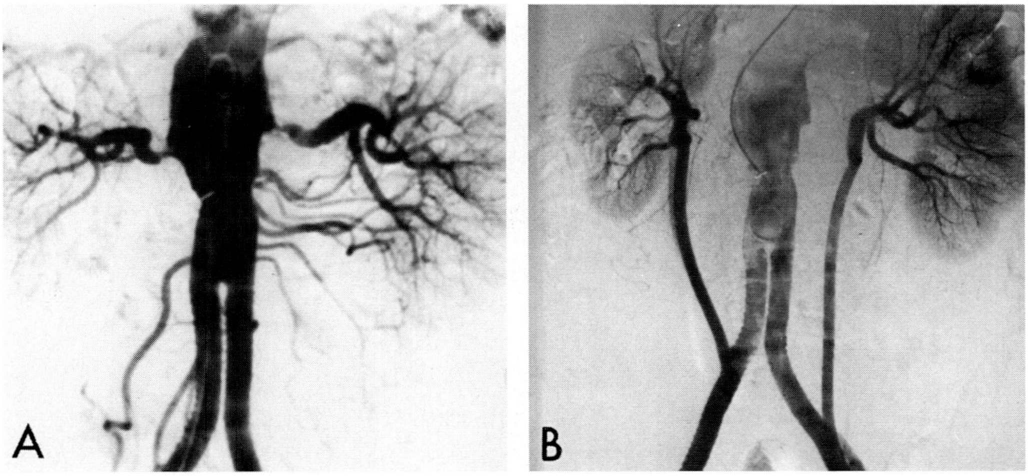

Figure 12–1. A. Preoperative arteriographic demonstration of bilateral severe orificial artery stenoses. B. Postoperative arteriogram of bilateral renal revascularization with ePTFE grafts originating from limbs of a previously placed aortobifemoral graft. Reprinted with permission from Messina LM, Zelenock GB, Yao KA, Stanley JC.[2]

conduit **(Fig. 12–1)**. To consider using the body of the graft as the origin of the bypass, or to perform an aortorenal endarterectomy in these circumstances, would entail dissection about the upper graft. The latter carries the risk of aortic anastomotic disruption that should obviously be avoided. In patients whose extensive aortic disease makes origination of the graft from the aorta hazardous and in those with severe compromise of cardiac function, revascularization procedures avoiding aortic clamping are appropriate. In such instances, nonanatomic renal revascularization such as iliorenal, splenorenal **(Fig. 12–2)**, or hepatorenal bypasses **(Fig. 12–3)** may be undertaken with satisfactory outcomes. Grafts with origins from the celiac circulation must only be placed when no proximal celiac artery entrapment or arteriosclerotic narrowing exists. When treating patients with bilateral disease or multiple renal arteries, an extensive aortorenal endarterectomy may be preferable to complex bypass reconstructions of multiple arteries with prosthetic or vein grafts. Lastly, when performing concomitant aortic reconstruction for either aneurysmal or occlusive disease, a transaortic aortorenal endarterectomy is viewed as an appropriate manner of treatment **(Fig. 12–4)**.

Patients with poorly controlled arteriosclerotic renovascular hypertension manifest by pulmonary edema and renal insufficiency do surprisingly well following aggressive interventional

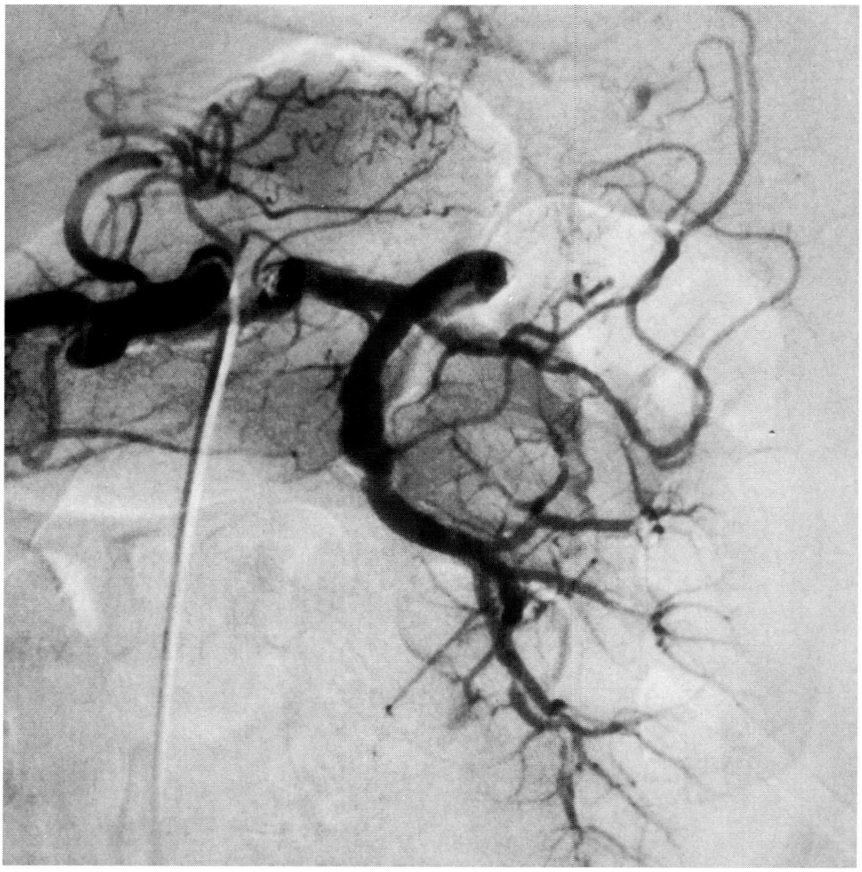

Figure 12–2. Splenorenal bypass, constructed by direct end-to-end anastomosis (arrow), of the left renal artery-to-splenic artery. This was accompanied by a right nephrectomy for irreparable renal ischemic injury to that kidney. Reprinted with permission from Stanley JC, Messina LM.[3]

therapy. In the Michigan experience at the time of hospital discharge, the mean postoperative blood pressure was 137/76 mm Hg and the number of drugs averaged 1.5 per patient. In regard to blood pressure control, two patients were classified as cured and 21 were improved. One patient whose blood pressure was improved had a severe underlying cardiomyopathy that prevented his discharge from the hospital and led to his eventual demise 4 months postoperatively. Improved renal function in this sample of patients was also evident with the mean postoperative serum creatinine being 1.8 mg/dl. Renal function improved in 18 patients, was unchanged in two patients and became worse in three patients, including the one patient who died. Dialysis was discon-

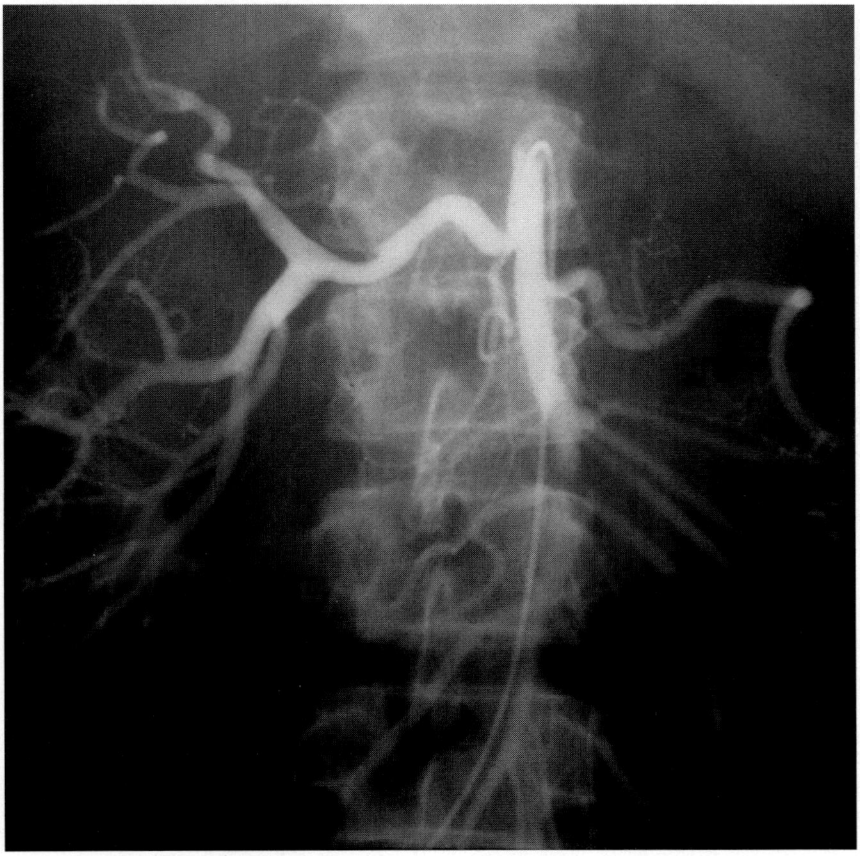

Figure 12–3. Hepatorenal bypass, constructed by direct implantation, in an end-to-side manner, of the right renal artery into a replaced common hepatic artery (arrow), originating from the superior mesenteric artery. A contralateral nephrectomy was also undertaken. Reprinted with permission from Stanley JC, Messina LM.[3]

tinued following operation in three of the five patients requiring dialysis preoperatively. Improved renal function appeared stable as evidenced by maintenance of the mean serum creatinine of 1.8 mg/dl at an average of 24 months followup (range 4 to 82 months). Only one patient exhibited renal function deterioration in late followup.

Although improvements in blood pressure control and renal function were important, the absence of pulmonary edema was the most dramatic benefit of operation in this group of patients. None of the Michigan patients experienced acute pulmonary edema in the early postoperative period. One patient who experi-

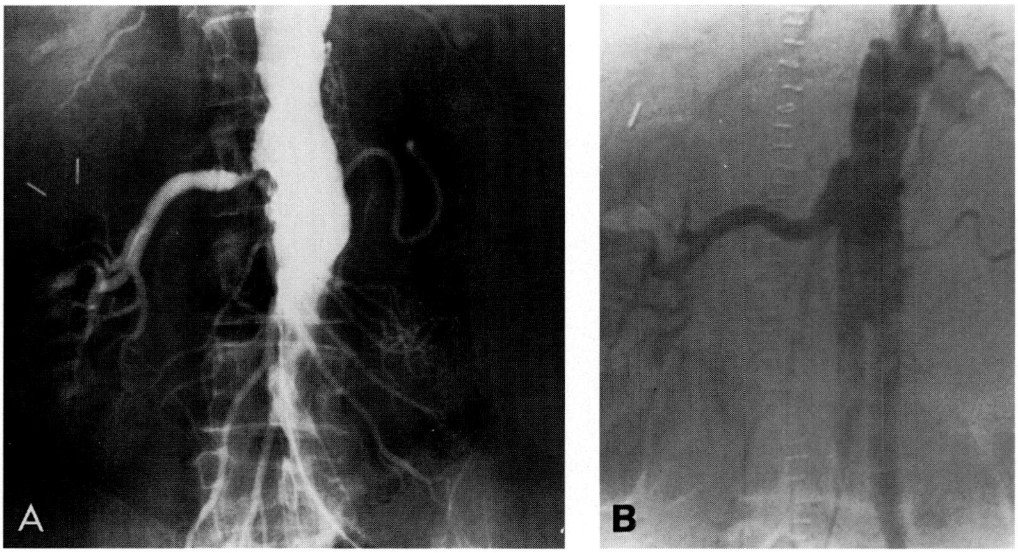

Figure 12–4. A. Preoperative arteriographic demonstration of occluded left renal artery, severe orificial stenosis of right renal artery, and aortic aneurysm. B. Postoperative arteriogram after left nephrectomy, transaortic right renal endarterectomy, and aortic aneurysmectomy with an aortofemoral bypass. Reprinted with permission from Messina LM, Zelenock GB, Yao KA, Stanley JC.[2]

enced pulmonary edema in late follow-up had known mitral insufficiency due to rheumatic heart disease.

DISCUSSION

Specific pathophysiologic events occur predictably in this subgroup of renovascular hypertensives.[5–8] Hemodynamically significant renal artery stenoses increase renin secretion and retention of sodium and water by the affected kidney. Renin release increases systemic angiotensin II concentrations, with subsequent vasoconstriction, decreased glomerular filtration, norepinephrine release from the adrenergic nervous system, and greater aldosterone production. Excess aldosterone causes further increases in sodium and water retention and results in excessive intravascular volume expansion, representing the volume component of renovascular hypertension. A normal contralateral kidney in such circumstances provides for a natriuresis that tends to restore euvolemia. Hypertension in this setting is primarily dependent on angiotensin II, representing the vasoconstrictive component of renovascular hypertension, and usually responds to administration of angiotensin-converting enzyme inhibitors. Unfortunately this subset of renovascular hypertensives rarely have a normal contralateral kidney. In this subset, the presence of bilateral renal artery stenoses, or unilateral stenosis in a patient with solitary kidney or a contralateral kidney exhibiting parenchymal disease, a compensatory natriuresis is impossible, and volume overload persists, becoming the dominant cause of hypertension.

Two factors appear central to the development of pulmonary edema in these patients. First is the presence of LVH, and second is actual intravascular volume overload. The former, manifest by concentric hypertrophy of the left ventricle was documented in 70% of the Michigan patients. Ventricular hypertrophy reduces myocardial compliance and may cause diastolic dysfunction.[9,10] The latter will cause increased left atrial pressures and may lead to pulmonary edema. Even modest volume overload can cause pulmonary edema in these patients. Such diastolic dysfunction may occur in the absence of systolic dysfunction, and may not be evident with routine clinical evaluations of ventricular function. The fact that 52% of the Michigan patients had normal ventricular ejection fractions supports this contention.

Aggressive antihypertensive drug therapy in this group of patients may exacerbate pulmonary edema by decreasing renal blood flow and increasing fluid retention. Treatment with loop diuretics may appear to be a logical strategy in these patients, but the severity of bilateral renal artery stenotic disease often limits the effectiveness of this form of therapy.

The fact that renal revascularization improved control of hypertension in all 23 of the Michigan patients was unexpected, and was clearly superior to outcomes generally anticipated in patients with arteriosclerotic renovascular hypertension **(Table 12–1)**.[11] The unanticipated improvement in control of arterial hypertension and renal function in this series suggests that recurrent pulmonary edema affects a distinct subset of patients with advanced renal artery occlusive disease whose clinical presentation reflects their obstructive renal artery lesions, with relatively protected kidney parenchyma unaffected by nephrosclerosis, which may not be the case in the majority of atherosclerotic renovascular hypertensives.

Contemporary antihypertensive drug therapy has resulted in major improvements in blood pressure control in many patients with high blood pressure. In fact, patients with unilateral renal artery stenosis and no manifestations of extrarenal arteriosclerosis are likely to be treated initially with drugs and are less likely to come to early renal revascularization, than are patients with bilateral renal artery disease, renal insufficiency, and multiple manifestations of extrarenal arteriosclerosis. The latter group

Table 12–1. Arteriosclerotic Renovascular Hypertension: Blood Pressure Response to Operative Intervention (Michigan Experience)

Subgroup	Outcome*			Operative†
	Cured (%)	Improved (%)	Failure (%)	Mortality (%)
Hypertension, Azotemia Pulmonary Edema (Present Series)	9	91	0	4
Hypertension, Clinically Overt Extrarenal Arteriosclerosis (11)	25	47	28	8.5
Hypertension, No Clinically Overt Extrarenal Arteriosclerosis (11)	33	58	9	0

* Hypertension was classified cured when no medications were required to maintain the blood pressure below 150/90 mmHg for at least 6 months, and improved if the blood pressure was maintained under 150/90 mmHg on fewer antihypertensive drugs (excluding ACE inhibitors). Patients with diastolic pressures greater than 90 mmHg, but less than 15% lower than preoperative levels, and all with diastolic pressures greater than 110 mmHg were classified as a failure of therapy.
† Mortality not included in Failure Category.

represent an ever increasing number of patients treated at most large medical centers.[12–14]

The timing of renal revascularization in these patients is often critical. They are usually elderly, severely ill, and are at high risk for any operation. The relatively common occurrence of malignant hypertension, hypertensive encephalopathy, dialysis for progressive renal insufficiency, and mechanical ventilation for respiratory failure, reflects the gravity of their illness. Unfortunately, prolonged efforts to improve the patient's operative risk are often met with a worsening of the patient's overall status.

Because many of these individuals are at high risk for operation, percutaneous transluminal angioplasty may be considered logical treatment, but its limitations must be recognized. Percutaneous transluminal renal angioplasty was performed in five of our patients. It was partially effective in only one patient, who subsequently required a nephrectomy for uncontrolled hypertension and recurrent pulmonary edema. It is not surprising that percutaneous transluminal angioplasty failure is common in these particular patients who have extensive aortic arteriosclerotic spillover renal artery disease. As a matter of fact, balloon angioplasty is likely to be unsuccessful in nearly two-thirds of such patients with bilateral ostial renal artery stenoses.

Surgical revascularization remains the standard means of treating this subgroup of renovascular hypertensives. This form of therapy may be provided with acceptable perioperative morbidity and good long-term results. It is important to attempt to retrieve all renal tissue at the time of initial operation. Thus, renal revascularization should be pursued even in instances of totally occluded renal arteries, provided the involved kidney does not have multiple infarctions and is greater than 7 cm length with a reasonable residual of cortical tissue. However, undertaking nephrectomy for a nonsalvageable kidney may be necessary to eliminate a source of persistent hypertension and improve the function of the remaining contralateral kidney.

Patients in the Michigan series most frequently underwent aortorenal bypass or transaortic endarterectomy. Nevertheless, nearly a third of the procedures were iliorenal bypasses, with the iliac artery or a limb of a previously placed aortic graft chosen as a safe disease-free conduit from which to originate a renal graft. Hepatorenal or splenorenal bypasses were also used in these patients. The low operative morbidity and mortality and excellent long-term outcomes in the Michigan experience support aggressive operative intervention in this subset of renovascular hypertensives. Clearly, documented pulmonary edema in a hypertensive patient with renal insufficiency should lead one to suspect this form of renal artery disease. In such a setting, early renal revascularization is likely to provide effective resolution of pulmonary edema, better control of the patient's hypertension, and improvement in renal function.

REFERENCES

1. Pickering TG, et al. Recurrent pulmonary edema in hypertension due to bilateral renal artery stenosis: treatment by angioplasty or surgical revascularization. *Lancet* 1988;2:551–2.
2. Messina LM, Zelenock GB, Yao KA, Stanley JC. Renal revascularization for recurrent pulmonary edema in patients with poorly controlled hypertension and renal insufficiency: A distinct subgroup of patients with arteriosclerotic renal artery occlusive disease. *J Vasc Surg* 1992;15:73–82.
3. Stanley JC, Messina LM. Renal revascularization for pulmonary edema in patients with poorly controlled renovascular hypertension and renal insufficiencey. In: Ueith FJ, ed. *Current Critical Problems in Vascular Surgery.* Volume 5. St. Louis: Quality Medical Publishing; 1994, pp.309–315.
4. Ying CY, Tifft CP, Gavras H, Chobanian AV. Renal revascularization in the azotemic hypertensive patient resistant to therapy. *N Engl J Med* 1984;311:1070–5.
5. Martinez-Maldonado M. Pathophysiology of renovascular hypertension. *Hypertension* 1991; A:707–19.
6. Palmer AH, Defeyter IR, Vandenbogaerde JF. Renal arterial stenosis as a cause of high output cardiac failure. *Int J Cardiol* 1989;22: 404–406.

7. Pickering TG. Renovascular hypertension: Etiology and pathology. *Sem Nucl Med* 1989;29:79–88.
8. Vensel LA, Devereux RB, Pickering TG, Herrold E McM, Borer JS, Laragh JM. Cardiac structure and function in renovascular hypertension produced by unilateral and bilateral renal artery stenosis. *Am J Cardiol* 1986;58:575–582.
9. deSimone G, Devereaux RB, Volpe M, Carnago MJF, Wallerson DC, Laragh JH. Relation of left ventricular hypertrophy, afterload, and contractility to left ventricular performance in Goldblatt hypertension. *Am J Hypertens* 1992;5:592–301.
10. Gaasch WH. Diastolic dysfunction of the left ventricle: Importance to the clinician. *Adv Int Med* 1990;35:311–40.
11. Stanley JC, Whitehouse WM Jr, Graham LM, Cronenwett JL, Zelenock GB, Lindenauer SM. Operative therapy of renovascular hypertension. *Br J Surg* 1982;69(Suppl):S63–S66.
12. Hansen KJ, Ditesheim JA, Metropol SH, Canzanello V, Graves J, Plonk GW Jr, Craven T, Dean RH. Management of renovascular hypertension in the elderly population. *J Vasc Surg* 1989;10:266–273.
13. Hansen KJ, Starr SM, Sands RE, Burkart JM, Plonk GW Jr, Dean RH. Contemporary surgical management of renovascular disease. *J Vasc Surg* 1992;16:319–331.
14. Libertino JA, Flam TA, Zinman LN, Ying CY, Breslin DJ, Swinton NW, Phelps MD, Tsapatsaris NP, Woods BO. Changing concepts in surgical management of renovascular hypertension. *Arch Intern Med* 1988;148:357–9.

13

Simultaneous Aortic Reconstruction and Renal Artery Revascularization

Richard P. Cambria

Clinical reports that detail patients treated with combined aortic and renal artery reconstruction contain a heterogeneous group of patients. Patient material is culled from two principle types of reports, namely those that detail experience with the combined operation from the standpoint of the procedure itself, and those that report experience primarily from the perspective of treatment of renovascular disease. These patients may present primarily for treatment of their renovascular disease, or their aortic lesion, and the renal artery reconstructions are not necessarily performed because of occlusive renal artery disease, but may be performed in the context of anatomic necessity during aortic surgery. In current practice combined procedures are being performed more frequently, irrespective of the demonstration of physiologic significance of the renovascular lesion. Factors contributing to this trend include an ever increasing safety of complex aortic reconstructions, the demonstrated durability of renal artery reconstruction,[1] and an increasing awareness of the role of renovascular disease in the development of chronic renal insufficiency.[2] In a review of contemporary series of large numbers of aortic reconstructions published over the last decade representing over 8,500 patients, some 5.7% of patients underwent combined procedures (range 2.1–18.7).[3] In the author's personal experience over the past five years, some 259 abdominal aortic reconstructions were carried out (80% for abdominal aortic aneurysms) and 12.3% of these procedures included a concomitant renal artery reconstruction. During the same interval, 50% of our total renal artery reconstructions were performed simultaneously with an aortic graft. As displayed in **Table 13–1,** data gathered from 15 representative series reported since 1980 indicates that a mean of 8.6% (range 3.2–18.5) of aortic grafts were supplemented by a renal artery reconstruction.

Table 13–1. Cumulative Experience with Combined Aortic and Renal Artery Grafting

Author	Number of Patients	AAA:AIOD	% of Aortic Surgery	Renal Graft Prophylactic (%)*	Renal Artery Surgery (%)			Early Failure (%)	Late Failure (%)	Operative Mortality (%)	5-Year Survival (%)
					Bilat	Endart	Bypass				
Branchereau (3) 1992	48	1:1.4	4.7	30	20	9	79	7	11	2	72
Chaikof (20) 1994	50	1.6:1	NA	0	40	2	98	NA	6	2	61
Cambria (1) 1994	129	2.9:1	12.2	6	9	10	90	2	7	8.5	71
Allen (13) 1993	102	1.5:1	8.2	31	14	12	55	NA	NA	4.9	77
Atnip (21) 1990	29	1.9:1	7.0	27	27	0	97	0	0	10.3	48
Stoney (16) 1989	44	1:1	NA	20	61	100	0	4†	2.7	4	NA
Tarazi (22) 1987	89	1.7:1	5	10	18	0	100	2.8	5.7	10	65
O'Mara (23) 1988	32	1:2.5	7	18	100	6	94	1.5	NA	3	60§
Stewart (25) 1985	63	1.2:1	9	8	46	0	100	1	3	3	NA
Sterpetti (26) 1984	39	NA	4.4	7.6	36	62	38	NA	NA	10	NA
Dean (27) 1984	50	1.4:1	18.5	0	18	10	80	NA	NA	12	NA
Stoney (4) 1984	90	1:1.6	16	11	53	67	33	NA	NA	9	89§
Shahian (28) 1980	39	1.3:1	3.2	7.6	15	0	97	NA	NA	10	74§
Kessler (29) 1984	102	2.2:1	NA	12	16	2	81	NA	NA	4	NA
Perry (30) 1984	60	2.3:1	NA	NA	5	8	74	6	9	5	NA
Totals Mean (Range)	966	1.3:1	8.6	13.4 (0–31)	24 (5–60)	19‡	72‡	4.0	—	6.5 (2–12)	68.5

* "Prophylactic" graft performed without hypertension or azotemia.
† 1/25 patients with routine post-op angio.
‡ Among series where both endarterectomy and bypass grafting used. Reimplantations excluded.
§ follow up 3–4 years.
NA = not available.

From a practical standpoint, the decision to proceed with a combined procedure may not be straightforward. Most would agree that a patient with a large aneurysm and a high-grade stenosis to a single functioning kidney would be best treated with a combined procedure. Alternatively, an octogenarian presenting with a large aneurysm and incidentally discovered to have a high-grade unilateral renal artery stenosis, normal serum creatinine, and no significant hypertension would appear to illustrate a circumstance where the renal artery lesion is best left alone. Clearly, between these two extremes is a wide spectrum of clinical scenarios wherein the following variables will enter into the decision-making relative to a combined procedure: 1. The indication for the aortic reconstruction i.e. absolute or relative. 2. The presence and severity of associated hypertension and the data providing either circumstantial, or definitive data that the renal artery lesion is functionally significant. 3. The level, if any, of renal insufficiency and the hope for reversal and/or stabilization of renal function by repair of the renal artery lesion. 4. Age, life expectancy, and associated comorbidity of the patient under consideration. 5. Surgical expertise and results with a variety of renal artery reconstructive techniques. Considering these clinical factors, the most common dilemma facing the vascular surgeon is when to proceed with a combined procedure for an incidentally discovered renal artery lesion in a patient presenting primarily for treatment of aortic pathology. Conversely, associated aortic atherosclerosis and/or aneurysm is frequently encountered in patients who present for treatment of renovascular disease and in some circumstances concomitant aortic reconstruction may be indicated to facilitate a site of inflow for the renal artery reconstruction. A review of the pertinent literature indicates that there is no consensus on either of these frequently encountered clinical scenarios, in particular the role of a “prophylactic” renal artery reconstruction in the case of an incidentally discovered and clinically silent renal artery stenosis during evaluation for aortic pathology. Those who emphasize a conservative posture to such patients cite the increased surgical risk of a combined reconstruction compared to either procedure performed independently. At the other end of the spectrum are those who advocate an aggressive posture toward the incidentally discovered renal artery lesion, emphasizing that current surgical results are favorable and the available natural history data of high-grade renal artery stenosis compares poorly with the expected durability of a renovascular reconstruction. Enthusiasm for extending this approach to all incidentally discovered renal artery lesions is tempered by a lack of natural history data for both patient and lesion in the circumstance where a clinically silent renal artery stenosis is found. Furthermore, multiple series including our own (1) appear to demonstrate that there is increased operative risk of the combined operation compared with isolated aortic reconstruction. In our experience during the interval 1976–91 with 129 patients, we found an impressive 8% mortality for the combined procedure. It is true that this operative mortality was both excessive when compared to that for isolated aortic reconstruction carried out over this time interval, and that such a mortality figure is neither acceptable in, nor representative of current practice. In the author's opinion comparison of surgical risk for the combined operation as opposed to isolated aortic reconstruction may be irrelevant. The reason for this consideration is the fact that patients treated with the combined operation have more diffuse atherosclerosis, more renal insufficiency, and in our experience more coronary artery disease when compared with a clinical risk file of patients treated with isolated aortic reconstruction.

PATIENT SELECTION FOR COMBINED PROCEDURES

Focusing for the moment on the patient who presents primarily for treatment of renovascular disease with either severe hypertension and/or renal insufficiency, it may occasionally be necessary to proceed with a combined procedure to afford an appropriate inflow site for an aorto-renal bypass graft. Our experience in patients with atherosclerotic renal artery lesions is that associated aortic atherosclerosis is the rule rather than the exception, and because of difficulty with originating a bypass from a heavily diseased aorta, we prefer to use alternate methods of renal artery reconstruction such as hepatorenal and splenorenal bypasses or transaortic endarterectomy in such circumstances.[1] However, associated stenotic disease of the celiac axis will preclude using its branches as a source of arterial inflow. In addition, these patients will occasionally have aortic pathology that would require repair on its own merits and in such circumstances we would proceed with a combined procedure. As a general rule, we avoid aortic replacement for the sole purpose of originating an aorto-renal bypass graft because of the availability of alternate methods of renal artery reconstruction as noted above, and the wish to limit the scope of surgery in these often poor risk patients. Although some have advocated prophylactic treatment of aortic atherosclerosis in this setting,[4] the available data mitigates against such a strategy. In my practice, the only anatomy wherein aortic grafting has been added for the patient presenting for renovascular surgery is the circumstance of infra-renal aortic occlusion.

The more commonly encountered scenario is that of the patient with anatomically significant renovascular disease discovered during evaluation for either abdominal aortic aneurysm or aorto-iliac occlusive disease. It is common knowledge that accessory and/or multiple renal arteries which may arise from the section of aorta where replacement is indicated can be seen in up to 25% of patients. An earlier report by Brewster et al from our institution indicated that nearly 25% of patients evaluated with routine preoperative arteriography before abdominal aortic aneurysm repair will be found to have significant renal artery pathology.[5] Olin et al studied nearly 400 patients with arteriography performed for either abdominal aortic aneurysm (AAA) or lower extremity occlusive disease and noted significant (>50%) renal artery stenosis in more than one third.[6] The detection of such renovascular pathology has been one rationale advanced for the routine evaluation of AAA patients with aortography. With respect to renovascular disease, several clinical and radiographic data point to the necessity for obtaining preoperative arteriography: 1. the suggestion of juxta-renal aneurysm anatomy on preoperative CT scan, 2. the detection of major asymmetry in kidney size indicating likely renal artery occlusion on preoperative CT scan, 3. clinically evident severe or recently accelerated hypertension, 4. preoperative azotemia in the absence of obvious renal parenchymal disease. Currently, contrast arteriography is required prior to making treatment decisions about renovascular lesions, although preliminary experience with magnetic resonance angiography suggests it may suffice for certain, as yet undefined, patients.

Is there any role for selective renal vein renin sampling at the time of arteriography in deciding the wisdom of renovascular repair? While a complete discussion of the value of functional studies relative to renovascular lesions is beyond the purview of this chapter, in the circumstance of surgical judgement as to the desirability of adding a concomitant renal artery reconstruction, renal vein renin information is seldom helpful. The single circumstance where I have found this of use is in the decision about whether to add a concomitant nephrectomy to an aortic reconstruction in the circumstance of a total renal artery occlusion and a small shriveled kidney. Impressively elevated renins in this circumstance would lead to a recommendation for nephrectomy.

The single most important variable with respect to the wisdom of proceeding with a combined procedure in a patient who would otherwise undergo an aortic resection is the paucity of our knowledge with respect to the natural history of such renovascular disease left untreated. Obviously, if a heretofore clinically quiescent renovascular lesion would remain so for the duration of the patient's lifetime a conservative posture would seem appropriate. Judgments about the wisdom of proceeding with a combined procedure are predicated upon knowledge of the natural history of both the lesion and the patient without repair of the renal artery stenosis. What information is available is generally obtained from

Table 13–2. Progression of Renal Artery Stenosis

Author	# Patients	Mode of Clinical Entry	Follow-up Months Mean (Range)	Progression of Lesion n (%)	Progression to Total Occlusion n (%)
Schreiber (9) 1984	85	RVH	52 (12–60)	37 (44)	14 (16)
Meaney (10) 1968	36	RVH	33 (6–84)	14 (39)	3 (8)
Wollenweber (11) 1968	30	RVH	28 (12–88)	21 (70)	NA
Dean (12) 1981	35	RVH	44 (6–102)	10 (29)	4 (11)
Tollefson (8)	27	AAA/AIOD	87 (15–276)	34 (71)	7 (15)
Zierler (7)	80	RAS SCREEN	12.7 (6–26)	7 (42)*	4 (11)†

* Those arteries with ≤ 60% @ start to ≥ 60%.
† Those > 60% at entry.
NA = not available; RVH = renovascular hypertension; RAS = renal artery stenosis; AIOD = aorto-iliac occlusive disease.

retrospective angiographic studies of highly selected patient groups. As summarized in **Table 13–2,** most of the earlier studies contained patients who were initially evaluated for hypertension with angiography, implying that many patients had, at the point of entry, functionally significant renovascular disease. Of the available studies, most have utilized serial contrast arteriography to assess renal artery disease progression except the recent report of Zierler et al wherein sequential duplex scanning was the imaging modality.[7] The study of Tollefson et al. is particularly germane to the subject of this chapter since it is the only available study where renal artery lesions were detected specifically during arteriography carried out for evaluation of aortic pathology.[8] These investigators studied 27 patients who had two or more arteriograms performed at a mean interval of 4.5 years between studies and with a clinical follow-up that averaged over 7 years. Despite the fact that the indications for patient entry were different than the earlier studies (aortic disease versus evaluation of renovascular hypertension) the data with respect to lesion progression was at the upper range of the reported earlier studies. The risk of progression to occlusion is remarkably similar to the range reported in the earlier studies **(Table 13–2)**. These investigators emphasized that most arteries which proceeded to occlusion harbored high-grade stenoses (~80%) at the time of initial evaluation, and that progression to occlusion was not necessarily accompanied by deterioration in renal function. Therefore, clinical parameters alone are unreliable in following high-grade renal artery lesions if the intent is to intervene prior to progression to total occlusion. Tollefson and Ernst cautiously recommended concomitant repair of high-grade renal artery lesions, particularly in patients with bilateral disease, at the time of indicated aortic surgery. The earlier studies summarized in **Table 2** emphasized the genuine risk of lesion progression and the threat of progression to total occlusion. The carefully conducted report of Schreiber et al also emphasized that progression to occlusion was significantly correlated with high-grade lesions at the time of initial study.[9] Seventy percent of patients with lesions of less than 50% stenosis showed no evidence of progression on follow-up study. This study did correlate lesion progression as a marker of clinical deterioration. In patients with lesion progression, over 50% had an increase in serum creatinine or increasing difficulty with blood pressure control. Meaney et al. demonstrated that neither age, sex, nor history of smoking had any positive predictive value with respect to renal artery lesion progression.[10] Wollenweber et al. were the first to emphasize the overall cardiovascular risk noted in patients with clinically significant renal artery stenosis. These investigators noted a five year actuarial survival of 66% in their patients followed with renovascular disease and emphasized that this was distinctly inferior to an age matched normal patient population.[11] Our own recently reported data detailed an actuarial five year survival of 75% in patients with surgically treated renovascular disease, suggesting that intervention for renovascular disease has a favorable effect on patient longevity. Similar to the report of Wollenweber et al., we also identified poor blood pressure control as a predictor of inferior long-term survival.[1] The only available data in the form of a randomized prospective study was reported by Dean and colleagues in 1981. They detailed the clinical course of 35 patients followed after initial randomization to medical therapy for angiographically documented renovascular hypertension. In addition to detailing lesion progression as outlined in **Table 13–2,** these investigators noted that nearly 50% of their patients followed on medical therapy had deterioration of renal function irrespective of the ability of medical therapy to control blood pressure.[12] The recently available report of Zierler and colleagues from the University of Washington detailed natural history data on 80 patients referred with either hypertension or renal insufficiency with a mean follow-up of one year. While disease progression was nil in initially normal arteries, the cumulative incidence of progression from $<60\%$ to $\geq 60\%$ renal artery stenosis was $42 \pm 14\%$ at 2 years. For arteries initially noted to have $\geq 60\%$ stenosis, the rate of progression to occlusion at 2 years was $11 \pm 6\%$. Disease progression was accompanied by poor control of diastolic blood pressure.[7]

From the available natural history information concerning renovascular disease, the following conclusions are justified: 1. Lesion progression and accompanying clinical deterioration is common in patients with high-grade ($\geq 80\%$ stenosis) renal artery lesions. 2. Following clinical parameters of blood pressure control and serum creatinine are unreliable predictors of renal artery lesion progression prior to occlusion, at least in part related to the functional status of the contralateral kidney. Clinical deterioration frequently will represent progression to total renal artery occlusion at which point some irreversible loss of functioning renal parenchyma has likely already occurred. 3. The natural history (i.e., durability) of a well-performed renal artery reconstruction compares favorably with the natural history of untreated high-grade renal artery stenosis. Displayed in **Figure 13–1** are life table patency data for our series of 140 aorto-renal bypass grafts performed with concomitant aortic grafting. Cumulative primary 5-year patency is nearly 90% and early perioperative failure occurred in just 2.1% of these reconstructions.[1] The interdependent variables that are considered in deciding the wisdom of a combined aorto-renal reconstruction include the functional significance, if any, of the renovascular lesion, the age, life expectancy, and associated comorbid factors present in the patient, the presence of unilateral versus bilateral disease, the presence or absence of renal insufficiency, and the severity of the lesion. Patients pre-

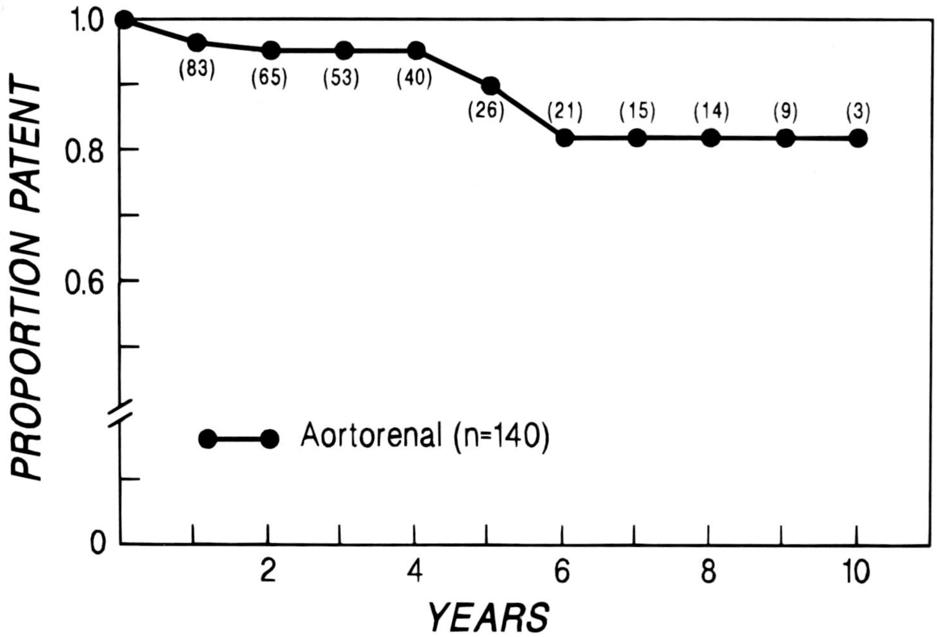

Figure 13–1. Life table graph demonstrating primary patency for 140 aortorenal bypasses performed in conjunction with a Dacron aortic graft during the interval 1976–91.

senting themselves for aortic surgery and in whom functionally significant renovascular lesions are discovered, should have a combined repair which may consist of a unilateral or bilateral reconstruction and/or a reconstruction and contralateral nephrectomy. As discussed in certain circumstances, patients with bilateral disease may be treated with a staged approach consisting of an initial unilateral renal artery reconstruction followed by subsequent aortic graft and contralateral renal artery reconstruction. In patients with high-grade renal artery stenosis who require aortic surgery but in whom the renal artery lesion is clinically silent, a combined procedure is entertained in accordance with a consideration of the variables noted above. After such consideration, current practice in our unit is consistent with that recently, albeit cautiously, advocated by others in favor of prophylactic renal artery reconstruction.[7,8,13] Simply stated, the current safety and demonstrated durability of adding a renal artery graft at the time of aortic surgery compares favorably with available natural history data for high-grade renal artery stenoses.

TECHNICAL CONSIDERATIONS

The reconstructive options available to the surgeon for renal artery repair are numerous. Many of the technical considerations that pertain to judgment in isolated renal artery reconstruction also pertain in the circumstance of combined procedures, with the exception, of course, of extra-anatomic bypass routes. The anatomic factors which mitigate on the decision as to which technique of reconstruction to use include the anatomy of the renal artery lesion itself including stenosis versus occlusion, and ostial as opposed to more distal renal artery stenosis, the proximal extent of the associated aortic lesion, which influences the position of cross-clamp placement, the presence of associated and/or clinically important mesenteric artery occlusive disease, and the elemental concern of whether a single or bilateral renal artery reconstruction is contemplated. In the circumstance of the totally occluded renal artery, reconstruction is often feasible and may retrieve an element of renal function depending on the status of the kidney subtended by the totally occluded artery. The single most important variable which indicates the feasibility of renal artery reconstruction is reconstitution of the main renal artery via collaterals on the delayed films of the diagnostic arteriogram.[14] Reconstruction of totally occluded renal arteries can provide important renal function salvage in certain patients and in our own experience some 16% of reconstructed renal arteries were found to be totally occluded at the time of diagnostic arteriography. Obviously, the extent to which the surgeon is willing to attempt revascularization of such compromised kidneys is influenced strongly by the overall level of renal function and the status of the contralateral kidney.

In the patient who is a candidate for a simultaneous aortic and bilateral renal artery reconstruction, the availability of extra-anatomic renal artery reconstructions (e.g., hepatorenal and splenorenal bypass) offers the surgeon the option of a staged approach. In patients with advanced levels of renal insufficiency and bilateral renal artery stenosis, a staged approach involving an initial right hepatorenal bypass, followed by an aortic reconstruction and concomitant left aorto-renal bypass has proven to be a convenient expedient.[15] In utilizing this method, the surgeon will limit the obligatory period of ischemic ATN to a single kidney at any one setting. In addition, atherosclerotic stenoses which extends a considerable distance in the right renal artery may present a technically challenging problem from an anterior approach because of the necessity of working on both sides of the root of the mesentery and inferior vena cava. It is worthwhile to note that in current practice, surgical techniques and overall operative safety have been sufficiently refined that the staged approach is only occasionally applied in patients with extreme renal insufficiency and/or those with special technical considerations which would indicate that a very distal bypass out onto the right renal artery would be required.

The general available to the surgeon for combined aortic and renal grafting are endarterectomy or bypass grafting. By far, the overwhelming majority of these procedures are aorto-renal bypass grafts performed with a side-arm graft originating from the aortic graft. Our data **(Fig. 13–1)** have proven that this is an extremely durable type of reconstruction. Furthermore, as shown in **Figure 13–2,** it is the most commonly employed technique for renal artery reconstruction in our practice. Several conduits have been used to perform this reconstruction but we could demonstrate no superiority for autogenous vein compared to prosthetic conduits, in particular Dacron. In our practice, a 6 mm Dacron side-arm graft is the most frequently used conduit, although there is no data nor reason to suspect that this is any better or worse than a PTFE prosthesis. Although we could not demonstrate a superiority for vein in this circumstance, my own preference is to use autogenous vein when particularly small and/or fragile renal arteries are encountered. This is largely for ease of workability rather than any conviction that it will afford superior long-term results. Presumably the high-flow within the renal arteries is the principal reason for excellent durability after a properly performed aorto-renal bypass graft. We have preferred an end-to-end anastomosis at the renal artery, believing that wide mobilization of the renal artery and deliberate end-to-end technique allows for a more precise reconstruction as compared to an end-to-side anastomosis on the renal artery. When the aortic lesion repaired is in the typical infra-

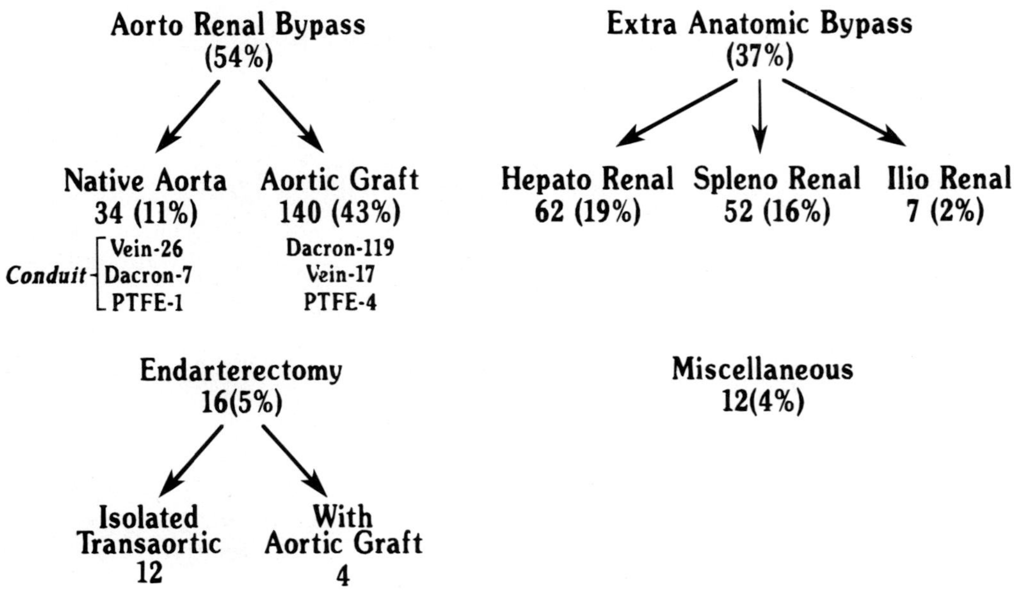

Figure 13–2. Reconstructive techniques used in 325 renal artery reconstructions in 285 patients during the interval 1976–91. Combined aortic and renal artery grafting was the most frequently used technique. (Reproduced with permission from Cambria et al.[1])

renal location and the clamp has always been infra-renal, the aortic reconstruction is generally completed first and as a final step in the procedure, the aorto-renal bypass is carried out. In circumstances where suprarenal or supraceliac clamping is necessary or when the aortic suture line itself is precariously close to a stenotic renal artery orifice, I prefer to perform the renal artery reconstruction immediately following the proximal aortic anastomosis.

Depending on individual patient anatomy, standard infra-mesocolic aortic exposure generally affords adequate exposure to sufficient length of renal artery to perform aorto-renal bypass grafting, particularly on the left side. We use a self-retaining retractor system during abdominal aortic surgery. In circumstances where large and/or juxta-renal aneurysms are encountered or when transaortic endarterectomy is contemplated (either isolated or in conjunction with an aortic graft), I prefer the so-called right-sided medial visceral rotation maneuver wherein the entire right colon is mobilized and the intestinal contents reflected up on to the patient's chest. As displayed in **Figure 13–3,** this converts the axis of orientation of the superior mesenteric artery from a 45° angle oriented toward the patient's right lower quadrant to a direct 90° perpendicular axis from the aorta. Deliberate sharp dissection of

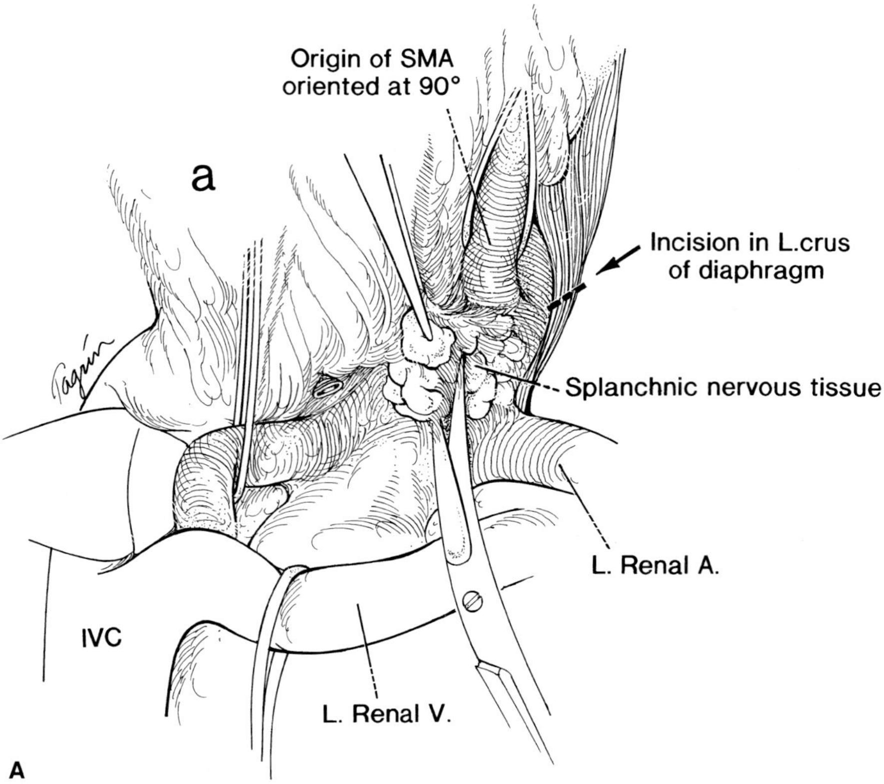
Origin of SMA
oriented at 90°
a
Incision in L.crus
of diaphragm
Splanchnic nervous tissue
L. Renal A.
IVC
L. Renal V.

A

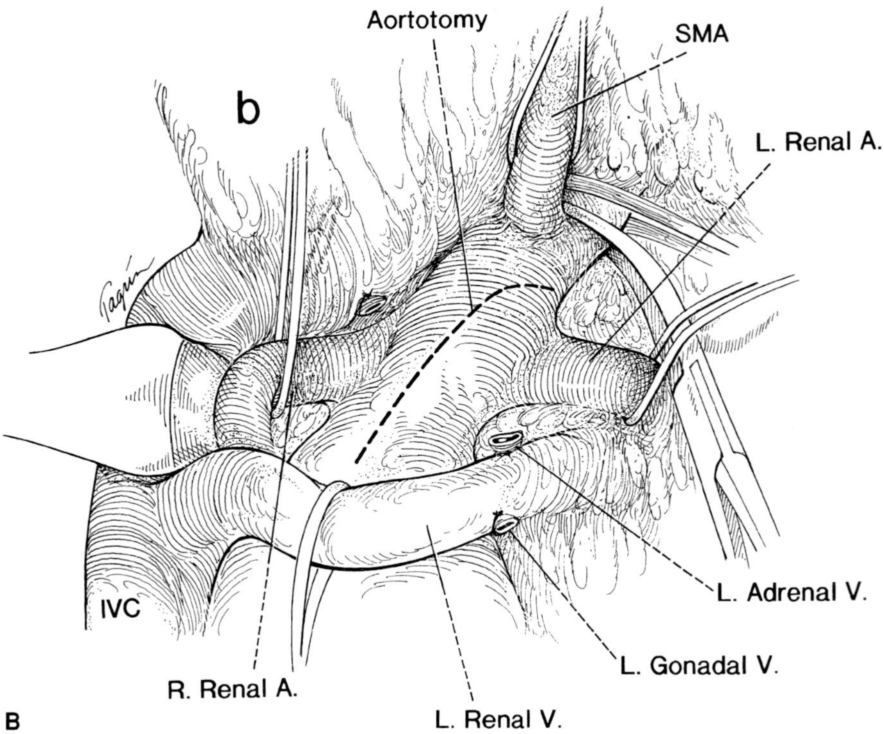
Aortotomy
SMA
b
L. Renal A.
IVC
L. Adrenal V.
L. Gonadal V.
R. Renal A.
L. Renal V.

B

the splanchnic ganglion and other densely adherent neural tissue at the origin of the superior mesenteric artery on the aorta will allow for circumferential dissection of the aorta and cross-clamping above the level of the superior mesenteric artery. This is required in the circumstance where transaortic endarterectomy is applied as there will frequently not be sufficient length between the origins of the superior mesenteric and renal arteries to comfortably accomplish this maneuver. The posterior aspects of the aorta at this level are deliberately exposed by incising the limbs of the diaphragmatic crura which is also necessary to control lumbar arteries in the region of the aortic cuff while the transaortic endarterectomy is carried out. Division of the left renal vein is avoided in virtually all circumstances, but the vein is widely mobilized by ligation of the adrenal and gonadal veins. Retraction of the inferior vena cava and/or working on both sides of the cava is easily accomplished in this exposure, although it is often necessary to divide lumbar veins on the posterior aspect of the cava. Aorto-renal bypass on the right side can generally be placed in an anatomic retrocaval position, particularly since the disease process is usually limited to the proximal main renal artery. However, in certain circumstances with disease extending far out into the right renal artery, working on both sides of the inferior vena cava and positioning the aorto-renal bypass anterior to the vena cava is acceptable. On the left side, the aorto-renal bypass is positioned posterior to the left renal vein.

The choice between endarterectomy and/or bypass graft to reconstruct the renal arteries is largely dictated by the anatomy of the lesion (lesions) and whether or not unilateral or bilateral reconstruction is carried out. When the aortic reconstruction is in a typical infra-renal location and a unilateral reconstruction is required, most surgeons would utilize a direct aorto-renal bypass graft and I would concur with this position. In the circumstance of bilateral simultaneous renal artery reconstruction combined with an aortic graft, consideration for endarterectomy is appropriate particularly when the renal artery lesions are limited to the aortic ostia or the very proximal renal arteries. In this circumstance, bilateral simultaneous endarterectomy can be accomplished with the exposure outlined in **Figure 13–3** with a renal ischemic time generally less than would be required for bilateral aorto-renal bypass grafts. Endarterectomy can be accomplished either by a transaortic route, requiring a longitudinal aortotomy

Figure 13–3. Surgical exposure for transaortic bilateral renal artery endarterectomy after right-sided medial visceral rotation maneuver. Dissection of the splanchnic nervous tissue anteriorly at the origin of the SMA and the limbs of the diaphragmatic crura posteriorly permit clamping above the SMA.

which is then carried laterally to either side of the aorta in a hockey stick fashion. Division of the aortic plaque posteriorly as the initial step will facilitate traction on the aortic plug augmented by eversion of the renal artery which has been circumferentially dissected for a considerable distance. Following clearing of the renal artery ostia, a 12 French irrigation catheter for installation of renal preservation solution is inserted into the renal arteries. Closure of the aortotomy is accomplished with running 4/0 monofilament suture and the now endarterectomized infra-renal aortic cuff can be cross-clamped with a soft-jawed clamp in order to allow restoration of renal artery perfusion. The infra-renal graft is then sewn in to the endarterectomized aortic cuff in the usual fashion. A second technique for aortic cuff endarterectomy uses an eversion method through the transected aortic stump as described by Stoney et al.[16]

These techniques all imply midline transperitoneal exposure for the aortic surgery. Use of a posterolateral retroperitoneal approach may be preferred by some surgeons for a majority of their aortic reconstruction, and in my own practice, I prefer this approach in certain circumstances of pararenal or suprarenal abdominal aortic aneurysms. Since the left kidney is elevated out of its bed in this exposure and the origin of the left renal artery on the aorta is an important landmark in this procedure, reconstruction of the left renal artery with a supplemental aorto-renal bypass is straightforward and simple with this exposure. Reconstructive options for the right renal artery from this approach are limited to orifice endarterectomy. In circumstances where multiple visceral vessel endarterectomy via a "trap-door" incision in the visceral aorta is required, the posterolateral retroperitoneal or a more proximal thoraco-abdominal approach is also preferred. Use of this anatomic exposure for certain complicated types of aneurysms has been championed by Williams and others.[17] I prefer this retroperitoneal approach if the aortic graft needs to be extended to the suprarenal aorta.

EXPERIENCE WITH COMBINED AORTIC AND RENAL GRAFTING

After considering surgical judgment and technical considerations as to when to apply the combined operation, a review of reported experience with the combined operation is appropriate. Summarized in **Table 13–1** are the major clinical series of the combined operation reported over the past decade. Only reports containing more than twenty-five patients and containing sufficient data on patients with a combined operation are included. Other contemporary reports such as that of Hallett et al from the Mayo Clinic,[18] and that of Hansen et al,[19] contain sufficient numbers of patients treated with the combined operation but are excluded only because they contained insufficient data on patients who underwent the combined operation as a specific subgroup. In contemporary practice, renovascular reconstruction concerns primarily patients with atherosclerotic disease since most patients with fibromuscular disease are adequately treated with balloon angioplasty. In this patient population with acknowledged diffuse vascular disease, most contemporary series of renovascular reconstruction contain a high percentage of patients who undergo combined aortic and renal reconstruction. Indeed, in our own series this figure was 43%, similar to the recent report from Dean's group (41%), and that from the Mayo Clinic (56%).[18,19] Reports that focus on the technique of combined aortic and renal revascularization may contain considerable numbers of patients in whom the renal artery lesion is functionally insignificant **(Table 13–1)**. The reports summarized in **Table 13–1** representing experience with nearly 1000 patients who underwent the combined operation indicate that a mean of 13.5% of the renal artery reconstructions were carried out for "prophylactic" indications, that is in patients without hypertension or renal insufficiency. This in no way implies that all patients with hypertension had a renovascular etiology for their hypertension. There is clearly a trend towards increasing aggressiveness to the so-called clinically silent or functionally insignificant renal artery stenosis in the patient who requires an aortic graft. Based on the previous discussions with respect to the natural history of renal artery stenosis, this trend may be entirely appropriate in settings where surgical expertise is proven. As expected, the presenting aortic pathology in patients who undergo the combined operation is more often an abdominal aortic aneurysm, although there is wide variability in the ratio of aneurysm to occlusive disease patients treated. Our own experience with a nearly 3 to 1 ratio of aneurysm to occlusive disease patients is the highest found in a review of the contemporary literature. It appears that the combined operation generally constitutes less than 10% of abdominal aortic reconstruction in most centers.

Aorto-renal bypass graft is the most frequently applied technique of renal artery reconstruction in patients who undergo combined operations. Many of the centers whose experience is represented in **Table 13–1** employ bypass grafting exclusively with the exception of the recent report of Stoney et al, which details experience with a specific endarterectomy technique.[16] Despite this preference for aorto-renal bypass evident in the literature, endarterectomy is enjoying a resurgence of popularity as a renal artery reconstructive technique, particularly among surgeons with extensive experience in renal artery reconstruction. As noted previously, I prefer to utilize transaortic endarterectomy in circumstances where a bilateral simultaneous reconstruction is carried out if the renal artery lesions are either ostial or in the proximal renal artery. The range of incidence of bilateral reconstruction (contralateral nephrectomy not included) at the time of the combined procedure is explained both by differing patient variables and surgeon's preference. For example, the 40% of the patients reported by Chaikof et al underwent bilateral reconstructions, but their report focused on ischemic nephropathy and was limited to patients with a serum creatinine greater than 1.8.[20] Similarly, the reports of Stoney et al[4,16] where endarterectomy has always been championed will contain a higher percentage of patients who undergo bilateral reconstructions because the transaortic endarterectomy is in my view better suited to a bilateral rather than a unilateral type of reconstruction. Many patients with renovascular disease will have bilateral stenoses. In our reported series, fully 40% of patients who underwent renal artery reconstruction had bilateral disease of at least 50% stenosis. However, in light of the natural history information summarized above, we believe only those renal artery stenoses of truly high-grade significance (i.e., ≥80%) are worthy of reconstruction.

Perioperative failure of renal artery reconstruction carried out with a concomitant aortic graft is unusual being noted in just 2% of our patients who underwent the combined operation. The figures cited in **Table 13–1** must be considered a minimum because few series contain routine early surveillance of the reconstructions. Similarly, the late failures are generally available only for those series with long-term clinical follow-up. Most failures of aorto-renal reconstruction occur in the early postoperative period and are therefore technical in nature.

Most surgeons accept that the inherent risk of combined aorto-renal grafting is higher than either procedure performed independently. Increased surgical risk is the principal component cited against so-called prophylactic aorto-renal grafting at the time of indicated aortic surgery. The mean operative mortality for the 15 series summarized in **Table 13–1** is 6.5% (range 2–12%). This operative mortality is clearly higher than that reported in a number of contemporary series of isolated aortic surgery including our own. In our unit, 567 elective abdominal aortic aneurysm operations were carried out between 1989–93 with an operative mortality of 2.3%. Although representing a substantially longer time interval with operations performed as early as 1976, we recently reported an 8.5% mortality for the combined operation and the corresponding figures for isolated renal artery reconstruction was 4%. However, over the past five years, mortality for the combined operation has been in the 3% range in our unit. Similar data can be obtained in comparing longitudinal experience from other centers. The 1984 report of Dean et al **(Table 13–1)** noted a 12% mortality for the combined operation while in their more contemporary ex-

Table 13–3. Clinical Features of 129 Patients Requiring Combined Aortic and Renal Reconstruction

Feature	% of 129 Patients
Poorly controlled hypertension	43
Serum creatinine > 1.5 mg/dl	51
Serum creatinine > 3.0 mg/dl	9
Diabetes	16
Clinically evident coronary artery disease	54
Reconstruction to a single functioning kidney	19

perience the corresponding figure has been less than 3%.[19] In the author's opinion, much of the stated comparisons of operative mortality between isolated aortic and/or renal reconstruction are not valid because the patient groups are not comparable. Detailed in **Table 13–3** are certain clinical features of 129 patients who underwent the combined operation in our unit. By way of comparison the clinical risk profile in a recently reported series of 202 patients who underwent isolated aortic reconstruction on our service was decidedly benign. This was true not only for the incidence and extent of renal insufficiency but also for coexistent coronary artery disease.[24]

SUMMARY

Combined aortic and renal artery atherosclerotic lesions are commonly encountered in an active practice of vascular surgery. In circumstances where both lesions require repair on their own merits a combined operation is the best approach in most circumstances. The question of when to repair renal artery lesions which are discovered during the course of evaluating aortic pathology is a common issue of surgical judgment. The available natural history data concerning high-grade renal artery stenosis would suggest that concomitant repair of these lesions at the time of indicated aortic grafting is worthwhile if it can be accomplished safely.

REFERENCES

1. Cambria RP, et al. The durability of different reconstructive techniques for atherosclerotic renal artery disease. *J Vasc Surg* (in press).

2. Rimmer JM, Grennari FJ. Atherosclerotic renovascular disease and progressive renal failure. *Ann Intern Med* 1993;118:712–719.
3. Branchereau A, et al. Simultaneous reconstruction of infrarenal abdominal aorta and renal arteries. *Ann Vasc Surg* 1992;3:232–238.
4. Stoney RJ, Skioldebrand CG, Ovarfordt PG, Reilly LM, Ehrenfeld WK. Juxtarenal aortic atherosclerosis: surgical experience and functional result. *Ann Surg* 1984;200:345–354.
5. Brewster DC, Retana A, Waltman AC, Darling RC. Angiography in the management of aneurysms of the aorta. Its value and safety. *N Engl J Med* 1975;292:822–825.
6. Olin JM, Melia M, Young JR, Graor RA, Risius B. Prevalence of atherosclerotic renal artery stenosis in patients with atherosclerosis elsewhere. *Am J Med* 1990;88:46–51.
7. Zierler RE, Bergelin RO, Isaacson JA, Strandness DE. Natural History of atherosclerotic renal artery stenosis: a prospective study with duplex ultrasound. *J Vasc Surg* 1994;19:250–8.
8. Tollefson DF, Ernst CB. Natural history of atherosclerotic renal artery stenosis associated with aortic disease. *J Vasc Surg* 1991;14: 327–31.
9. Schreiber MJ, Pohl MA, Novick AC. The natural history of atherosclerotic and fibrous renal artery disease. *Urol Clin North Am* 1984;11: 383–92.
10. Meaney TF, Dustan HP, McCormack LJ. Natural history of renal artery disease. *Radiology* 1968;91:881–7.
11. Wollenweber J, Sheps SG, Davis GD. Clinical course of atherosclerotic renovascular disease. *Am J Cardiol* 1968;21:60–71.
12. Dean RH, et al. Renovascular hypertension: anatomic and renal function changes during drug therapy. *Arch Surg* 1981;116:1408–15.
13. Allen BT, Rubin BG, Anderson CB, et al. The simultaneous surgical management of aortic and renovascular disease. *Am J Surg* 1993; 166:726–33.
14. Dean RH, Lawson JD, Hollifield JW, et al. Revascularization of the poorly functioning kidney. *Surgery* 1979;85:44–52.
15. Brewster DC, Moncure AC. Hepatic and splenic artery for renal revascularization. In Bergan JJ and Yao TST, ed. Arterial surgery: New Diagnostic and operative techniques. New York: Grune and Stratton, Inc. 1988;389–405.
16. Stoney RJ, Messina LM, Goldstone J, Reilly LM. Renal endarterectomy through the transected aorta: a new technique for combined aortorenal atherosclerosis. *J Vasc Surg* 1989;9:224–33.
17. Williams GM, Ricotta J, Zinner M, Burdick J. The extended retroperitoneal approach for treatment of extensive atherosclerosis of the aorta and renal vessels. *Surgery* 1980;88:846–54.
18. Hallett JW Jr, Fowl R, O'Brien PC, Bernatz PE, Pairolero PC, Cherry KJ Jr, et al. Renovascular operation in patients with chronic renal insufficiency: do the benefits justify the risks? *J Vasc Surg* 1987;5: 622–7.
19. Hansen KJ, Star SM, Sands RE, Burkhart JM, Plonk GW, Dean RH.

Contemporary surgical management of renovascular disease. *J Vasc Surg* 1992;16:319–31.
20. Chaikof EL, Smith RB, Salam AA, Dodson TF, Lumsden AB, Kosinski AS, Coyle KA, Allen RC. Ischemic nephropathy and concomitant aortic disease: a 10-year study. *J Vasc Surg* 1994;19:135–48.
21. Atnip RG, Neumyer MM, Healy DA, Thiele BL. Combined aortic and visceral arterial reconstruction: risks and results. *J Vasc Surg* 1990; 12:705–15.
22. Tarazi RY, Hertzer NR, Beven EG, O'Hara PJ, Anton GE, Krajewski LP. Simultaneous aortic reconstruction and renal revascularization: Risk factors and late results in eighty-nine patients. *J Vasc Surg* 1987;5:707–14.
23. O'Mara CS, Maples MD, Kilgore TL. Simultaneous aortic reconstruction and bilateral renal revascularization. *J Vasc Surg* 1988;8: 357–66.
24. Cambria RP, Brewster DC, Abbott WM, et al. The impact of selective use of dipyridamole thallium scan and surgical factors on the current morbidity of aortic surgery. *J Vasc Surg* 1992;15:43–51.
25. Steward MT, Smith RB, Fulenwider JT, Perdue GD, Wells JO. Concomitant renal revascularization in patients undergoing aortic surgery. *J Vasc Surg* 1985;2:400–4005.
26. Sterpetti AV, Schultz RD, Feldhaus RJ, Peetz DJ. Aortic and renal atherosclerotic disease. *Surg Gynecol Obstet* 1986;163:54–59.
27. Dean RH, Keyser JE, Dupont WD, Nadeau JH, Meacham PW. Aortic and renal vascular disease: factors affecting the value of combined procedures. *Ann Surg* 1984;200:336–343.
28. Shahian DM, Najafi H, Javid H, Hunter JA, Goldin MD, Monson DO. Simultaneous aortic and renal artery reconstruction. *Arch Surg* 1980;115:1491–1497.
29. Kessler AR, Mulherin JL, Edwards WH. Combined aortic and renal arterial reconstruction. *South Med J* 1984;77:155–158.
30. Perry MO, Silane MF. Management of renovascular problems during aortic operations. *Arch Surg* 1984;119:681–685.

PART III

SURGICAL TECHNIQUE FOR RENOVASCULAR HYPERTENSION AND RENAL SALVAGE

14

Renal Revascularization: Overview of Surgical Technique and Exposure

Richard H. Dean

A variety of operative techniques have been advocated for treatment of renovascular disease. Principal among these methods are renal artery bypass, thromboendarterectomy, and renal artery reimplantation. Bypass techniques include direct aortorenal bypass with autogenous artery, saphenous vein or synthetic conduits and extra-anatomic bypasses using hepatorenal, splenorenal, ileorenal or even mesenteric renal bypasses. Currently, these latter extra-anatomic techniques are gaining broad popularity. Nevertheless, the preferential benefit or even comparative value of such procedures is yet unproven.

PREOPERATIVE PREPARATION

Antihypertensive medications are reduced during the preoperative period to the minimum necessary for blood pressure control. Frequently, patients requiring large doses of multiple medications for control will have significantly reduced requirements while hospitalized. If continued therapy is required, then α-methyldopa or vasodilators (e.g., Procardia) are the drugs of choice. There is little effect on hemodynamics when these agents are combined with anesthesia. We have also commonly continued low-dose propranolol therapy as well without any adverse effects. If the patient's diastolic blood pressure is 120 to 140 mm Hg, it is essential that the pressure be brought under control and that operative treatment be postponed until this is accomplished. Recently, if blood pressure has been difficult to control, we have transferred the patient to the intensive care unit, where intravenous nitroprusside therapy with continuous intraarterial monitoring of blood pressure is instituted for the 24 hours before operation. Similarly, if the patient has a significant history of heart disease, pulmonary artery wedge pressure and cardiac output are monitored to maintain optimal cardiac hemodynamics and recognize and correct adverse changes before they become clinically significant.

OPERATIVE TECHNIQUES

Certain measures are applicable in almost all renal arterial operations. Mannitol, 12.5 mg, is administered intravenously at least 10 min before renal crossclamping and heparin, 100 units/kg, is given intravenously. Occasionally, protamine is required for reversal of the heparin at the end of the reconstruction. Finally, accurate monitoring of blood loss and fluid replacement during the operation is mandatory, because episodes of hypotension are especially detrimental to renal function under these circumstances.

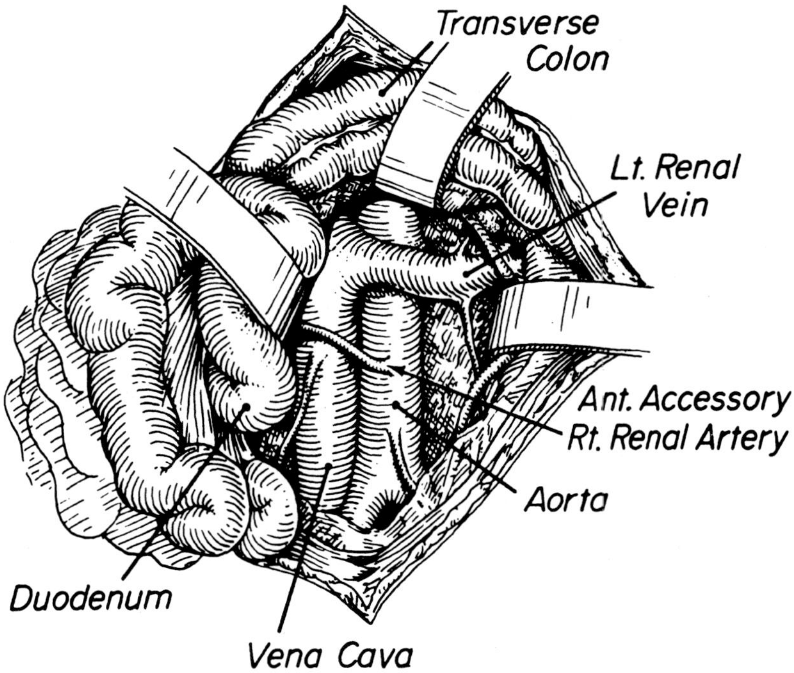

Figure 14–1. Exposure of the left renal hilum through the base of the mesentery. The adrenal, lumbar and gonadal veins must be ligated and divided to give adequate visualization of the renal artery. Note the anterior accessory right renal artery. This uncommon right lower pole artery traverses anterior to the vena cava and can easily be traumatized if its presence is not recognized.

Exposure

Adequate exposure is the most difficult but important aspect of renal artery surgery. A midline incision from the xiphoid to the pubic symphysis provides excellent access to either renal artery. This incision is carried to the side of the xiphoid process to gain an additional 3–4 cm of proximal exposure. To expose the left renal artery, the posterior peritoneum overlying the aorta is incised longitudinally and the duodenum is reflected to the patient's right. By extending the posterior peritoneal incision to the left along the inferior border of the pancreas, an avascular plane behind the pancreas can be entered. This allows excellent exposure

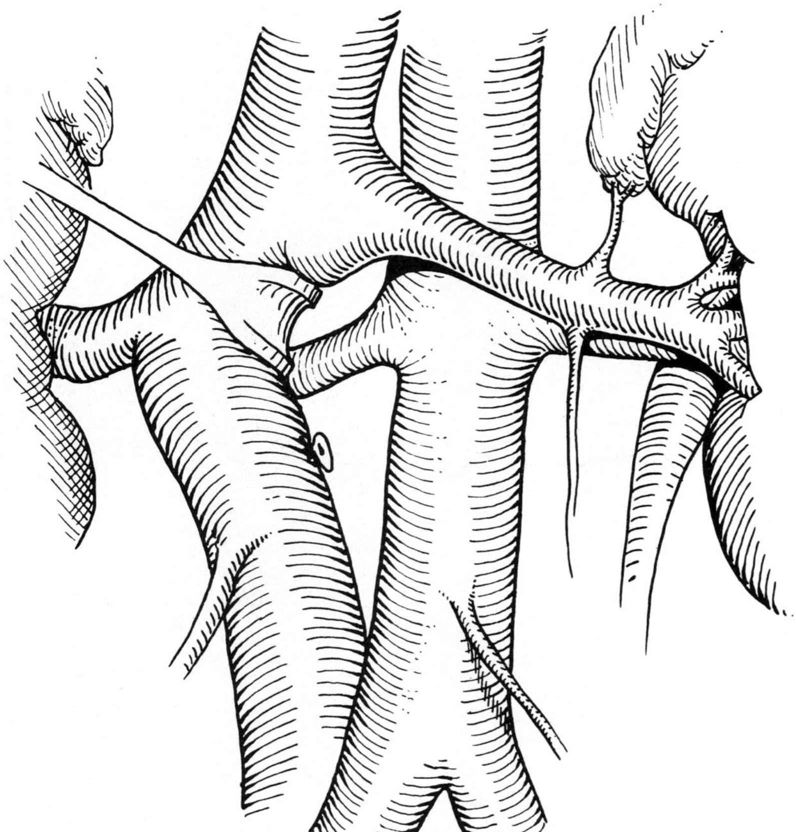

Figure 14–2. Exposure of the proximal right renal artery through the base of the mesentery. Two pairs of lumbar veins have been ligated and divided, and the vena cava is retracted to the right. Proximal right renal artery lesions can be visualized adequately through this approach.

of the entire renal hilum on the left and is of special significance when distal lesions are to be managed **(Fig. 14–1)**. The renal artery lies behind the left renal vein. In some cases it is easier to retract the vein cephalad to expose the artery. In others, caudal retraction of the vein provides better access.

The gonadal and adrenal veins which enter the left renal vein must be ligated and divided to facilitate exposure of the artery. Another frequent tributary is a lumbar vein that enters the posterior wall of the left renal vein and is easily avulsed unless special care is taken in mobilizing the renal vein. After dividing the left adrenal and gonadal veins, the entire length of the left renal artery can be visualized behind the renal vein.

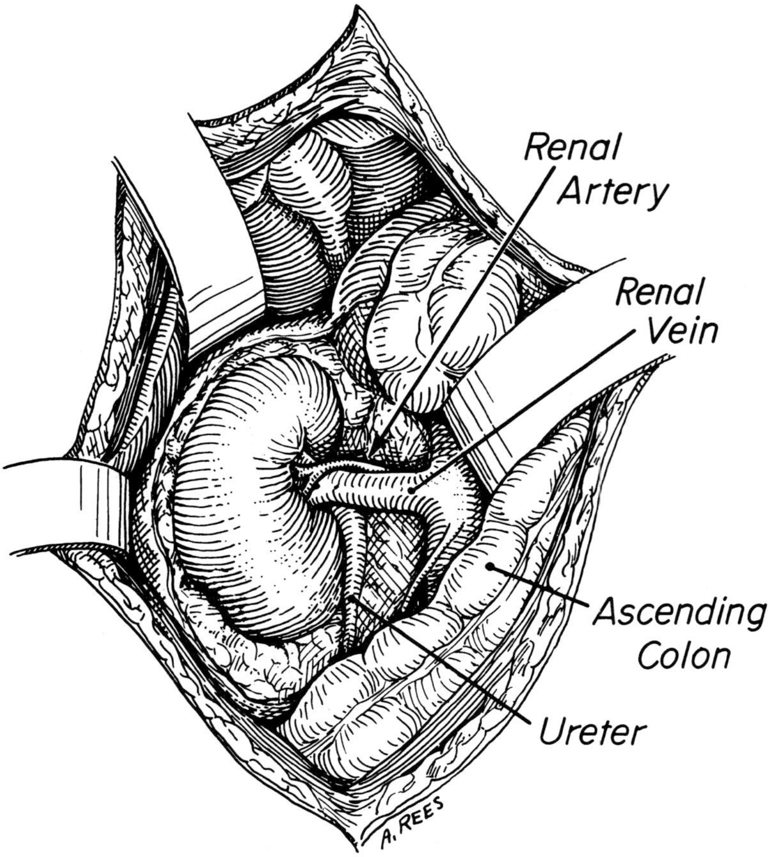

Figure 14–3. Exposure of the right renal artery following reflection of the duodenum and right colon to the left. The distal right renal artery and its branches are best visualized by this technique.

The proximal right renal artery can be exposed through the base of the mesentery by ligating two or more pairs of lumbar veins and retracting the vena cava to the patient's right and the left vein cephalad **(Fig. 14–2)**. The distal right renal artery is best exposed, however, by mobilizing the duodenum and right colon medially **(Fig. 14–3)**. The right renal vein is mobilized and is usually retracted cephalad to expose the artery.

When bilateral simultaneous procedures such as bilateral endarterectomies are performed we routinely mobilize the aorta to a level above the superior mesenteric artery for supramesenteric aorta crossclamping. Division of the diaphragmatic crura as they wrap around the aorta facilitates this exposure. Similarly, total

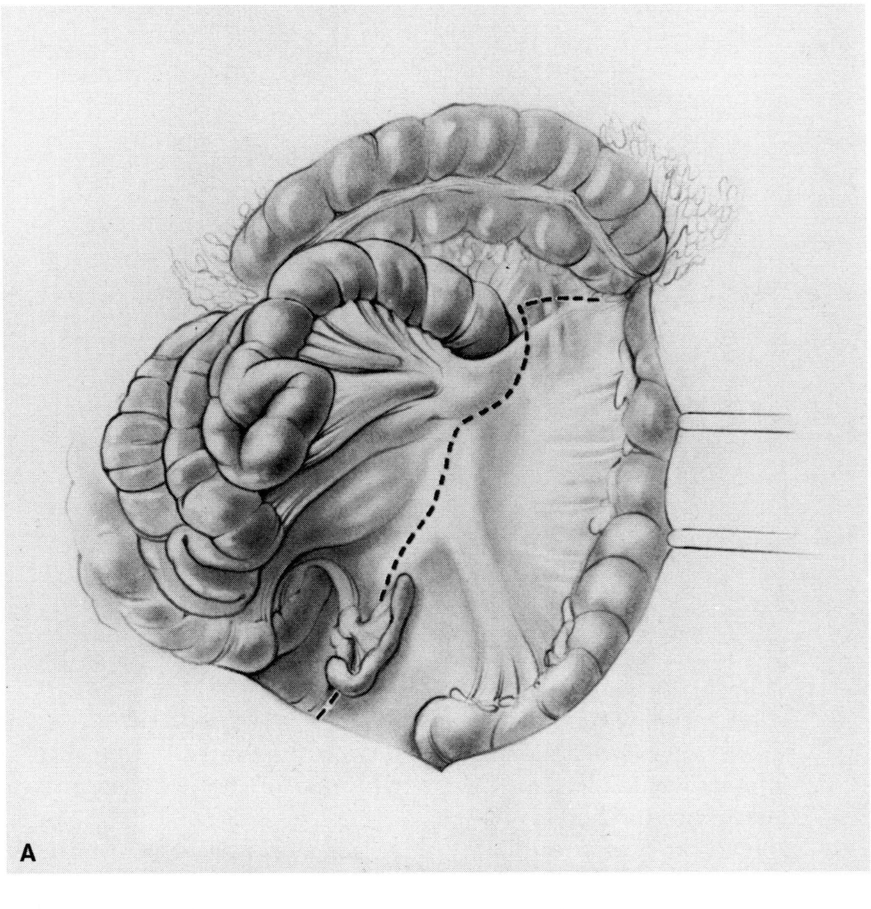

A

Figure 14–4. Drawing of incisions (A&B) and exposure (C) that is used for crossclamping above the superior mesenteric artery for bilateral renal artery endarterectomies.

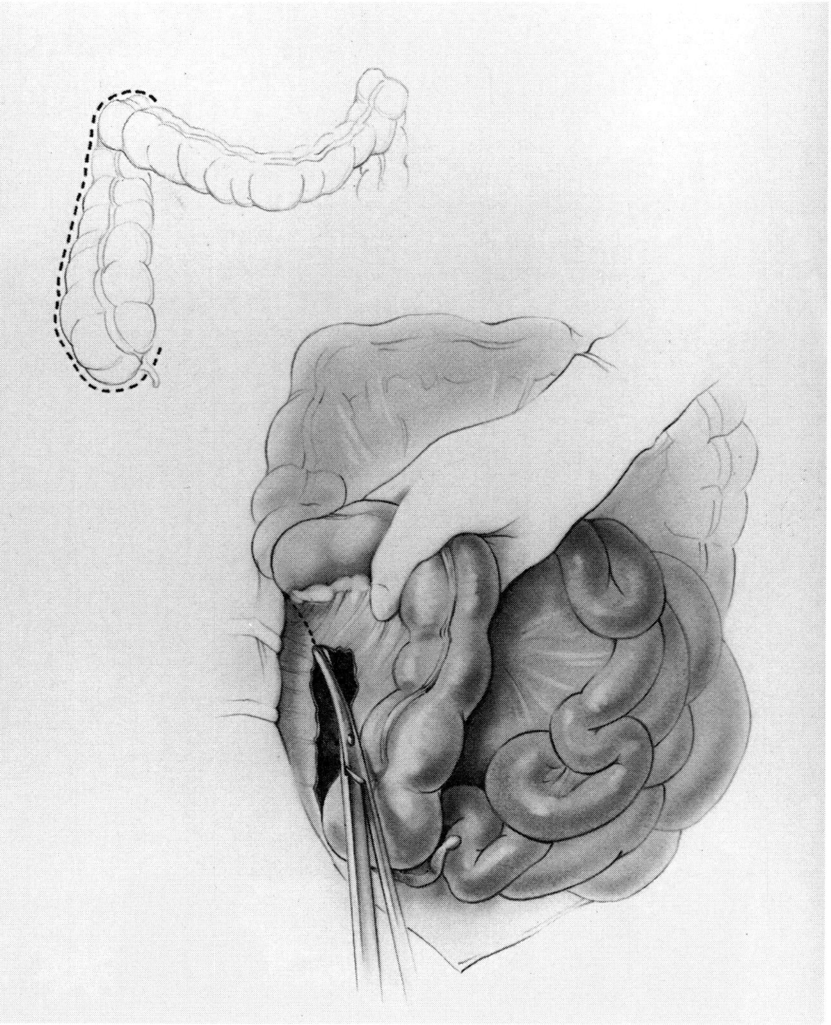

B

Figure 14–4. *(continued)*

mobilization of the right colon and small bowel with placement of these viscera onto the chest wall provides the wide exposure to enhance visualization of the entire area of the juxtamesenteric and juxtarenal aorta.

Incision begins at the base of the mesentery and continues around the cecum and up the right lateral mesocolon peritoneal reflection. Using this technique, the entire small bowel and right colon is eviscerated to expose the entire juxtarenal aorta and both renal arteries **(Fig. 14–4)**.

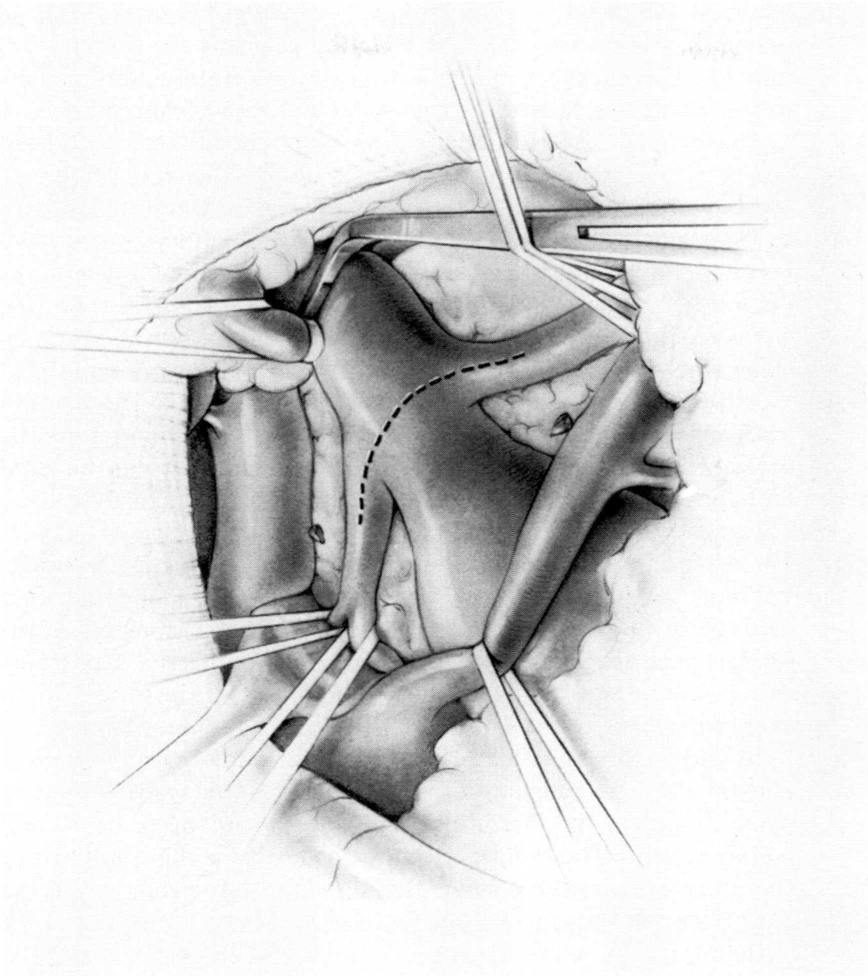

C

Figure 14–4. *(continued)*

AORTORENAL BYPASS

Technique

Three types of graft are usually available for aortorenal bypass: autogenous saphenous vein, autogenous hypogastric artery and synthetic prostheses. Arterial autografting using hypogastric artery has great theoretical appeal in that autogenous tissue is utilized which matches in size and consistency the affected renal arteries. Despite these advantages, however, the added risk of pelvic dissection and the fact that the hypogastric artery itself may be atherosclerotic or the source of important collateral flow to the intestines seem to mitigate against its widespread use.

Expanded polytetrafluoroethylene (6 mm in diameter) has been our preferred material when a synthetic prosthesis is preferred. We have found it to be technically superior to Dacron in regard to the ease of suturing to small vessels. Although long-term studies are not available to assess its durability, we believe it compares favorably to Dacron in this regard. Nevertheless, we have limited our use of such grafts to instances of proximal atherosclerotic lesions where the distal renal artery is large (4 mm in diameter).

Although circumstances may require the use of these other graft materials, autogenous saphenous vein has emerged as the preferred graft material donor in most centers. It can be used for bypass in atherosclerotic disease and fibromuscular dysplasia. The advantages of autogenicity and flexibility allow the use of very fine suture for direct anastomosis to branch vessels, if necessary. Further, the procurement of a short segment of saphenous vein through a separate groin incision adds little to either operative time or post operative morbidity. Nevertheless, if the saphenous vein is small (less than 4 mm in diameter) or if it has been previously sacrificed, other sources of graft material must be used.

In end-to-side renal artery bypass, the renal artery-vein graft anastomosis should be performed first. Since this is generally the most difficult anastomosis, it is much easier if the graft is completely mobile. The length of the arteriotomy in the renal artery should be at least three times the diameter of the renal artery to guard against late suture line stenosis.

Before the anastomosis is created, each of the branches of the renal artery is gauged with renal artery dilators. Since branch stenosis in patients with fibromuscular dysplasia may be missed on angiography, this maneuver may be diagnostic as well as therapeutic. A 6/0 or 7/0 monofilament polypropylene (Prolene) suture material is employed with loop magnification. A continuous suture line is used to allow the greatest exposure for the placement of sutures at the distal end of the arteriotomy. Greatest emphasis is placed on the placement of these four or five sutures. If these are placed deeply or with an inappropriate advancement, a stenotic outflow for the graft is created and there is the risk of later graft thrombosis.

After the renal artery anastomosis is complete, heparinized saline is injected and the suture line is checked for leaks. The occluding clamps and slings are then removed from the renal artery and an atraumatic small bulldog clamp is placed across the vein graft adjacent to the anastomosis. The aortic anastomosis is then performed.

The aorta is cross-clamped below the renal arteries and a wedge of aortic wall is excised to create a large orifice for the vein graft. This is especially important if the aorta is thickened or calcified by extensive atherosclerosis. Again, the anastomotic diameter should be at least three times the vein graft diameter to prevent later suture line stenosis and subsequent thrombosis. The graft is usually brought behind the renal vein on the left and behind the vena cava on the right. However, there are instances in which the anatomy of the renal arteries is such that a course anterior to the left renal vein or to the vena cava on the right seems more appropriate.

In contrast to the end-to-side bypass technique, we usually first construct the proximal (aortic) anastomosis when performing an end-to-end renal artery bypass. After the proximal anastomosis is completed the renal artery is ligated proximally and transected. The renal artery and graft are then spatulated to provide an anastomotic diameter at least three times the diameter of the renal artery. Again, a continuous suture line using 6/0 or 7/0 monofilament polypropylene is employed for this anastomosis.

THROMBOENDARTERECTOMY

In some cases of bilateral atherosclerotic occlusions of the renal artery origins, simultaneous bilateral endarterectomy may be the most applicable procedure. Although transaortic endarterectomy is used with increasing frequency we most commonly employ a transverse incision in most instances. This arteriotomy is carried across the aorta and along the renal artery to a point beyond the stenosis **(Fig. 14–5)**. With this method, the distal intima can be assessed directly and tacked down with mattress sutures under direct vision if necessary. Following completion of the endarterectomy, the arteriotomy is closed. In most patients this closure is performed with a vein patch to ensure that the proximal renal artery is left widely patent.

We use transaortic endarterectomy in patients with multiple renal arteries that are involved with orificial stenoses. In this instance we will proceed with a longitudinal aortotomy and endarterectomy of the aorta and renal arteries. We also use this technique in patients who also require simultaneous aortic graft replacement. In this circumstance the endarterectomy is done through the transected aorta. In both of these instances it is important to have adequate mobilization of the renal arteries to allow eversion of the vessel into the aorta to visualize the distal component of the renal artery endarterectomy. Duplex ultrasonography is used to examine the end point after completion of the endarterectomy in all patients.

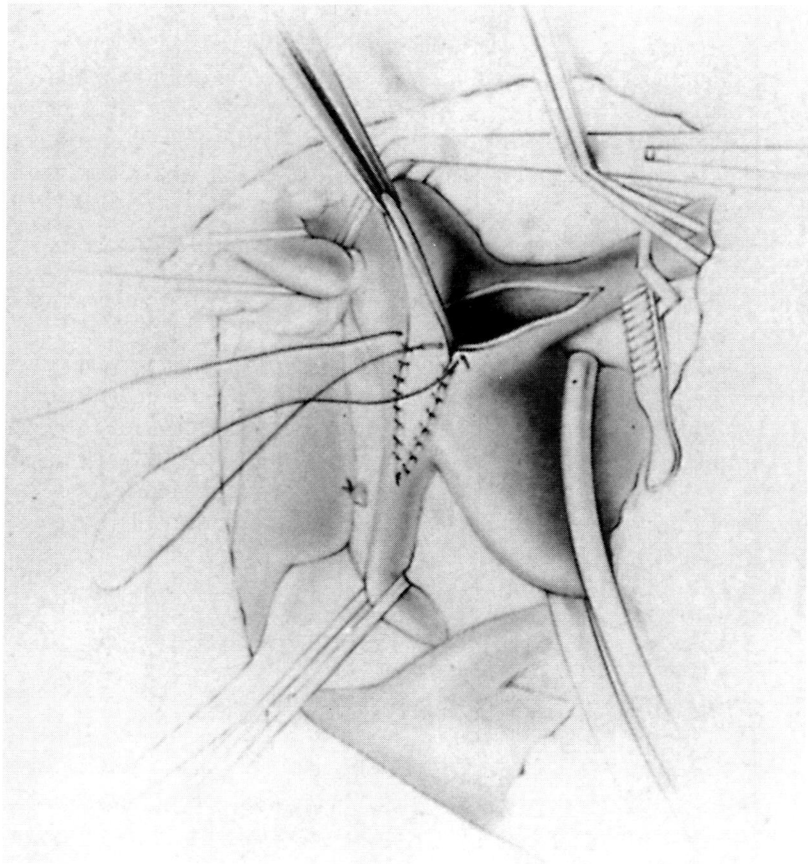

Figure 14–5. Incision closure after transverse aortotomy and renal artery endarterectomy showing the use of a patch to widen the orifice of the renal arteries.

RENAL ARTERY REIMPLANTATION

Many patients will have a somewhat redundant renal artery after it has been dissected from the surrounding retroperitoneal tissue. When renal artery stenosis is limited to its origin and the vessel is redundant, the renal artery can simply be transected and reimplanted, after spatulation, into the aorta at a slightly lower level **(Fig. 14–6)**. Occasionally this can even be done in small children and thereby abolish the necessity of using a graft **(Fig. 14–7)**. Renal implantation is performed by suture ligation of the origin of the renal artery after transection. After excising a button of aorta just below the renal artery, the renal artery is spatulated and reattached to the aorta using 6/0 monofilament polypropylene sutures.

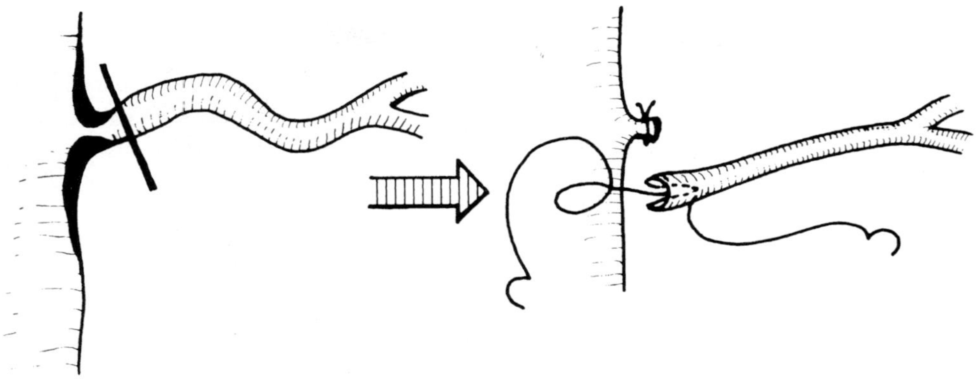

Figure 14–6. Site of aortotomy and renal artery transection for renal artery reimplantation.

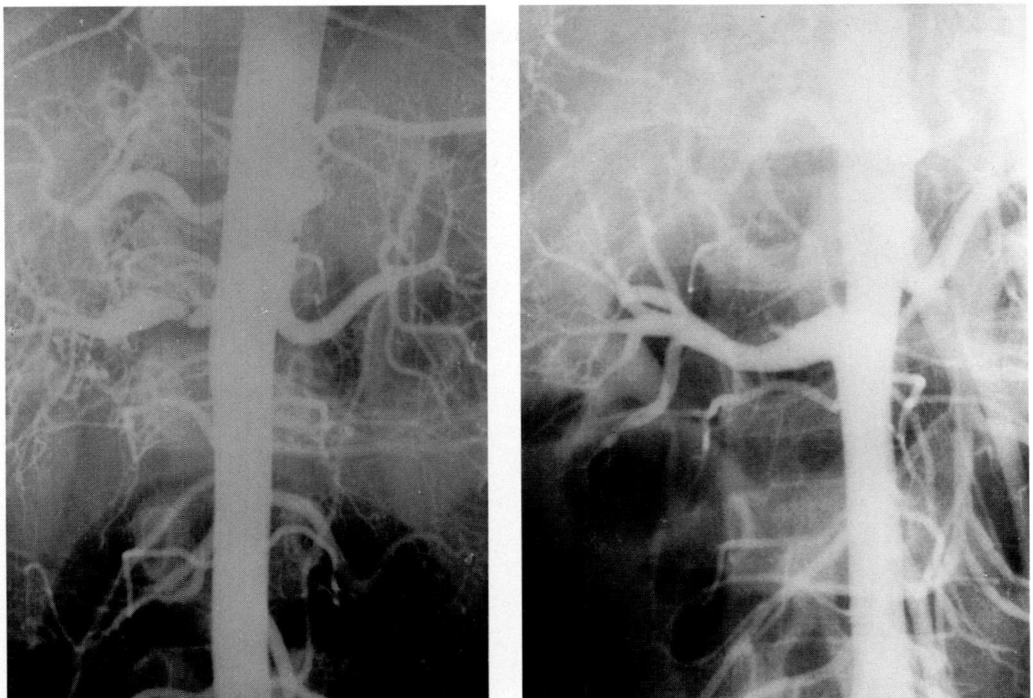

Figure 14–7. Preoperative (left) and postoperative (right) arteriogram before (left) and after (right) renal artery reimplantation in a five-year-old male with a proximal renal artery stenosis.

EXTRA-ANATOMIC BYPASSES

Extra-anatomic procedures have received increased use and popularity as an alternative method of renal revascularization in the high-risk patient. The authors do not believe that these procedures are comparable to direct reconstructions, but they are useful in a highly selected subgroup of high-risk patients.

Hepatorenal Bypass

A right subcostal incision is usually used to perform the hepatorenal bypass. The hepatoduodenal ligament is incised, and the common hepatic artery both proximal and distal to the gastroduodenal artery origin is encircled **(Fig. 14–8)**. Next, the descending duodenum is mobilized by Kocher's maneuver, the inferior vena cava is

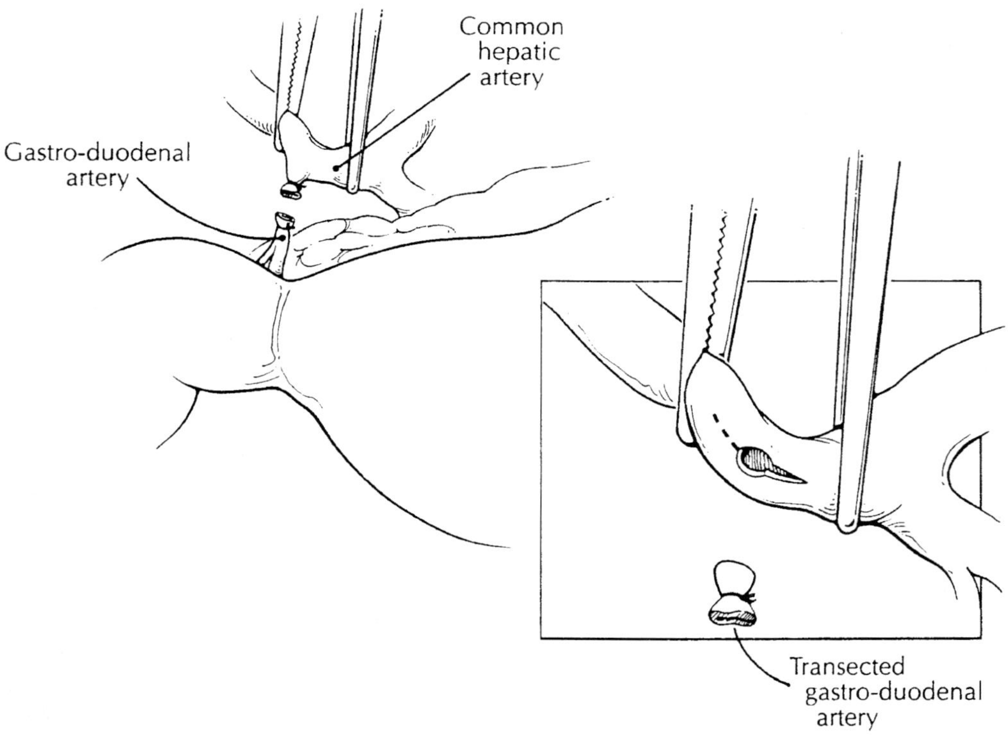

Figure 14–8. Exposed common hepatic artery and the proximal gastroduodenal artery after excision of the hepatoduodenal ligament.

identified, the right renal vein is identified, and the right renal artery is encircled where it is found, either immediately cephalad or caudad to the renal vein.

A greater saphenous vein graft is usually used to construct the bypass. The hepatic artery anastomosis of the vein graft can be placed at the site of the amputated stump of the gastroduodenal artery or proximal to this branch when it must be saved as a collateral to gut perfusion. After completion of this anastomosis, the renal artery is transected and brought anterior to the vena cava for anastomosis end-to-end to the graft.

Splenorenal Bypass

Splenorenal bypass can be performed through a midline or a left subcostal incision. The posterior pancreas is mobilized by reflecting the inferior border cephalad. When the retropancreatic plane has been entered, the splenic artery can be mobilized from the left gastroepiploic artery to the level of its branches. The left renal artery is exposed as described earlier. After the splenic artery has been completely mobilized, it is divided distally, spatulated, and anastomosed end-to-end to the transected renal artery **(Fig. 14–9)**.

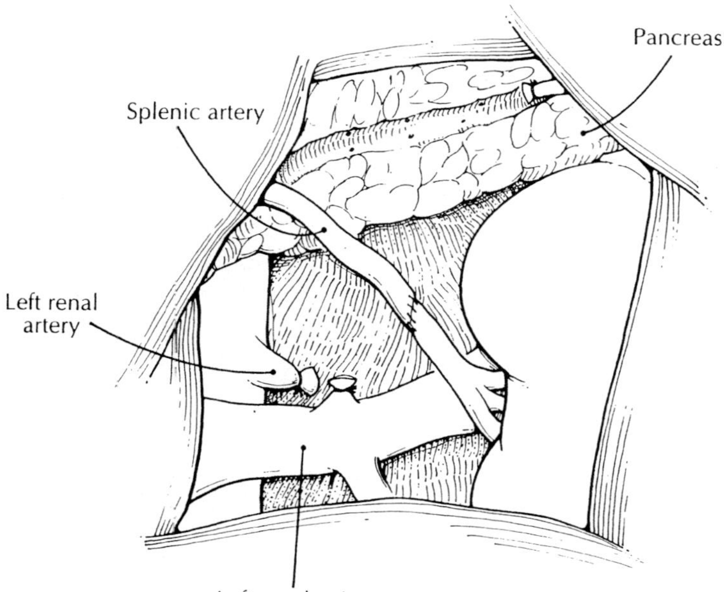

Figure 14–9. Transected splenic artery that has been anastomosed end-to-end to the transected left renal artery.

SUMMARY

In conclusion, many techniques are useful for the revascularization of the ischemic kidney. None of these techniques are useful in all cases. Any one of these procedures may be the most ideal given an individual patient's anatomy and associated risk factors. Knowledge of each of the techniques and their proper application will maximize results of operative management.

15

Transaortic Renal Endarterectomy and Antegrade Aortorenal Reconstruction

Linda M. Reilly, Laurie M. Kuestner, and Ronald J. Stoney

Pararenal aortic atherosclerosis produces a variable degree of narrowing of the renal artery ostia, either alone or in combination with aortic aneurysmal degeneration or obstruction. Renal ischemia resulting from significant renal artery stenosis or occlusion may cause or accelerate diastolic hypertension, impair renal function or produce progressive renal ischemia resulting in irreversible infarction and/or atrophy. These threatening clinical consequences mandate early detection and treatment to relieve reversible symptoms and prevent progressive organ threatening events. The pattern and distribution of atherosclerosis in this region may be repaired by direct operation or palliated in some circumstances by minimally invasive catheter based interventional techniques of angioplasty and stent placement. This chapter will discuss operative techniques to review the obstructing plaque from the renal arteries (transaortic renal endarterectomy) and antegrade aortorenal bypass from the supraceliac aorta.

Endarterectomy was first performed by dos Santos in Lisbon, Portugal in 1946,[1] and pioneered in the United States by Wylie in San Francisco in 1951.[2] His first operation was an aortoiliac endarterectomy, but within a year he successfully performed the first renal and aortic endarterectomy.[3] Later, Freeman reported a similar operation.[4] Transaortic endarterectomy evolved at UCSF under Wylie and was extended later to the major visceral arteries as well. The approach is based on the distribution of the disease to be removed. The disease begins within the aortic intima spreads or "flows" into the renal artery ostia. Removal is best begun in the aorta and continued into the renal arteries where the disease terminates in a predictably smooth tapered end-point or transition to more normal intimal lining. Our early attempts at transrenal artery removal were not consistently able to remove the aortic based component of the plaque. That method was abandoned in favor of the transaortic procedure.

The technique is applicable to nearly all patterns of pararenal aortic atherosclerosis, and the site of origin and the number of renal arteries involved. Perhaps, aneurysmal degeneration of the proximal renal artery itself, a rare finding, would constitute a true contraindication to this technique.

TECHNIQUE

Pararenal Aortic Occlusive Disease

The patient is positioned supine and the abdomen is opened through a full length mid-line incision. The pararenal aorta can be exposed through an infracolic posterior peritoneal approach with displacement of the pancreas cephalad. This provides unrestricted access to the upper abdominal aorta. The exposure to be used is maintained using a table mounted self-retaining retraction system (Omni-Tract Surgical, St. Paul, Minn).

The aorta is mobilized from the superior to the inferior mesenteric artery origin. Circumferential mobilization requires dividing the diaphragmatic crura to free the aorta from the spine. The renal arteries are dissected well beyond the distal extent of palpable or visible disease. Paired posterior branches are exposed for temporary control. Supramesenteric dissection for aortic clamp control is necessary when the distance between the SMA and renal artery origin is less than half the vertebrae (~2 cm).

Mannitol is used to establish a diuresis and the patient is anticoagulated with 3,000 units of heparin. Proximal and distal aortic clamps are applied. All intervening branches are controlled by clamps. The aorta is opened by an 8 cm longitudinal aortotomy curved to the left to avoid the SMA origin **(Fig. 15–1)**. The disease is bilateral in the majority of patients, so a bilateral procedure is usually required. The endarterectomy plane is established in the outer media on the edge of the aortotomy with the thickest lesion. A Halle dissector, or battery powered Autosector (Omni-Tract) is used to develop the plane circumferentially both proximally and distally. The specimen is transected inferiorly and superiorly with scissors at the edge of the plane avoiding loosened flaps of the remaining aortic intima. The aortic specimen is gently retracted to the patient's left with forceps and centrifugal dissection of the right renal artery specimen is performed with the dissector **(Fig. 15–2)**. Displacing the right renal artery clamp toward the aorta prolapses the renal artery into the aorta to facilitate visualization

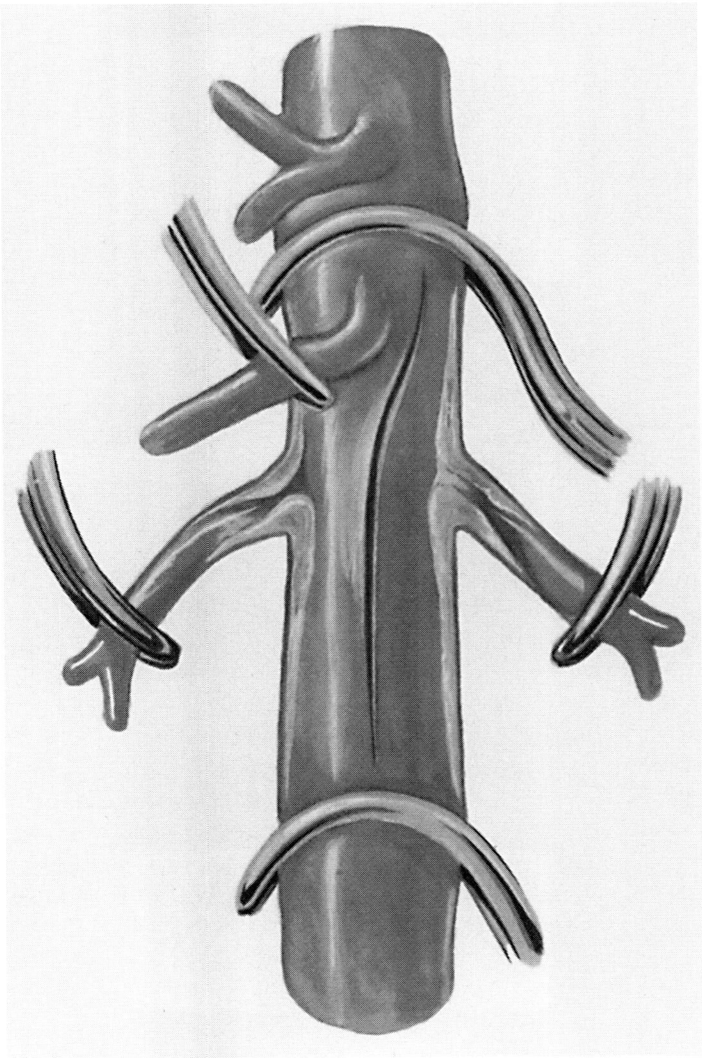

Figure 15–1. The pararenal aorta and branches have been isolated and controlled with clamps. The paravisceral aorta is the site of proximal clamping. A longitudinal aortotomy is outlined in the midline with an extension to the left side of the origin of the superior mesenteric artery. Note the presence of significant bilateral pararenal atherosclerosis.

of the critical end-point. The media is gently pushed away from the core or specimen until the feathered end-point finally separates. This maneuver is repeated for the left renal artery and is facilitated by the surgeon performing this maneuver from the right side of the patient. The entire aortic core with projecting renal orifice lesions is removed, usually as a single specimen **(Fig. 15–3)**. After thorough flushing with dilute heparin solution and back bleeding by successive release of the occluding renal artery clamps, the aortotomy is closed with a continuous 4-0 suture. After release of the clamp and restoration of aortic and renal flow, the

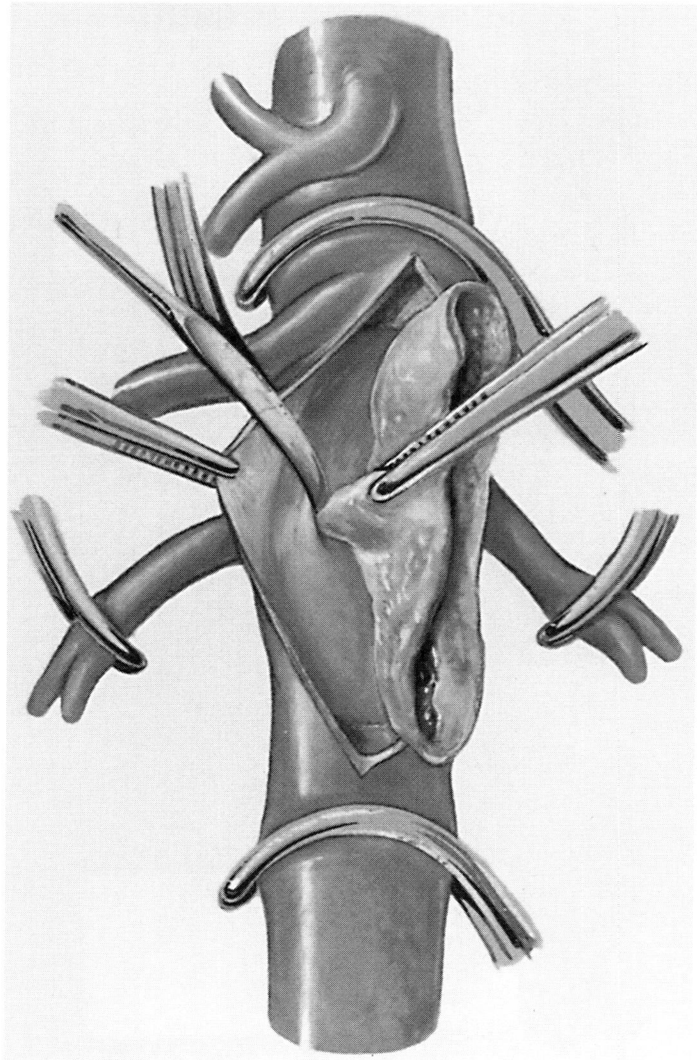

Figure 15–2. Extraction endarterectomy of the right renal artery. Note that the dural elevator is being used to displace the artery away from the plaque as it is delivered from the renal artery.

endarterectomized segments are noted to be slightly dilated without a palpable edge where the transition to normal renal artery intima begins.

An adequate endpoint is confirmed by direct inspection of the prolapsed renal artery through the aortotomy prior to wound closure after the reconstruction using duplex sonography to characterize the flow profile **(Fig. 15–4)**.

If only unilateral endarterectomy is required for a unilateral lesion or a solitary kidney, a disc of thickened aortic intima surrounding the diseased renal orifice is freed and then the same

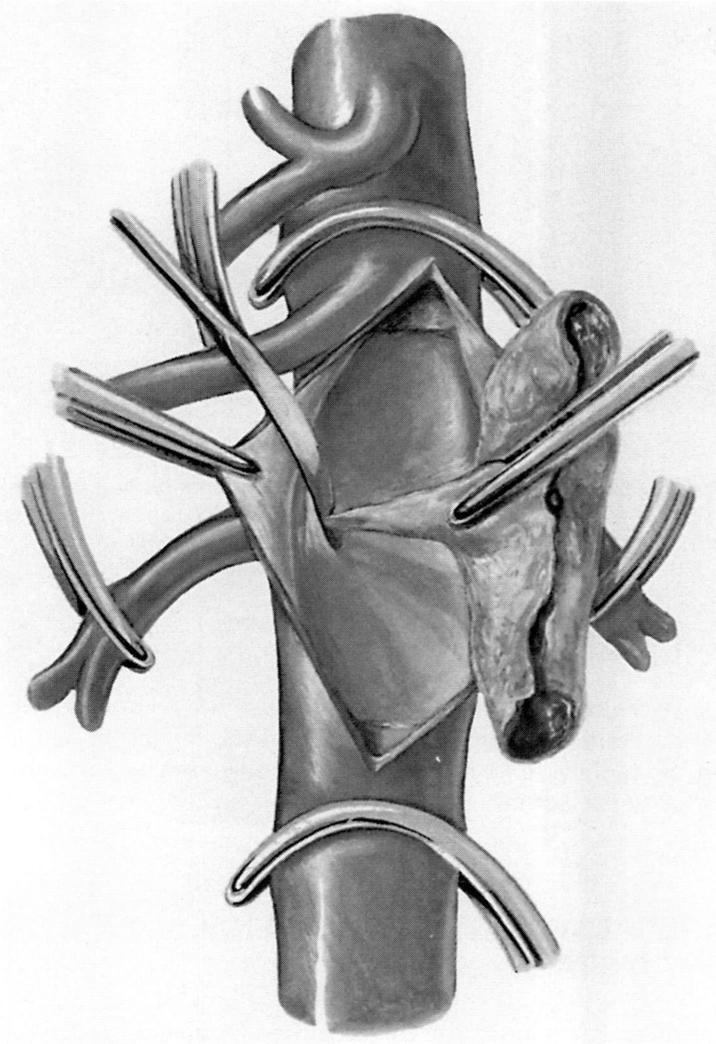

Figure 15–3. The endarterectomy specimen is removed from the aorta after completion of the renal endarterectomy.

centripetal dissection of the renal artery specimen proceeds as described.

When multi-renal arteries are involved, the aortotomy is extended to span the length of the aorta, giving origin to the branches. The technique, employing sleeve removal of the aortic intima and bilateral multiple renal endarterectomies is rapid and effective. This technique, transaortic renal endarterectomy, has several advantages over other revascularization methods. It permits an autogenous revascularization of all renal arteries in one maneuver with a brief 20–30 minute period of ischemia. The only

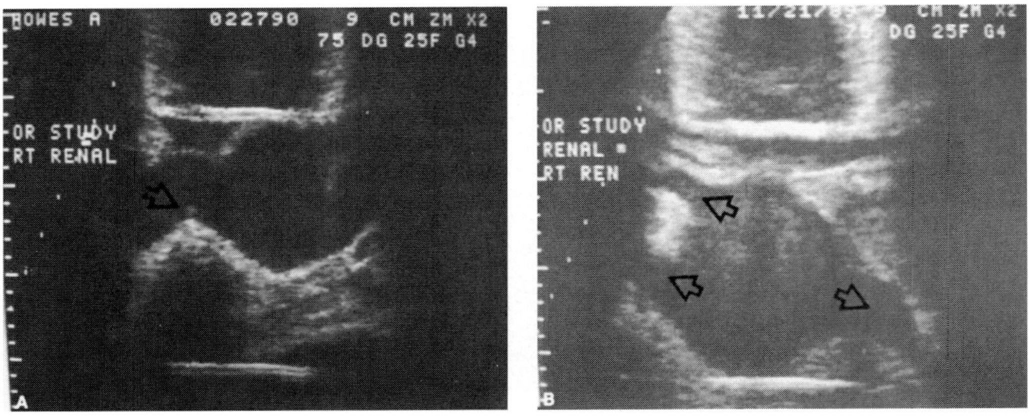

Figure 15–4. A. Intraoperative duplex scan in transverse view after transaortic renal thromboendarterectomy. The aorta and right renal artery are well visualized. There is a minor defect due to residual disease (arrow). B. Transverse intraoperative duplex scan showing two patent right renal arteries and a single left renal artery after transaortic renal thromboendarterectomy.

disadvantages are the time it takes to acquire the technical proficiency with extraction endarterectomy and the length of time to perform the tedious dissection required to prepare the pararenal aorta prior to the actual endarterectomy.

PARARENAL ANEURYSM WITH RENAL ARTERY DISEASE

When pararenal aneurysm disease requires inclusion grafting in association with symptomatic renal artery disease, the approach can be changed to a left medial visceral rotation.[5] This approach is employed when exposing aneurysms of the upper portion of the abdominal aorta. It offers unrestricted exposure since the pancreas and overlying viscera are displaced medially and to the right. Longitudinal division of the left crus of the diaphragm and reflection of the autonomic ganglion overlying the upper aorta exposed the renal and visceral arteries which can be mobilized as needed. When graft replacement of a pararenal aneurysm is required, occasionally one renal orifice can be preserved in the diagonally transected proximal aortic cuff **(Fig. 15–5)**. Transaortic renal endarterectomy is performed as previously described through the aortotomy. Then the beveled graft is anastomosed and unilateral renal blood flow restored by relocating the aortic clamp to the graft. The other renal artery orifice is removed from

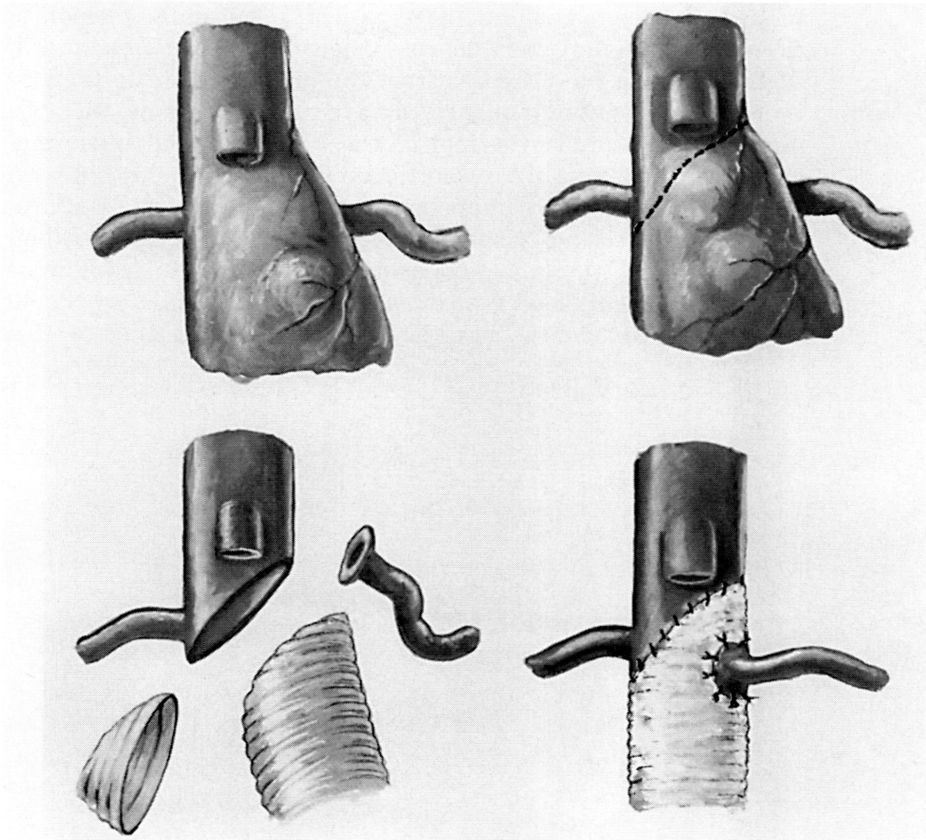

Figure 15–5. A pararenal aneurysm primarily involving the left side of this aortic segment. The proposed line of bevelled aortic transection is outlined. The residual aorta and left renal artery are shown after removal of the aneurysmal aorta. A beveled graft is attached end-to-end to the pararenal aorta with a continuous suture. The left renal artery is reimplanted on a Carrel patch to the side of the graft.

the aneurysmal aortic wall as a Carrell patch **(Fig. 15–5)**. Prior to reattachment to an appropriately sized defect in the graft, extraction renal endarterectomy can easily be performed on this renal orifice if required.

COMBINED RENAL AND AORTIC DISEASE

The association of pararenal atherosclerosis producing renal ischemic consequences and aortic aneurysm or occlusive disease is being recognized frequently now that more complete imaging techniques are used to evaluate these patients. Concomitant repair of the aorta and renal artery disease is now feasible when indicated. Although aorta renal bypass from the prosthetic aortic graft or remote bypass to the renal arteries are surgical options, we favor direct reconstruction (in-line) of the pararenal and infrarenal aorta. The technique of transaortic renal endarterectomy has been modified so it can be accomplished through the transected juxtarenal aorta prior to anastomosis of the prosthetic aortic graft.[6] When the proximal aortic clamp is relocated on the proximal graft, mesenteric and renal blood flow is restored in approximately 30–40 minutes. Then the distal graft or graft limbs are attached to sites

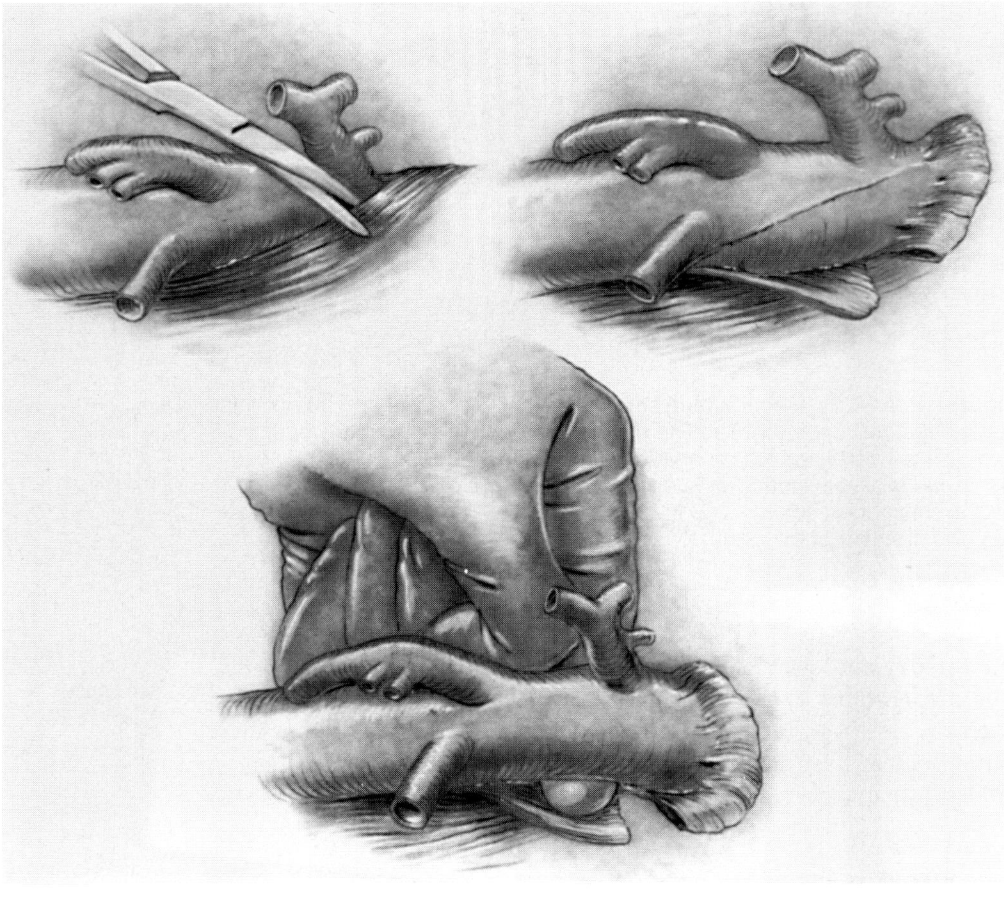

Figure 15–6. Lateral view of pararenal aortic mobilization. The crura of the diaphragm are divided with scissors and the aorta is elevated. Blunt finger dissection separates the posterior surface of the aorta from the anterior lumbar spine.

appropriate for treating the underlying aortic aneurysmal or occlusive problem.

The infracolic approach is suitable in these situations, unless a reoperation is necessary. Dense scarring in these circumstances can be avoided by using left medial rotation with exposure of the pararenal aorta through previously unoperated tissue planes. The only difference in the preparation and exposure and mobilization of the pararenal aorta from that already described for the longitudinal transaortic renal endarterectomy is the extent of the retroaortic mobilization. Proximal index finger dissection behind the aorta provides the ability to elevate the pararenal segment away from the spine. When the juxtarenal aorta is transected, the elevated proximal end of the aorta is clearly visible which facilitates the endarterectomy.

After transabdominal infracolic exposure of the pararenal aorta, the pancreas is retracted upward and the renal vein mobilized. The division of the diaphragmatic crura permits the dissection of the retroaortic space **(Fig. 15–6)**. The autonomic ganglia

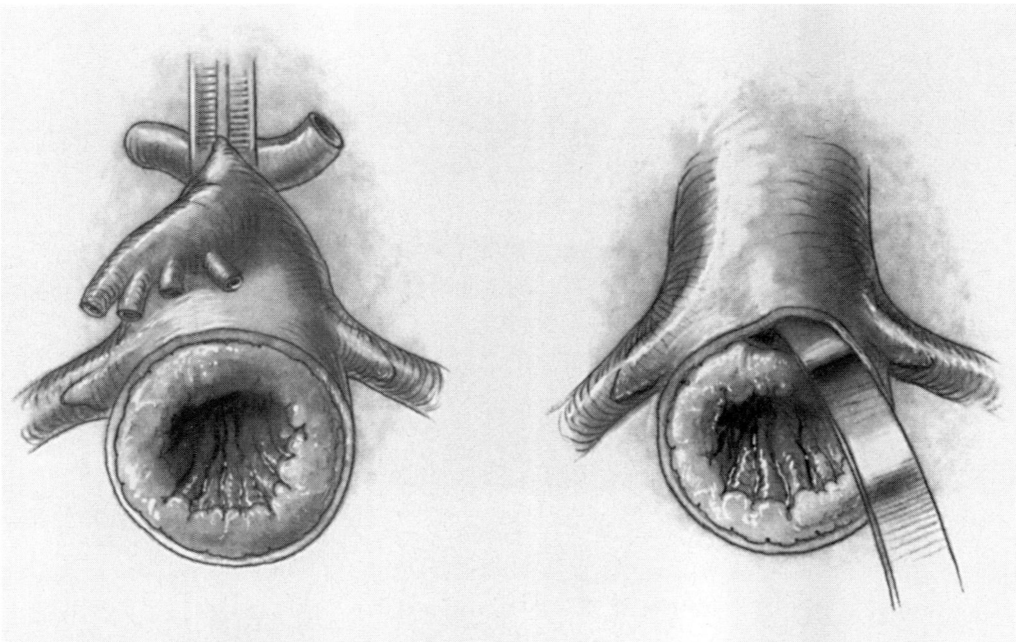

Figure 15–7. The pararenal aorta from the front. The proximal clamp is placed between the celiac axis and the superior mesenteric artery, allowing visualization of a thickened aortic atheroma with bilateral renal artery extensions. The Halle dural elevator is used to initiate the dissection plane between the underlying aortic media and the intimal lesion.

tissue is incised and reflected to expose the upper aortic branches as well as the renal arteries. After determining the extent of the infrarenal aortic disease which is to be concomitantly treated, diuresis is induced with mannitol, and anticoagulation instituted. The aorta is clamped usually just proximal to the SMA origin and distal to the renal level **(Fig. 15–7)**. The intervening renal mesenteric and intercostal vessels are controlled and the aorta transected just below the renal origin. The mobile aortic stump is angled anteriorly for better visibility **(Fig. 15–8)**. The endarterectomy plane is established at the edge of the aorta and the continued separating the plaque from the uninvolved media. When this has been completed to the level of the SMA origin, traction to the right allows centrifugal dissection of the left renal artery plaque as the renal artery is prolapsed into the aorta **(Fig. 15–9)**. The endpoint is separated under direct vision. This is repeated for the

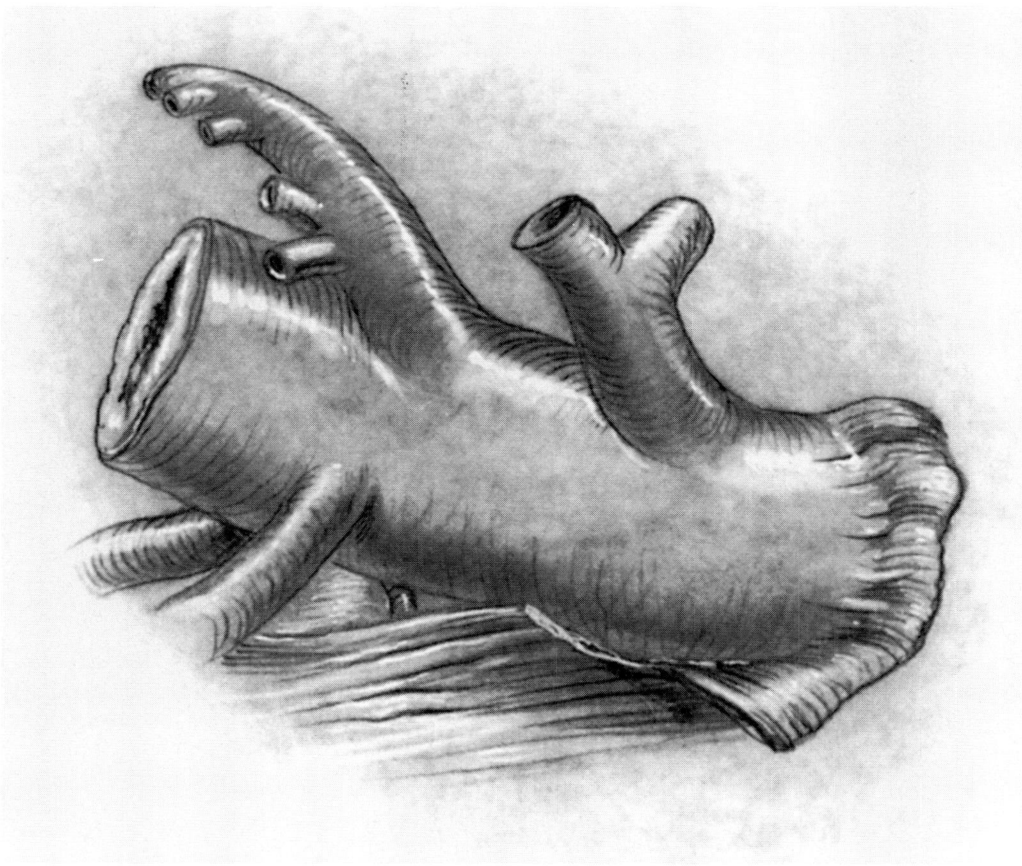

Figure 15–8. The mobilized and elevated pararenal aortic segment.

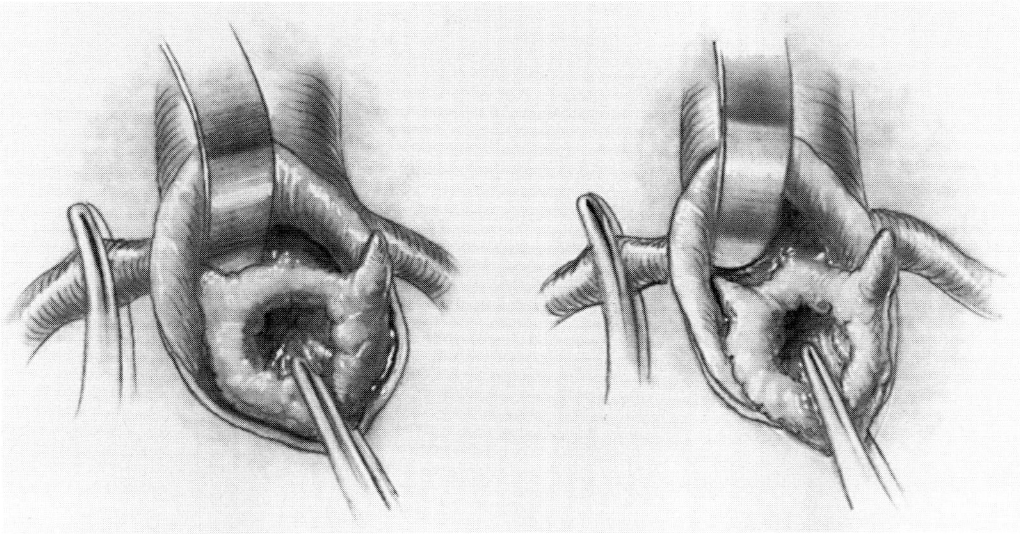

Figure 15–9. The extraction endarterectomy of the left renal artery has been completed. The procedure is being carried out on the right side. The elevator separates the atheroma from the residual normal renal artery media.

right renal artery endarterectomy. The aortic plaque is transported proximally and removed. The stump is irrigated. The renal arteries individually back bled and flushed with heparin saline solution. The aortic graft is then anastomosed end-to-end to the aorta with continuous synthetic suture and the proximal clamp replaced on the proximal graft. Renal and mesenteric flow is restored **(Fig. 15–10)**. This requires 30–40 minutes of ischemia. This distal prosthetic reconstruction is dictated by the underlying aneurysm or occlusive disease. Prompt resumption of urine flow is evidence of perfused functioning in renal parenchyma. Duplex scanning confirms an adequate technical result prior to closure.

ANTEGRADE AORTORENAL BYPASS

Alternate methods of renal revascularization utilize bypass grafts from a variety of inflow sites. We prefer antegrade grafts originating from the supraceliac aorta since they have improved flow characteristics and originate from the predictably undiseased inflow site. They are used for reoperations to avoid scarring from prior failed revascularizations of the aorta and renal arteries. The supraceliac aorta can be exposed by a transabdominal transcrural

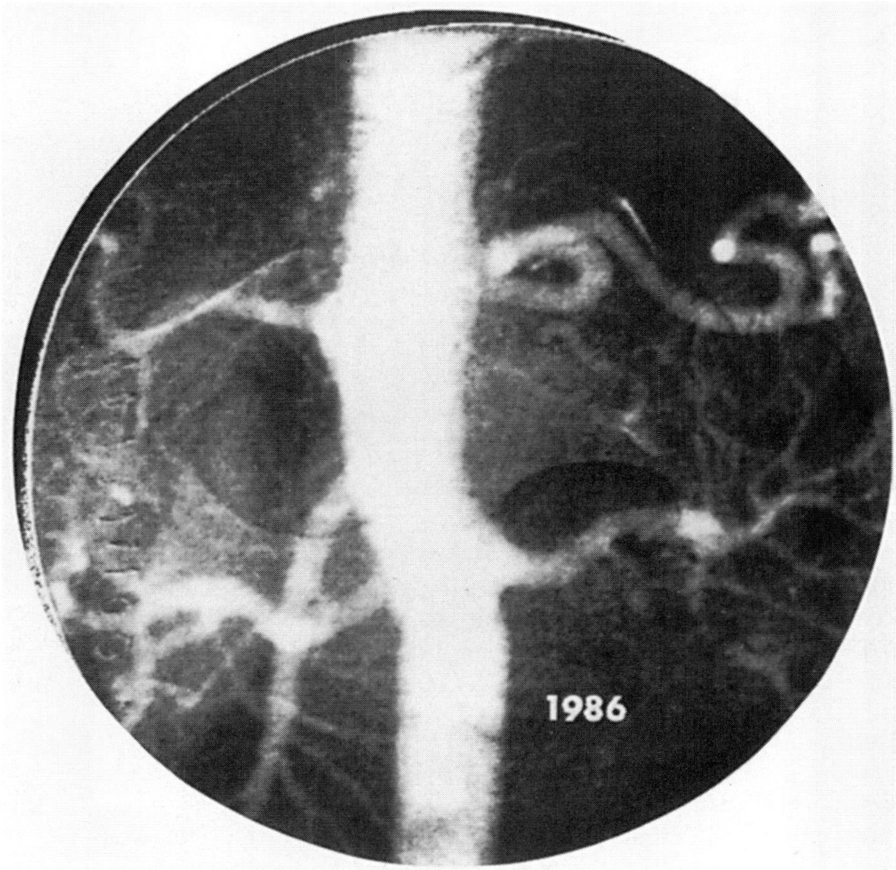

Figure 15–10. Postoperative aortogram after transverse aortorenal endarterectomy and prosthetic infrarenal aortic graft.

route or by left medial visceral rotation. The transcrural exposure is simpler, but requires indirect tunnelling to both renal arteries. Left medial visceral rotation simplifies graft routing to the left side and more thorough mobilization of the aorta.

The aorta is mobilized circumferentially for a distance of 4–6 cm by the celiac origin. This allows either cross-clamping in the aorta to isolate a segment for graft anastomosis to an elliptical anterior aortotomy **(Fig. 15–11)**. A bifurcated or straight graft is used depending on the number of kidneys requiring revascularization.

On the right, the tunnel is made behind the head of the pancreas towards the renal hilum. Depending on the extent of scarring from the prior operation, the right renal artery may be exposed by a modified right medial visceral rotation. Gentle finger

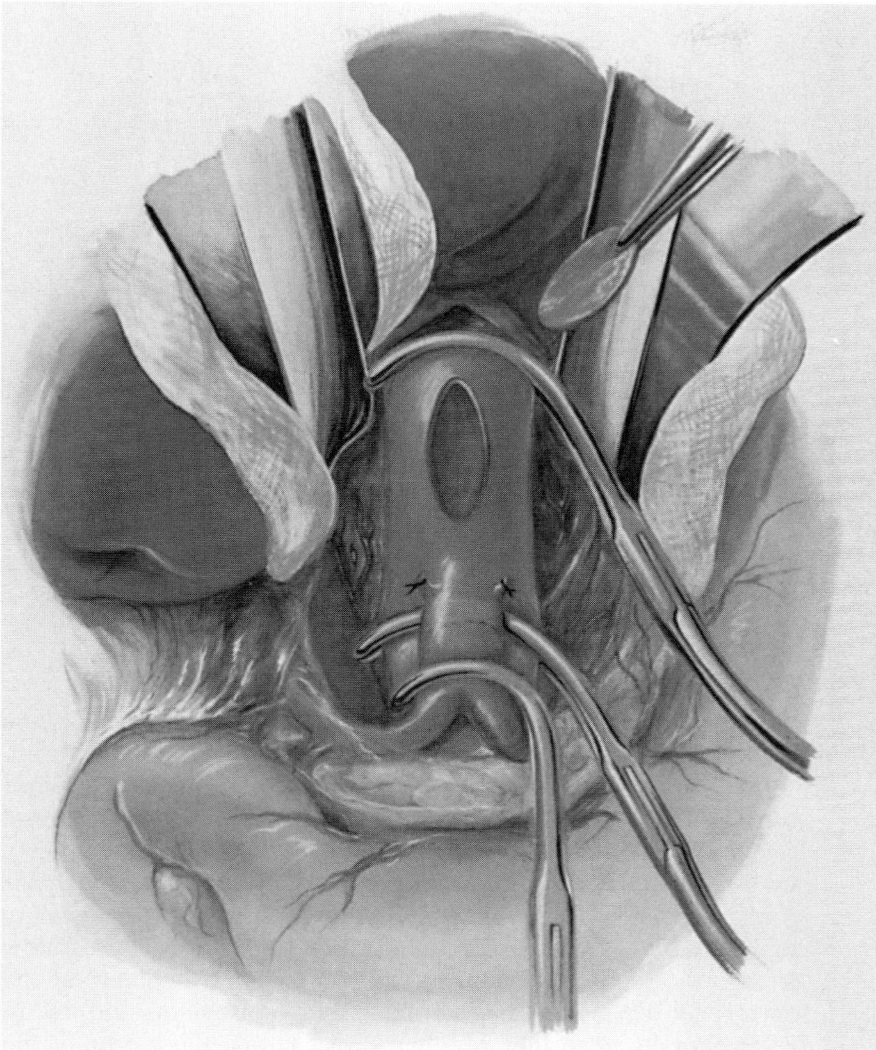

Figure 15–11. The supraceliac aorta is controlled between two aortic clamps, and the elliptical aortotomy is created.

dissection completes the graft tunnel and the right limb of the attached bifurcation graft is routed through this space. End-to-end anastomosis of graft to renal artery are preferred and require approximately 20 minutes of renal ischemia **(Fig. 15–12)**.

The left tunnel is created behind the body of the pancreas. The left renal hilus can be exposed using a modified left medial visceral rotation approach. After the left renal graft is positioned and oriented, a similar anastomosis restores left renal perfusion **(Fig.**

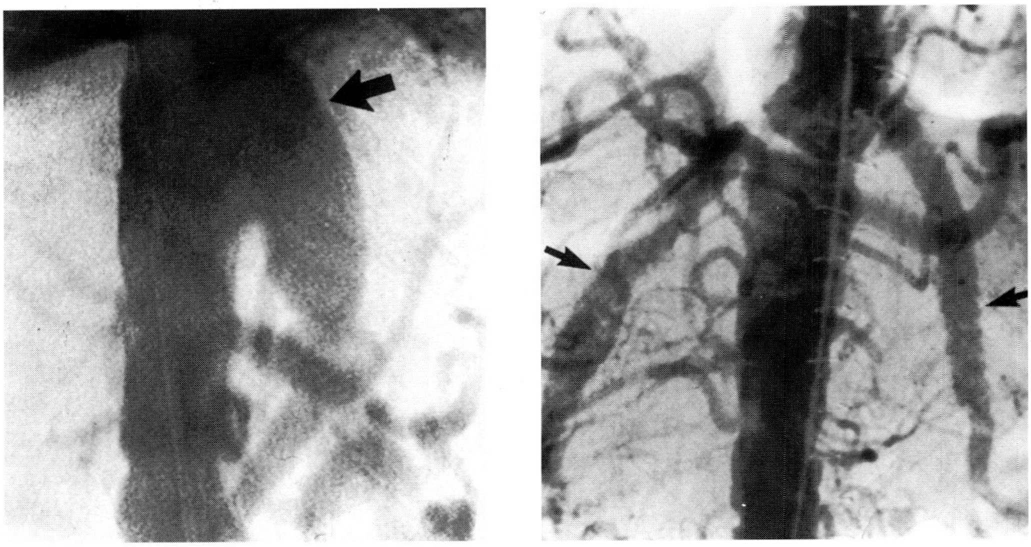

Figure 15–12. Postoperative angiogram of antegrade aortorenal bypass.

15–12). Duplex scanning confirms the technical adequacy of the bypass.

The antegrade aortorenal bypass is used infrequently. Reoperations and occasional renal revascularization for thoracoabdominal coarctation (Middle Aortic Syndrome) are the usual indications. Like the antegrade aortovisceral bypass, the aortorenal bypass grafts are short, high flowing conduits. They are preferred to extra-anatomical reconstructions which use less certain inflow from the celiac branches or the iliac arteries. The safety of the aortorenal bypass in hazardous reoperative problems and its durability make it our choice when direct revascularization of the native renal arteries is not feasible.

REFERENCES

1. Dos Santos JC. Sur la desobstruction des thromboses arterielles anciennes. *Mem Acad Chir* 1947;73:409–411.
2. Wylie EJ, Kerr E, Davies O. Experimental and clinical experiences with the use of fascia lata applied as a graft about major arteries after thromboendarterectomy and aneurysmorrhaphy. *Surg Gynecol Obstet* 1951;93:257–272.
3. Wylie EJ, Perloff DL, Stoney RJ. Autogenous tissue revascularization techniques in surgery for renovascular hypertension. *Ann Surg* 1969; 1970:416–428.

4. Freeman EF, Leeds FH. Operations on large arteries. Application of recent advances. *Calif Med* 1952;77:229–233.
5. Sauer L, Stoney RJ. Transabdominal exposure of the pararenal aorta and medial visceral rotation. *Sem Vasc Surg* 1989;2(4):209–213.
6. Stoney RJ, Messina LM, Goldstone J, Reilly LM. Renal endarterectomy through the transected aorta: A new technique for combined aortorenal atherosclerosis—A preliminary report. *J Vasc Surg* 1989; 9:224–233.

16

Renal Revascularization: Splenic and Hepatic Arteries as Inflow Vessels

Ashby C. Moncure and
David C. Brewster

Surgical renal artery reconstruction is effective and durable therapy for patients with poorly controlled hypertension and/or deterioration of renal function secondary to atherosclerotic renal vascular disease.[1–5]

A variety of alternatives are available to accomplish renal artery revascularization. Aortorenal bypass grafting, using autogenous vein, arterial autografts, or prosthetic conduits, has been the preferred method of renal revascularization because of the predictability of high inflow, relative simplicity of the operation, and well documented durability of result. Substantial aortic atherosclerosis is also frequently present as well, and may make difficult the originating of the graft from the native aorta. Transaortic thromboendarterectomy, a more complex procedure, has been more widely utilized in the recent past and is felt particularly applicable to patients with bilateral renal artery disease. Renal artery reimplantation may be a very useful procedure, particularly in combination with replacement of a diseased distal aorta with Dacron graft, but is difficult to successfully achieve in the presence of a diseased aorta. Percutaneous transluminal angioplasty has not proven to be a durable procedure in the presence of disease at or near the renal artery ostia, the commonest location of atherosclerotic disease leading to renal artery stenosis or occlusion.

Hepato- and splenorenal bypass grafts have been utilized in the Vascular Surgical Unit at the Massachusetts General Hospital for more than 20 years and our favorable experience with these conduits has been previously reported.[6] Although originally employed in desperate situations such as in renal artery trauma or periaortic infection, further experience with the procedures has lead to a broadening indication for their use. This approach has been frequently used to avoid a diseased or scarred aorta from previous aortic operation, to allow a staged approach to correction of bilateral renal artery stenoses or multiple vascular lesions; as a "lesser operation" for medically poor risk patients; and also, more rarely, for complex problems including aortic dissection, renal artery aneurysm and renal artery involvement with thoracoabdominal aneurysm as well as aortic infection and trauma. Favorable experience with this approach has evolved such that hepato- and splenorenal bypass graft are frequently the procedure of choice in the elderly patient with atherosclerotic renovascular disease, avoiding the hemodynamic effects of aortic crossclamping and the difficulties frequently encountered in originating a graft from a diseased aorta.

HISTORICAL PERSPECTIVES

The first reported use of splenorenal arterial anastomosis as a method of renal artery reconstruction, although not successful, was by Thompson and Smithwick[7] in 1952. In 1953 Hurwitt, et al[8] reported a series of successful splanchnic artery switches in dogs and suggested clinical application of these techniques in human beings for various disease processes. The first splenorenal grafts were described by Hurwitt et al[9] and DeCamp, Snyder and Bost[10] in 1956 and 1957, respectively. Since that time, scattered reports have appeared; large series have been reported by Novick et al[11] and Moncure et al.[6]

Use of the hepatic circulation for operative management of right renal artery disease was originally described by Libertino et al[12] in 1976 and in 1979 Novick et al[13] reported their experience in an experimental and clinical setting. In 1984 large series of right renal artery reconstructions with the hepatic circulation used for inflow was reported by Chibaro, Libertino, and Novick[14] and by Moncure et al[6] in 1986.

Preoperative Preparation

The preoperative evaluation necessary to employ hepato- and splenorenal arterial reconstruction includes midstream biplane aortography demonstrating the origin of the celiac axis as well as the origin of the superior mesenteric artery. Because the gastroduodenal artery is usually divided in the course of hepatorenal grafting, the patency of the superior mesenteric artery should be ensured because it would be unwise to interrupt a major collateral source if ostial disease of the superior mesenteric artery is present. Angiography is also used to document anatomic variations involving the celiac axis and superior mesenteric arterial circulation.

In addition to excellent preoperative angiography, other aspects of preoperative preparation should be directed at ensuring a stable cardiac status and as optimal renal function as is possible to achieve. Cardiac consultation should be obtained, the patient's medication program reviewed, and any abnormalities corrected, as feasible. Adequate hydration is important. Operation should be postponed for a period after diagnostic angiography to ensure that any element of contrast induced renal failure is not present or that it has cleared.

OPERATIVE MANAGEMENT

Technique of Hepatorenal Reconstruction

The patient is placed supine with the legs externally rotated, and the abdominal wall, groins and medial thighs prepared and draped as a sterile field. A right subcostal incision extending medially across the midline and laterally to the tip of the right eleventh rib **(Fig. 16–1A)** allows excellent access to the porta hepatis and the right renal artery. The hepatoduodenal ligament is incised **(Fig. 16–1B)**, and the common hepatic artery both proximal and distal to the gastroduodenal artery origin is encircled **(Fig. 16–1C)**.

The descending duodenum is mobilized by Kocher's maneuver **(Fig. 16–2A)**, and dissection is carried down along the gastroduodenal artery, which serves as a constant and helpful reference point. If the gastroduodenal artery is 3 cm in length before its bifurcation and appears to have an internal diameter of 3.5 mm. after dilatation, the surgeon may consider use of this vessel for primary end-to-end anastomosis to the right renal artery. In many instances, however, the gastroduodenal artery will not be of sufficient length or adequate caliber after gentle dilatation with a #3 Fogarty catheter. The surgeon must then be prepared to harvest the proximal greater saphenous vein to lead a graft from the hepatic artery, usually at the gastroduodenal artery origin, down to the right renal artery.

After the Kocher maneuver, the inferior vena cava and the right renal vein are readily located. The right renal artery is identified as it emerges from behind the vena cava, usually just above or below the renal vein **(Fig. 16–2B)**. Frequently, the most favorable part of the renal artery with which to work is that part involved with post-stenotic dilatation, found immediately distal to the area of stenosis, which is usually at the renal artery ostium. To make this area available for anastomosis as well as to acquire as much length of renal artery as possible, the inferior vena cava may be mobilized and the proximal right renal artery isolated subjacent to it, along the left border of the vena cava. To assure the appropri-

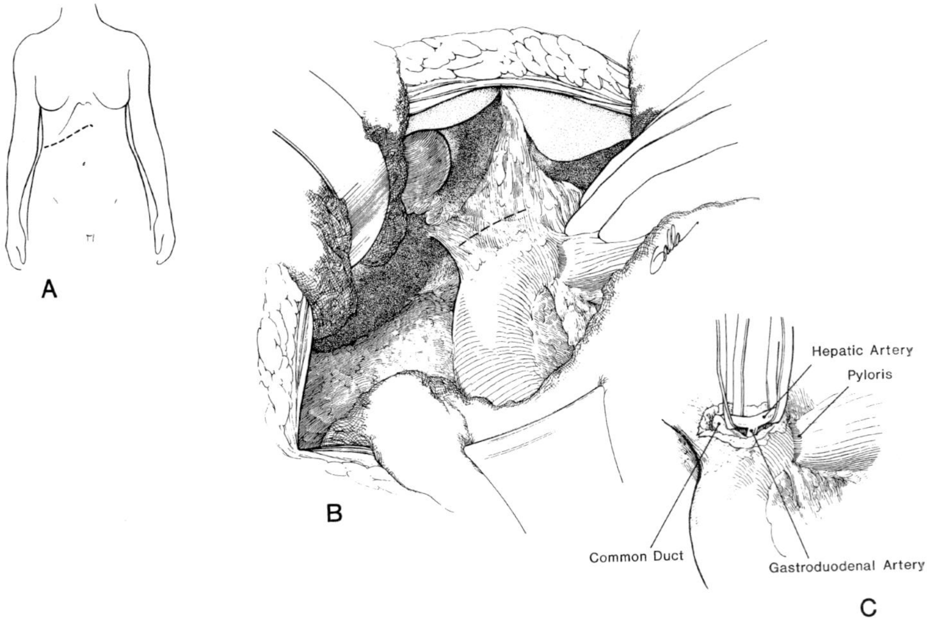

Figure 16–1. Technique of hepatorenal reconstruction. A. Right subcostal incision extending medially across the midline and laterally to the tip of the right eleventh rib allows access to the porta hepatis and the right renal artery. B. The hepatoduodenal ligament is incised. C. The common hepatic artery is encircled both proximal and distal to the gastroduodenal artery origin.

ate axial orientation of the right renal artery as it is rotated up for end-to-end anastomosis to the gastroduodenal artery or saphenous vein graft, an adventitial stripe of fine silk suture material may be passed along the cephalad border of the renal artery.

If the gastroduodenal artery is to be used primarily **(Fig. 16–4)**, the origin of the gastroduodenal artery is occluded with a fine bulldog clamp and the gastroduodenal artery transected at its bifurcation, ligated distally, and thereafter a #3 Fogarty embolectomy catheter is passed through the end of the gastroduodenal artery up into the hepatic artery, the balloon inflated with 0.6 cc. of sterile injectable saline, and then brought back through the gastroduodenal artery in the inflated position. The gastroduodenal artery is elastic and can usually be safely dilated without inflicting harm on the artery. The occluding bulldog clamp at the origin of the gastroduodenal artery may be released subsequently to assess the adequacy of flow through the artery. The right renal artery is then divided just beyond palpable disease and, after probing, its end is spatulated and the artery is rotated up and anasto-

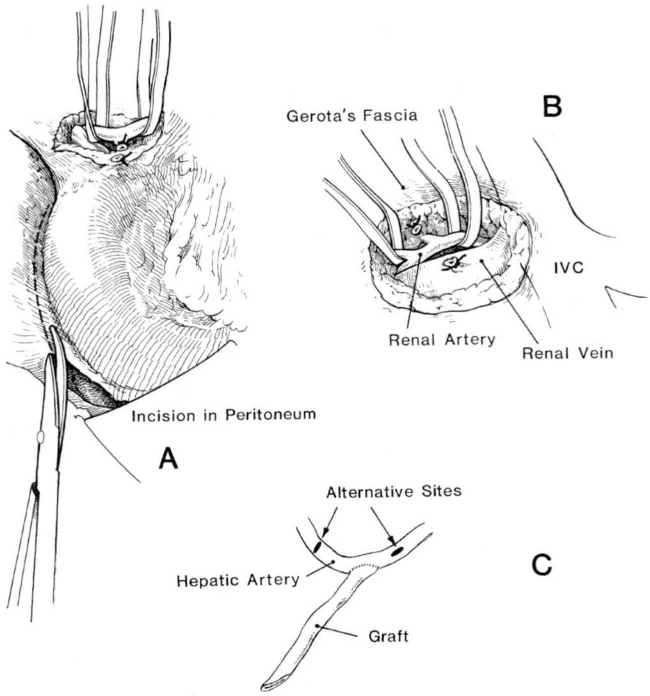

Figure 16–2. Technique of hepatorenal reconstruction. A. The descending duodenum is mobilized by Kocher's maneuver, and dissection is carried down along the gastroduodenal artery, which serves as a constant and helpful reference point. B. The inferior vena cava and the right renal vein are identified, and the right renal artery encircled where found, either immediately cephalad, behind, or caudad to the renal vein. C. A segment of reversed greater saphenous vein is anastomosed to the hepatic artery after it is occluded proximally and distally, the site of proximal anastomosis usually lying at the origin of the gastroduodenal artery at its takeoff from the hepatic artery.

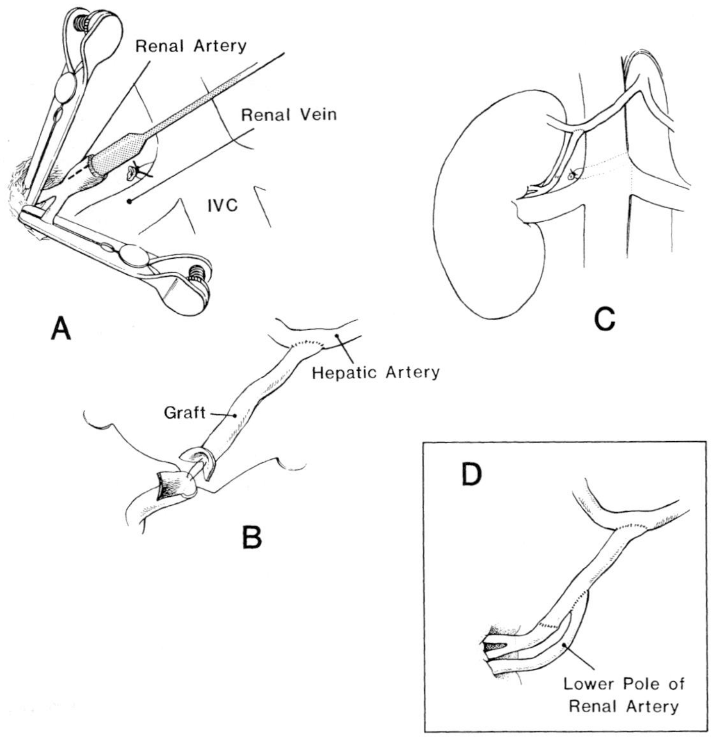

Figure 16–3. Technique of hepatorenal reconstruction. A. The right renal artery is ligated at its origin, divided, profused with chilled heparinized Ringer's lactate solution, and gently dilated with graduated coronary probe. B. The distal right renal artery is spatulated on its superior surface and anastomosed end to end with the spatulated end of the reversed greater saphenous vein graft with an oblique anastomosis of 6-0 Prolene. C. The completed hepatorenal vein graft is illustrated. D. If a lower pole renal artery is present, it is anastomosed into the side of the vein graft.

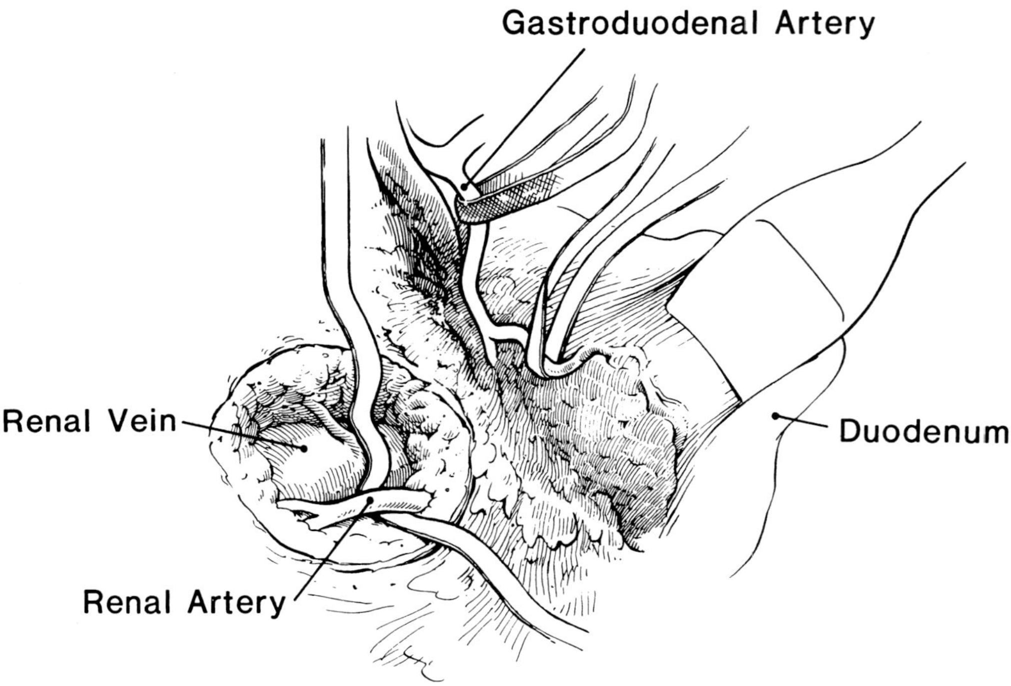

Figure 16–4. Technique of hepatorenal reconstruction. If the gastroduodenal artery appears of large size and is relatively long at evaluation of the arteriogram, it should be considered for use as the conduit. It is dissected from its origin from the hepatic artery to its bifurcation or entry into the pancreas at which time it is divided, dilated with a #3 Fogarty catheter and if it probes to 3.5 mm internal diameter and is of sufficient length, it should be considered as an in situ conduit.

mosed to the spatulated end of the gastroduodenal artery **(Fig. 16–5)**.

If the gastroduodenal artery is not believed to be adequate to serve as source for inflow, a segment of reversed greater saphenous vein is anastomosed to the hepatic artery after it is occluded proximally and distally, the site of proximal anastomosis usually lying at the orgin of the gastroduodenal artery at its takeoff from the hepatic artery **(Fig. 16–2C)**.

The right renal artery is then ligated at its origin, and divided beyond all palpable occlusive disease. The distal renal artery is profused with chilled heparinized Ringer's lactate solution, and gently dilated with graduated coronary probes **(Fig. 16–3A)**. It is not wise to dilate this vessel with a Fogarty catheter because the intima is easily split. When rotated cephalad, the right renal ar-

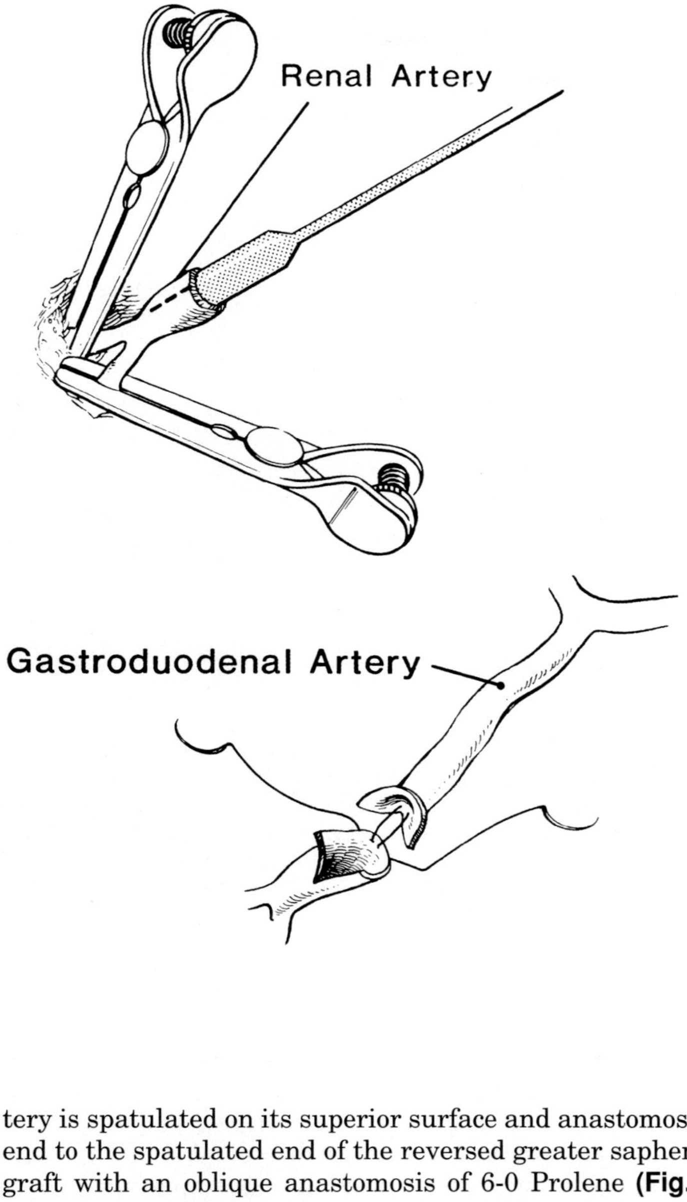

Figure 16–5. Technique of hepatorenal reconstruction. After the renal artery is divided beyond the palpable disease, it is dilated with graduated coronary probe and if length is sufficient, the spatulated ends of the gastroduodenal artery and right renal artery are anastomosed using an oblique anastomosis of 6-0 Prolene.

tery is spatulated on its superior surface and anastomosed end to end to the spatulated end of the reversed greater saphenous vein graft with an oblique anastomosis of 6-0 Prolene **(Fig. 16–3B)**. After release of clamps, the pulse can be assessed within the distal vein graft on the right renal artery **(Fig. 16–3C)**. If a lower pole renal artery is present, it may be anastomosed into the side of the vein graft. **(Fig. 16–3D)**

Technique of Splenorenal Arterial Anastomosis

The patient is placed in a modified right lateral decubitus position with the left flank elevated approximately 45 degrees from hori-

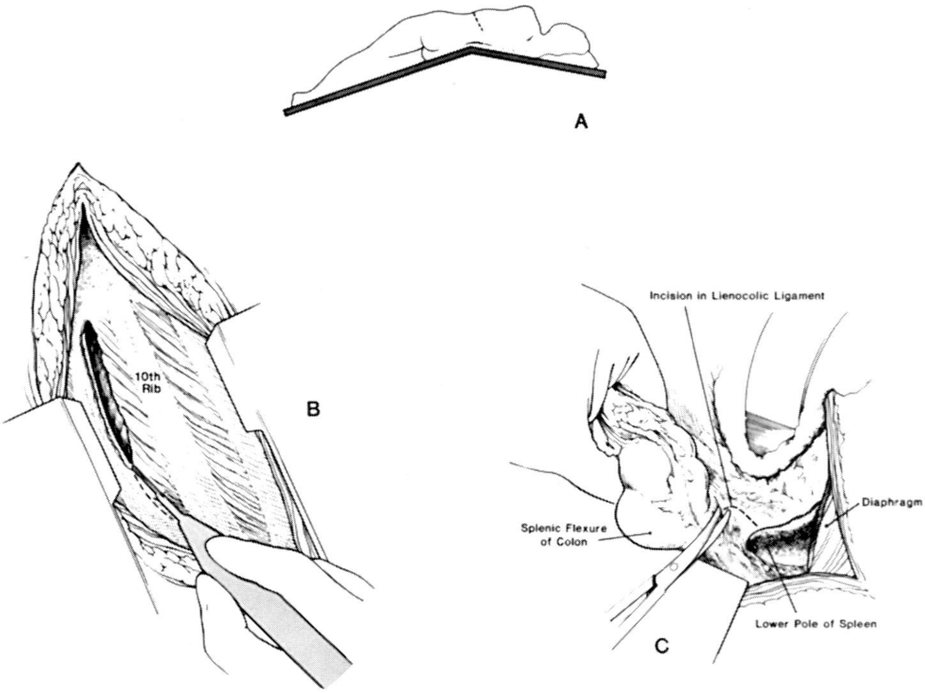

Figure 16–6. Technique of splenorenal arterial anastomosis. A. Patient positioned in modified right lateral decubitis position with left flank elevated 45 degrees from horizontal. B. Thoracoabdominal incision, beginning at lateral border of upper left rectus sheath is carried obliquely into left tenth interspace. C. Diaphragm is incised radially for short distance, and lienocolic ligament is incised, allowing splenic flexure of colon to decrease caudally.

zontal **(Fig. 16–6A)** and the upper abdomen and left side of the chest are prepared and draped. The medial right thigh is also prepared and draped for saphenous vein harvest, if its use is later found necessary for grafting. A thoracoabdominal incision, beginning at the lateral border of the upper left rectus sheath, is carried obliquely into the left tenth interspace, detaching the intercostal muscles from the upper border of the anterior eleventh rib **(Fig. 16–6B)**. The diaphragm is incised radially for a short distance to allow the incision to be opened widely and the lienocolic ligament is incised **(Fig. 16–6C)**, which allows the splenic flexure of the colon to fall caudally and the pancreas to be approached along its inferior margin.

The posterior surface of the pancreas is exposed by turning the inferior margin of the pancreas anteriorly, leaving the spleen in its normal location **(Fig. 16–7A)**. Gerota's fascia overlying the left

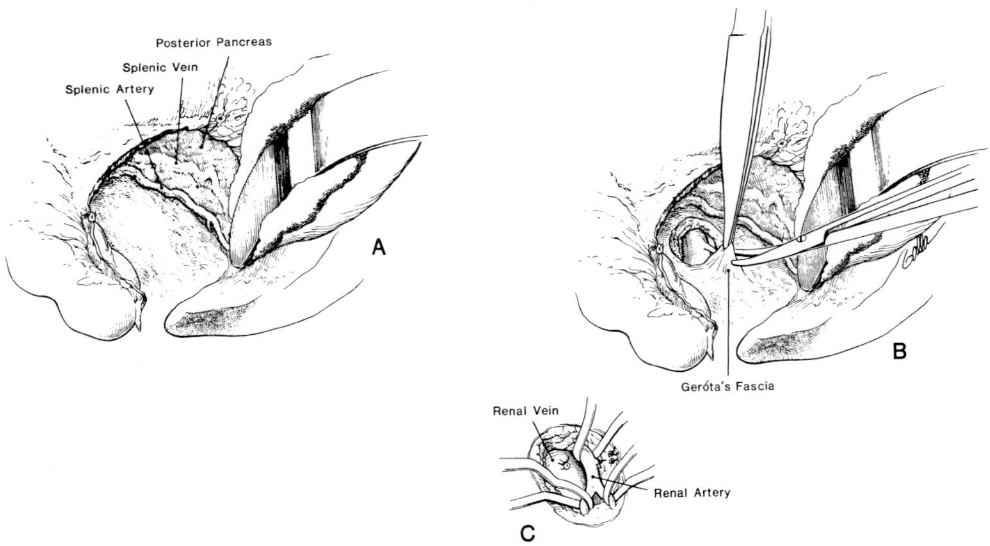

Figure 16–7. Technique of splenorenal arterial anastomosis. A. Posterior surface of pancreas is exposed by turning inferior margin of pancreas anteriorly, leaving spleen in its normal location. B. Gerota's fascia overlying left renal hilum is incised, exposing left renal vein. C. Left renal artery adjacent to vein is identified and encircled.

renal hilum is incised **(Fig. 16–7B)**, the left renal vein is identified, and the left renal artery encircled **(Fig. 16–7C)**, dividing the left adrenal vein between ligatures.

The splenic artery is encircled immediately proximal to the left gastroepiploic artery origin **(Fig. 16–8A)** and dissection is carried proximally, separating the splenic artery from the pancreas; any branches at this level are divided. The splenic artery, after bulldog occlusion at its origin, is divided at about the level of the left gastroepiploic artery **(Fig. 16–8B)**, spatulated on its inferior surface **(Fig. 16–8C)**, and a #3 Fogarty embolectomy catheter is passed through the artery, into the aorta, and brought back with its balloon in the inflated position **(Fig. 16–8D)**, to overcome the severe spasm that frequently occurs at the time of dissection. If inflow is considered inadequate, the splenic artery should be transected in stages, more proximally until inflow is found adequate. If residual length of the splenic artery is not adequate, reverse saphenous vein graft can be interposed to reach the renal artery. This may occasionally be necessary.

The left renal artery is clamped at its origin after gentle bulldog clamps occlude it distally **(Fig. 16–9A)** and, after division, is li-

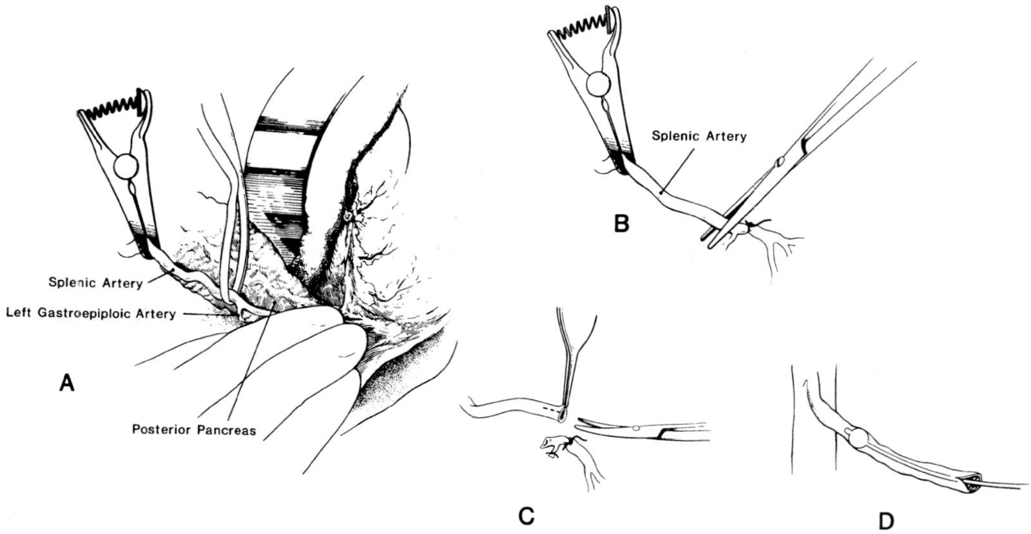

Figure 16–8. Technique of splenorenal arterial anastomosis. A. Splenic artery is encircled immediately proximal to left gastroepiploic artery and cleared of branches proximally. B. After proximal occlusion, splenic artery is divided at level of left gastroepiploic artery. C. Splenic artery is spatulated on its inferior surface for short distance. D. Fogarty embolectomy catheter (No. 3) is passed into aorta and backed out through proximal splenic artery with balloon inflated.

gated proximally with heavy silk. Distally the lumen is probed with successively larger coronary dilators to overcome spasm **(Fig. 16–9B)**. An oblique end-to-end anastomosis is accomplished, after the superior surface of the renal artery is spatulated **(Fig. 16–9C)** with 6-0 Prolene; the reconstruction lies posterior to the pancreas. The spleen may be left in situ, being adequately supplied by blood flow from the short gastric vessels **(Fig. 16–9D)**. The length of splenic artery needed to reach the end of the left renal artery rarely exceeds 5 cm, in that the renal artery rotates up towards the splenic artery after it is divided.

Although patients are not systemically anticoagulated, the splenic artery is filled with chilled heparinized Ringer's lactate to safely extend the period of tolerable renal ischemia.

RESULTS

In the Massachusetts General Hospital series of 66 hepatorenal and 56 splenorenal arterial reconstructions for atherosclerotic

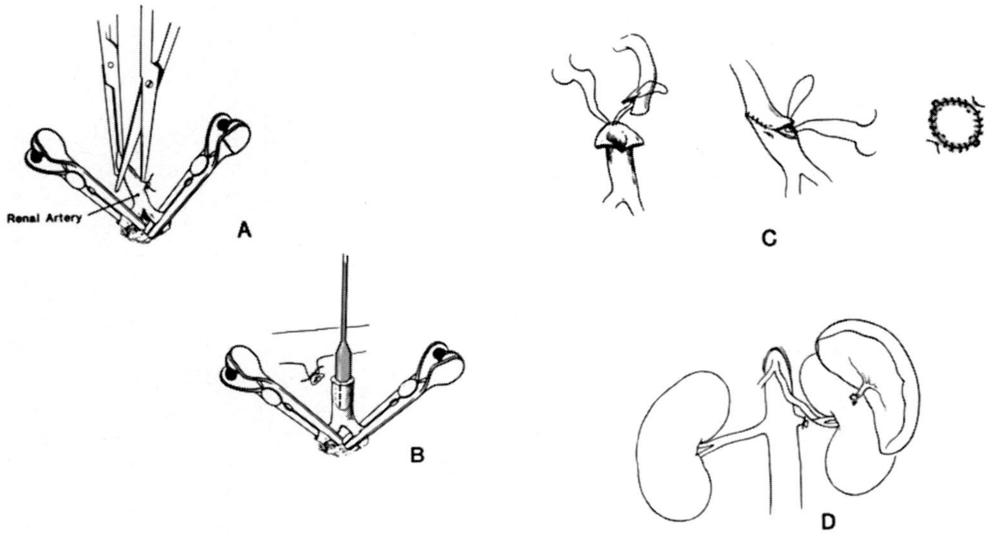

Figure 16–9. Technique of splenorenal arterial anastomosis. A. Left renal artery is occluded proximally and distally and transected near its origin. B. Coronary dilators are used to probe renal artery lumen. C. Superior surface of renal artery is spatulated and end-to-end anastomosis of splenic and left renal arteries is carried out with oblique anastomosis interrupted at four quadrants. D. Spleen is left in place, and path of splenic and renal arteries lies posterior to pancreas.

renal artery disease, the operative mortality rate was 4.1% with 5% early graft failure (≤30 days) and major post-operative complication rate of 11%. Cure or improvement in hypertension was achieved in 84% of patients in whom this represented the major indication for renal artery reconstruction (total cure in 12%) Peri-operative deterioration of renal function was predictive of early graft failure and was also seen in bilateral simultaneous renal artery reconstruction. Stabilization or improvement of excretory function was accomplished in 85% of patients in whom this represented the major indication for renal revascularization. Cumulative patency at five years was found to be 82%. In no instance of hepatorenal reconstruction was post-operative hepatic dysfunction seen.

SUMMARY

A wide variety of alternatives are available to accomplish renal artery revascularization. Any given operative technique may not

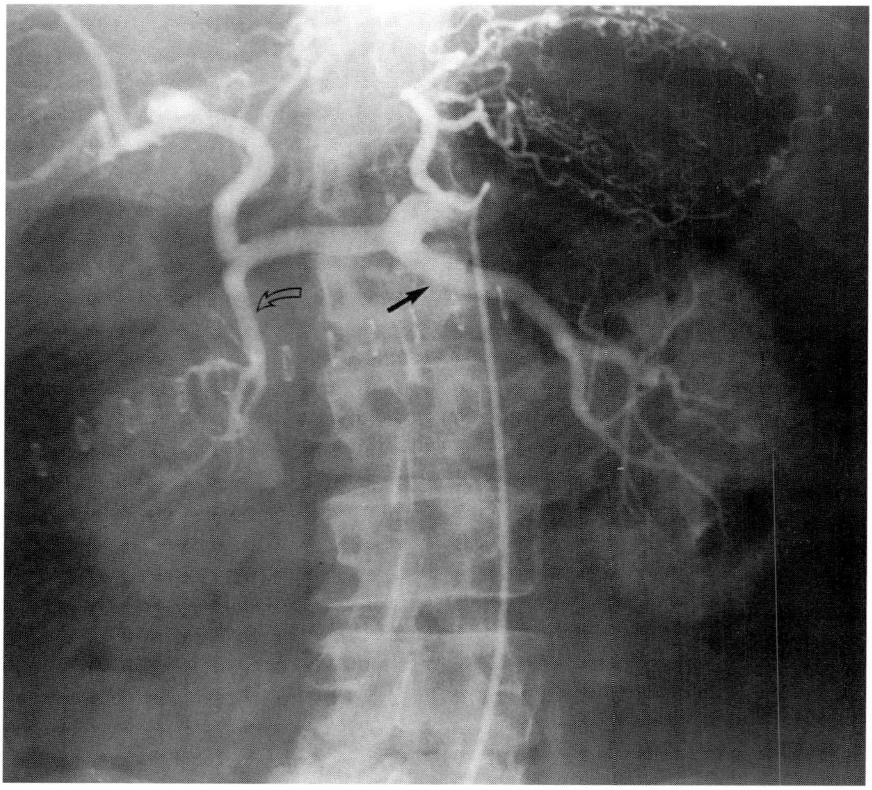

Figure 16–10. Post-operative selective celiac arteriogram after bilateral renal artery revascularization using the hepatic (open arrow) and splenic (closed arrow) arteries.

be applicable in all clinical situations, and thus the surgeon must carefully select the method of renal revascularization appropriate to each patient, considering the general condition of the patient, body habitus and the patient's individual anatomy. Since late failure of all forms of surgical renal artery reconstruction are uncommon, an appropriate operation tailored to the above variables and specifically intended to avoid early technical problems appears the most important factor in obtaining a durable result. The use of the hepatic or splenic circulation for inflow for renal revascularization may be a preferable alternative to conventional renal artery reconstructive techniques (aortorenal bypass grafts, transaortic thromboendarterectomy) in selected circumstances in patients requiring renal artery reconstruction for renovascular hypertension or preservation/retrieval of renal function.

REFERENCES

1. Dean RH, Krueger TC, Whiteneck JM, et al. Operative management of renovascular hypertension: Results after a follow-up of fifteen to twenty-three years. *J Vasc Surg* 1984;1:234–42.
2. Stanley JC, Fry WJ. Surgical treatment of renovascular hypertension. *Arch Surg* 1977;112:1291–97.
3. Lawrie GM, Morris Jr GC, Soussou ID, et al. Late results of reconstructive surgery for renovascular disease. *Ann Surg* 1980;191:528–33.
4. Novick AC, Pohl MA, Schreiber M, et al. Revascularization for preservation of renal function in patients with atherosclerotic renovascular disease. *J Urol* 1983;129:907–12.
5. Cambria RP, Brewster DC, L'Italien GJ, et al. The durability of different reconstructive techniques for atherosclerotic renal artery disease. *J Vasc Surg* (in press).
6. Moncure AC, Brewster DC, Darling RC, et al. Use of the splenic and hepatic arteries for renal revascularization. *J Vasc Surg* 1986;3:196–203.
7. Thompson JE, Smithwick RH. Human hypertension due to unilateral renal disease with special reference to renal artery lesions. *Angiology* 1952;3:493–505.
8. Hurwitt ES, Altman S, Borow M, et al. Intraabdominal arterial anastomoses. *Surgery* 1953;34:1043–60.
9. Hurwitt ES, Seidenberg B, Haimovici H, et al. Splenorenal arterial anastomoses. *Circulation* 1956;14:532–9.
10. DeCamp PT, Snyder CH, Bost RB. Severe hypertension due to congenital stenosis of artery to solitary kidney: Correction by splenorenal arterial anastomosis. *Arch Surg* 1957;75:1023–6.

17

Ex Vivo Reconstruction of the Renal Artery for Aneurysm and Other Abnormalities of Renal Vascular Anatomy

Kenneth L. Brayman,
Yevgeniy Gincherman, Mark M. Levy,
Amit Patel, Jeffrey Carpenter, Ali Naji,
and Clyde F. Barker

Since the reports by Marshall et al[1] and Ota et al[2] of the first successful ex vivo human renal artery reconstructions, the clinical indications for this procedure have been expanded and further refined. In cases of renal artery aneurysm or multiple arteries in renal allografts, ex vivo surgery is the preferred technique to reconstruct renal vascular anatomy prior to auto- or allotransplantation of the organ. Ex vivo renal reconstruction requires nephrectomy followed by hypothermic perfusion of the kidney with a heparinized renal preservation solution. Following ex vivo microvascular repair of the renal artery, the kidney can be autotransplanted to an aortic or iliac position. While many renal artery lesions (e.g. stenosis) are amenable to correction by conventional in situ surgical techniques, extracorporeal techniques are advantageous when complex or poorly accessible hilar lesions are present, or when multiple renal arteries or renal artery branches require reconstruction.

There are two circumstances when renal artery reconstruction ex vivo is most successfully employed. First, when renal ischemia time is projected to exceed 45 minutes to 1 hour, preservation infusion and ex vivo reconstruction are recommended. Second, when dissection of small vasculature is required, the in situ technique provides inadequate exposure. Other indications for extracorporeal renal artery surgery includes those circumstances following failed percutaneous transluminal renal angioplasty for renal artery stenosis, reconstruction of complex renal artery aneurysms, renal arteriovenous fistulas, and renal arterial dissections. In this chapter, we will review the history of ex vivo surgery of the renal artery with reference to both auto- and allotransplantation of the kidney. A contemporary view of the surgical techniques used will be discussed. Finally, the University of Pennsylvania experience with ex vivo surgery of the renal artery will be reviewed.

Renal Autotransplantation

Hardy was the first to describe the successful use of renal autotransplantation in humans,[3] using this technique to repair high ureteral injuries. The description of this seminal work paralleled technical success following renal allotransplantation in humans. The applicability of ex vivo surgery and renal autotransplantation to renal artery reconstruction was pursued vigorously in selected centers worldwide thereafter. Ota et al[2] were the first to describe a series of successful ex vivo renal artery reconstructions in dogs. Repaired renal arteries remained patent and excellent renal function was obtained in eighteen of twenty dogs studied (two animals died from renoarterial thrombosis). A similar technique of ex vivo renal artery repair was applied by these authors to a 39-year-old male presenting with renovascular hypertension due to right renal artery stenosis. The right kidney was revascularized ex vivo using a saphenous vein graft, and the patient remained well and normotensive beyond two years of follow-up.

The 1970s were replete with reports of large and small series of ex vivo renal artery reconstruction. Belzer and associates[4] in 1970 described the use of pulsatile perfusion of the kidney during ex vivo renal artery reconstruction in dogs. They argued that continuous pulsatile extracorporeal perfusion of the kidney, in contrast to simple cold storage, permitted more time to perform the delicate microvascular repair of the more distal renal arteries. The technique of anastomosing two renal arteries together to form a common channel that could subsequently be anastomosed to another vessel was described. This surgical technique is now commonly used for revascularization of renal allografts with multiple renal arteries of comparable size. However, simple cold storage of the explanted kidney rather than pulsatile perfusion is commonly used for renal preservation.

Employing Belzer's renal pulsatile perfusion technique, Corman et al[5] reported the first small series of ex vivo renal artery reconstructions performed in human subjects. They reported three patients, two with bilateral renal artery stenosis, and one with a unilateral renal artery laceration secondary to a stab wound. In the later case, at the time of vascular reconstruction, the kidney was anuric. Following surgery, the kidney resumed function, obviating the need for dialysis.

In 1974, Belzer et al[6] reported the first two clinical cases of sequential bilateral ex vivo renal artery reconstruction for bilateral renal artery stenosis. They used hypogastric and splenic arteries as arterial grafts. The authors monitored renal vein renin levels, and stressed that these levels alone could not be used to diagnose renovascular hypertension in patients with bilateral disease. Although the authors divided the ureter prior to reimplantation into the iliac fossa, they suggested that the dissecting platform could be placed above the abdominal cavity, leaving the ureter intact. The technique of preserving ureteral continuity or ureteral re-implantation (ureteroneocystostomy) are both used.

Husberg et al,[7] 1 year later, reported five more patients who underwent ex vivo renal artery repair. Included in this series was the first description of an ex vivo excision of a renal cell carcinoma followed by renal autotransplantation. Ex vivo renal artery reconstruction was carried out concomitantly with tumor resection in a patient who had previously undergone a contralateral nephrectomy. An intravenous pyelogram obtained four months after surgery demonstrated satisfactory renal function. In a second case reported by Husberg, a 6-year-old boy with congenital uropathy requiring bilateral nephrostomies presented with a non-functioning right kidney and a compromised and hydronephrotic left kidney. An autotransplantation of the left kidney with ex vivo ureteral and vascular repairs was performed with excellent results. This case represents the first pediatric experience with ex vivo renal artery reconstruction.

Putnam et al[8] presented the successful application of ex vivo renal repair to two novel clinical scenarios. They used the ex vivo surgical approach to resect complex staghorn calculi from a solitary kidney. Ex vivo perfusion of the kidney was employed, and the renal pelvis and parenchyma was bivalved to remove the calculi. Adequate renal function returned after revascularization of the kidney of this patient. The authors also described bilateral renal autotransplantation after nephrectomy and temporary ex vivo perfusion performed to repair an extensive abdominal aortic aneurysm.

In 1975, Belzer et al[9] reported a total of ten patients who were treated by a variety of different approaches that included bilateral ex vivo reconstruction, unilateral in situ and contralateral ex vivo repair, and unilateral ex vivo reconstruction and contralateral nephrectomy. Hypogastric, splenic, common and external iliac arteries were used as arterial autografts. The ureter was either left intact or transected. No significant complications were reported in this series postoperatively.

Several additional series of extracorporeal renal artery reconstructions reported excellent outcomes (9-22C). Novick et al[17] reviewed 108 patients who underwent renal autotransplantation for renal artery disease (n = 67), ureteral replacement (n = 27), or renal cell carcinoma (n = 14). Of these patients, 54 patients required branch renal artery reconstruction, and a successful clinical outcome was achieved in 96% of these cases.

The management of complex renovascular disease in 68 consecutive patients, most with fibromuscular dysplasia, was reported by Murray et al.[22] They reported fifty-two ex vivo procedures with no operative deaths or graft failure documented (follow-up 6 months to 18 years). Renal function was improved or unchanged in forty-eight of these patients during a mean follow-up of 7.5 years. Successful correction of aneurysmal disease was accomplished in all eleven cases presented in this report.

Jordan et al[25] reported the largest series of ex vivo renal artery reconstruction in pediatric patients. They reported the use of renal revascularization in 16 patients, 15 for severe hypertension, and 1 for aneurysmal disease. Revascularization was successful in fourteen patients, but three required low-dose antihypertensive medication post-operatively. Two post-operative complications (hydrothorax and retroperitoneal fluid collection) resolved without sequelae following appropriate treatment. Van Bockel and coworkers[26] evaluated their short and long term results of extracorporeal renal artery reconstruction in sixty-five patients (five children) with renovascular hypertension who were treated from 1974 through 1989. Fibrodysplasia (n = 54) predominated as the etiology of hypertension. Extracorporeal renal artery surgery was performed on seventy-eight kidneys among sixty-five patients. In most cases, autologous artery was used for reconstruction. Only one death (1.5%) occurred in the preoperative period. A beneficial blood pressure response occurred in 53 (82%) over the short term (mean 7.9 months) and in 49 (80%) over the long term (mean 5.9 years). Renal function improved in all patients with preoperative renal dysfunction.

At the University of Pennsylvania, we have performed ex vivo renal artery repair and renal autotransplantation on fourteen kidneys in thirteen patients. Indications have included aneurysmal disease of the aorta involving the renal artery,[3] renal artery stenosis with severe atherosclerotic aortic disease,[4] peripheral renal artery stenosis,[3] renal artery aneurysm[7] and renal artery rupture following angioplasty.[1] Complications have included one perioperative death, one patient requiring postoperative dialysis, and one patient requiring vein graft dilatation. Renal salvage was accomplished in 13 of 14 organs.

Allotransplantation of Renal Grafts with Multiple Arteries

The presence of multiple renal arteries were at one time considered a contraindication to the use of a kidney from a living donor. However, the increasing shortage of donor kidneys has broadened the role of ex vivo renal artery reconstruction techniques in renal transplantation.[27,28]

In 1979, Novick et al[29] reported the transplantation of twenty-one kidneys with multiple renal arteries (14 cadaver and 7 living-related). They compared clinical outcomes in this group with a control cohort of 79 recipients of renal allografts with a single artery. The authors reported no difference in initial or long-term allograft function between these two groups and emphasized three basic surgical techniques readily applicable to most anatomic variations encountered. These techniques included use of a conjoined arterial anastomosis, end-to-side anastomosis, and use of various autologous vascular grafts to fashion a single main renal artery for anastomosis to the recipient. No cases of arterial thrombosis, stenosis or hemorrhage were reported in this series.

Chin reported 40 cases of ex vivo renal artery reconstruction in kidney allografts.[30] Arterial anastomotic revision of one graft was required using the recipient hypogastric artery. They reported no immediate or delayed hemorrhage and two intraoperative deaths (due to myocardial infarction and severe sepsis). An expanded series was reported in 1990,[31] with ten additional cases including one renal autotransplantation following ex vivo repair of a renal artery aneurysm. No additional complications were reported.

Talbot-Wright et al[32] reported a 15-year experience from Barcelona, Spain with ex situ vascular repair and/or reconstruction of the renal artery and vein. Twenty-one ex vivo renal artery reconstructions were performed, with no significant complications reported. Rossi et al[33] presented their experience with fifty-seven living-related donor kidneys with multiple arteries. No significant surgical complications were documented in donors or recipients, but three patients suffered irreversible acute rejection after transplantation. Again, a comparison made between renal recipients of grafts with multiple renal arteries with patients who received kidneys with a single renal artery was done and no differences were documented in renal function, blood pressure control or graft or patient survival between the two groups.

The experience at the University of Pennsylvania with ex vivo reconstruction of donor renal allografts with multiple arteries from cadaveric and living donor sources is extensive. Between 1966 and 1994, more than two thousand renal transplants have been performed at our institution including more than eight hundred from living donors. Roza et al reviewed our series of renal artery reconstructions from living donors and described forty-one reconstructions performed between 1966 and 1987. Immediate complications **(Table 17–1)** (within 30 days of procedure) included urinary leak,[6] arterial bleeding,[3] acute tubular necrosis,[4] perirenal abscess,[1] and hemorrhage from a peptic ulcer.[1] Postoperative hypertension was documented in nine patients (two cases at-

Table 17–1. Renal Artery Reconstructions: Ex Vivo Repair in Living Donor Allografts. University of Pennsylvania Experience

	1966–87	1987–1994
Patients	41	11
Donors # Arteries		
Double	39	11
Triple	2	0
Reconstructions		
End-Side (main renal)	32	9
End-End (branch hypogastric)	7	0
Common Channel	1	1
Unknown	1	1
Complications (30 days)		
Urinary Fistula	5	0
Obstruction	3	0
Arterial Bleed	2	0
Occlusion	1	1
ATN	3	0
Abscess	1	0
Bleeding Peptic Ulcer	1	0
Hypertension	9	1
Renal Artery Stenosis	2	* No w/u for RAS
Due to Rejection	7	
Follow up		
48 Patients		
Mean 5 years		
Range 6 months to 14 years		

tributed to renal artery stenosis, seven due to rejection). Since the report by Roza et al[34] in 1987, 11 additional cases of renal artery reconstruction in living donor allografts have been performed. One case of post-operative hypertension and one case of arterial occlusion has been documented. Thus in the recent series, the overall rate of complications has decreased dramatically.

OPERATIVE TECHNIQUE

For renal autotransplantation, a flank incision is used to obtain extraperitoneal exposure of the affected kidney. The incision can be kept lateral and just inferior to the twelfth rib or can be extended anteriorly and inferiorly to facilitate exposure of the ureter and iliac vessels for the purposes of re-implantation. Gerota's fascia is incised and opened along the long axis of the kidney. The renal pedicle is then dissected to define all renal arteries and veins. Most patients will have undergone imaging studies (e.g., arteriogram, digital subtraction angiogram, magnetic resonance angiogram or spiral computed tomography) in an effort to define renal anatomy preoperatively. However, angiographically occult polar vessels must be identified and preserved, especially inferior polar arteries, ligation of which can comprise the blood supply to the ureter. Gonadal and adrenal veins are ligated and divided to obtain the greatest possible length of renal vein. The ureter is dissected from surrounding retroperitoneum, but not skeletonized, so as to preserve the collateral descending blood supply.

Prior to nephrectomy, diuresis should be encouraged by adequate fluid replacement and the use of intravenous mannitol and loop diuretics. Some authors use systemic heparinization prior to clamping the renal artery and vein. We generally do not find this to be necessary and include heparin in the renal preservation solution. The renal vessels are clamped near their junction with the aorta and vena cava and transected distal to the clamp maximizing length for subsequent reconstruction. The renal vessels are then perfused. With the clamps in place, the renal artery and renal vein stumps are suture ligated and oversewn, using fine continuous nonabsorbable suture (5–0 or 6–0 Prolene). After adequate hemostasis has been assured, moistened laparotomy sponges are placed in the wound while the ex vivo repair takes place.

If the ex vivo reconstruction can be conveniently performed by elevating the kidney on the anterior abdominal wall or on a sterile platform, the ureter may be mobilized in a limited fashion, but without transection. However, better exposure and more controlled ex vivo conditions are frequently obtained by dividing the ureter and entirely removing the kidney from the operative field. This permits reconstructive surgery to be performed at the bench with appropriate cooling and magnification.

Kidney Preservation

An atraumatic cannula is inserted into the renal artery, and the explanted kidney is flushed with cold Eurocollins solution (containing 5000 u heparin/liter;[35–37] until no blood is noted to return from the renal vein and the renal parenchyma is homogenously pale. The kidney is then wrapped with gauze and placed in a basin filled with Eurocollins solution at 4 degrees Celsius. Periodic flushing of the kidney ensures optimal cooling of the organ but is often not necessary.

Continuous pulsatile perfusion is not routinely performed.[38] It is updated so that all branches of the renal artery can be flushed. Small cannulae are often required for small individual renal arteries and we favor 22, 24 or higher gauge intracaths for this purpose. When introducing the catheter into the small renal artery, care must be taken not to disrupt the delicate intima.

Arterial Reconstruction

Ex vivo reconstruction is optimally performed on a separate back table under optimal conditions of lighting, magnification and surgeon comfort. The delicate vascular dissection and suturing are best performed while in a sitting position, with elbows at table height. The kidney may rest in a shallow basin of cold preservation solution during reconstruction. Under these conditions, it is possible to accurately dissect the main renal artery, and obtain adequate visualization and control of renal artery branches. The type of arterial reconstruction to be performed should be chosen based upon the individual anatomy of the various renal arteries. Microsurgical techniques are utilized and anastomoses are performed with fine monofilament polypropylene suture (7-0 or 8-0). Ligation of vessels should be avoided to prevent postoperative renovascular hypertension. The diseased arterial segments are resected and reconstruction is then begun.

The most common arterial reconstruction to be performed involves an end-to-side anastomosis of a small renal artery branch to the main renal artery. This pattern of reconstruction is often used to manage multiple renal arteries of allografts prior to transplantation **(Fig. 17–1)**. A second pattern of reconstruction involves side-to-side anastomosis of two small renal arteries to create a common inflow channel with a single lumen of larger diameter. This common channel can then be anastomosed to an arterial or venous graft **(Fig. 17–1,** arteries 3 and 4) or directly to the external iliac artery.

The size and branching pattern of the hypogastric artery make it an ideal arterial autograft to reconstruct a single conduit from multiple renal arteries **(Fig. 17–2)**. In such circumstances, the renal branches are divided beyond the diseased segment and anastomosed end-to-end to the hypogastric autograft. In addition, multiple renal artery branches can be managed with end-to-side anastomoses to the hypogastric artery. Autologous vein, divided into segments, may be constructed into bifurcating or trifurcating grafts, using end-to-side anastomoses **(Fig. 17–3)**. Venous autografts may also be used to reconstruct multiple renal arteries from a living donor **(Fig. 17–4)**. Use of venous autografts mandates frequent post-operative surveillance to detect aneurysmal changes in the graft. Use of prosthetic grafts in ex vivo renal artery

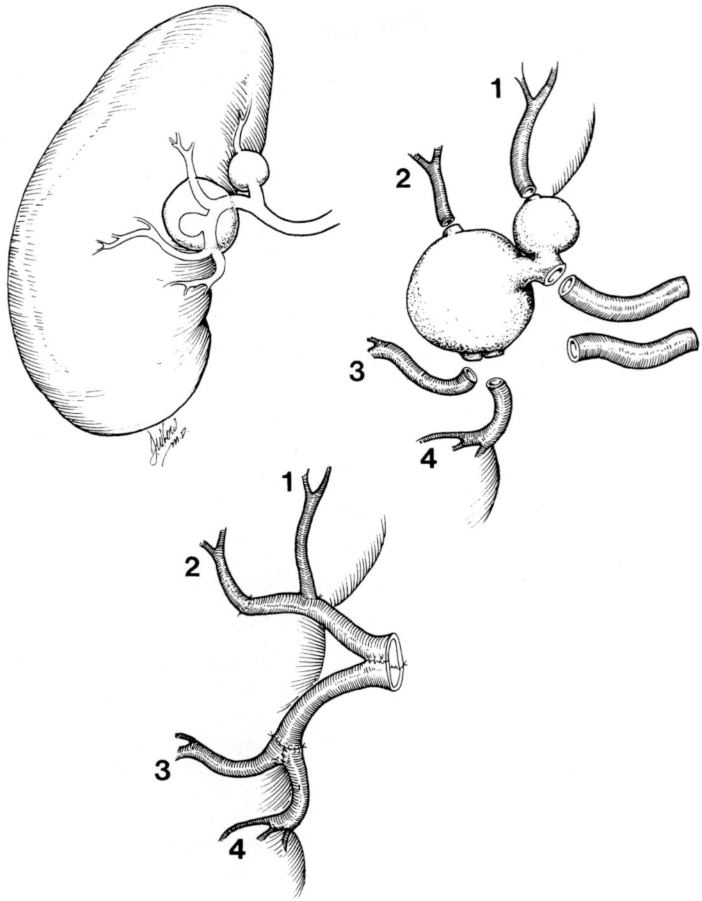

Figure 17–1. Ex vivo reconstruction of renal artery following resection of multiple distal renal artery aneurysms. Resection of the aneurysm left four distal renal artery branches. Successful reconstruction involved two short segments of hypogastric arterial autograft, with which a final common channel was constructed using side-to-side technique. End to end, end to side, and common channel techniques were used to anastomose the renal artery branches to the hypogastric arterial autograft.

reconstruction is best reserved for cases where autologous tissue is not available and is not favored.

Reimplantation

The kidney is frequently reimplanted into the iliac fossa with vascular anastomoses performed end to side to the external iliac artery and vein. Preparation of the iliac vessels involves complete clearance of perivascular lymphatics. Lymphatic tissue must be meticulously ligated and divided to avoid post-operative lymphocele formation in the retroperitoneum.

The reconstructed kidney is removed from the cold basin and returned to the operative field. The organ is oriented in the patient's iliac fossa to minimize the risk of vessel kinking secondary

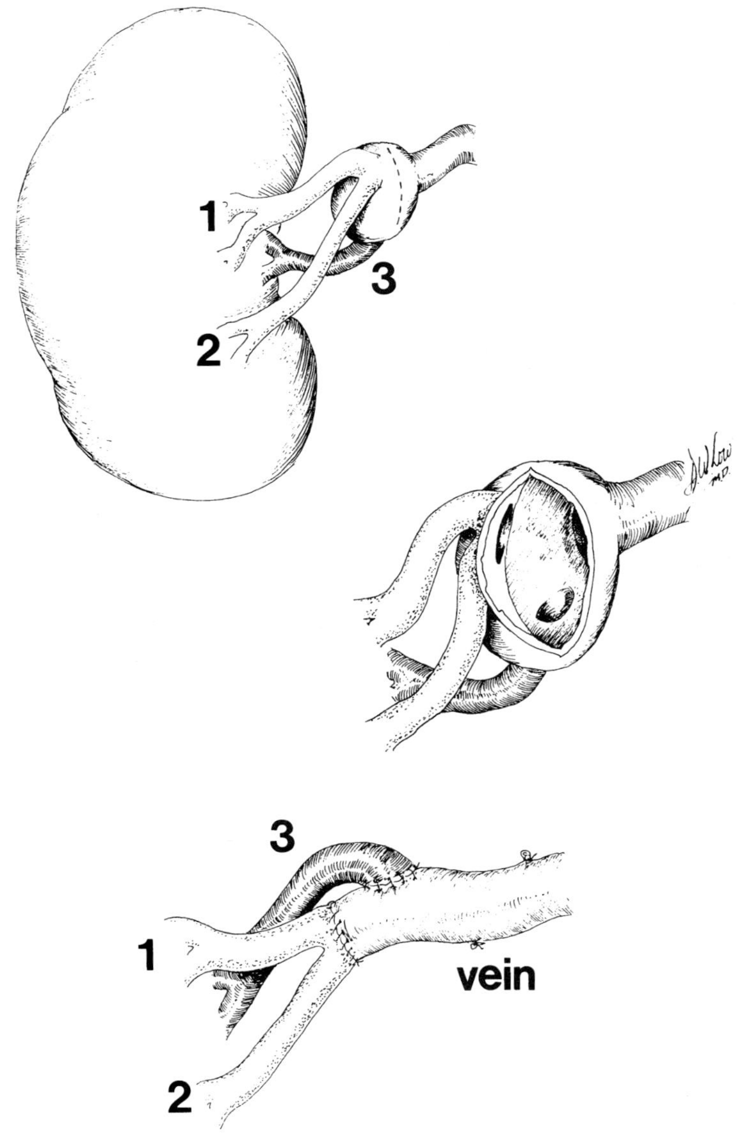

Figure 17–2. Ex vivo reconstruction of a renal artery following resection of a renal artery aneurysm occurring at the junction of the main and secondary renal arteries. A single arterial conduit constructed from autologous saphenous vein provided the necessary length to replace the resected arterial segment. End-to-end and end-to-side anastomoses between the distal renal arteries and the venous autograft are demonstrated.

to rotation and with the ureter of the kidney pointing towards the bladder. Following placement of vascular clamps, end-to-side anastomoses are constructed between renal vasculature and the external iliac vein and artery (5-0 and 6-0 polypropylene suture, respectively). The vascular clamps are released initially from the vein and then from the artery. Rapid and uniform return of color to the autograft indicates a patent reconstruction, and anastomotic patency may be assessed using Doppler ultrasound. Evidence of

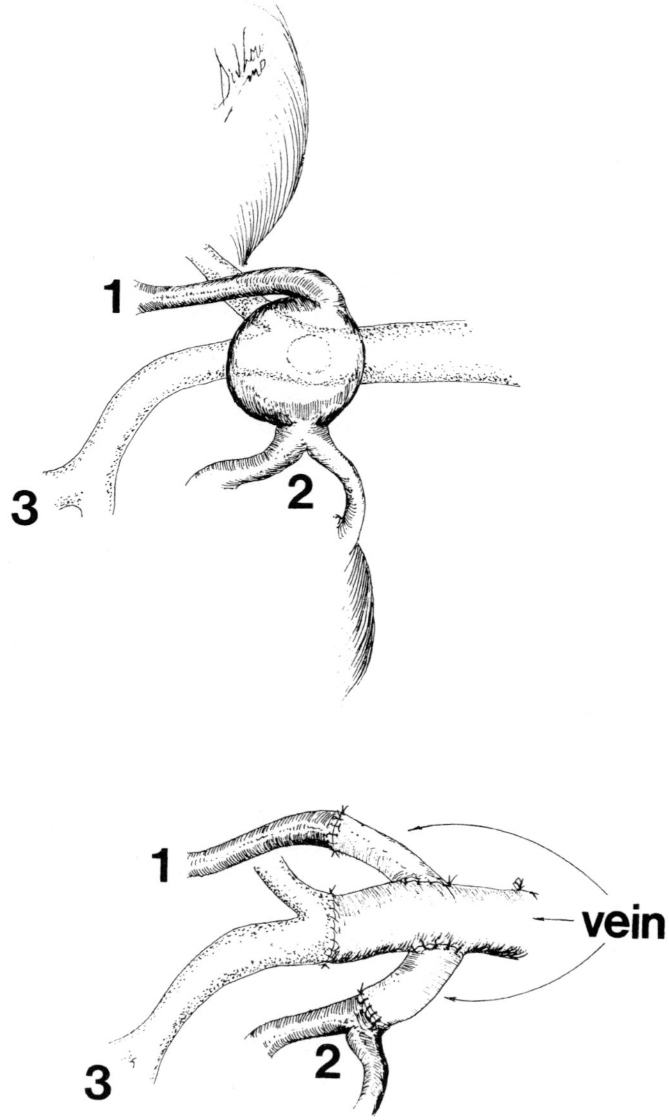

Figure 17–3. Ex vivo reconstruction of renal artery following the resection of a renal artery aneurysm that involved three major renal artery branches. Successful reconstruction of this renal artery used autologous saphenous vein fashioned into a trifurcation to provide a single arterial inflow.

arterial insufficiency requires immediate revision. With vascular anastomosis intact and hemostasis achieved, an extravesical ureteroneocystostomy is constructed in cases that involved ureteral transection. The anastomosis is performed in one layer using absorbable 6-0 PDS suture. The bladder musculature is then approximated over a small length of a ureter to prevent reflux (4-0 PDS). Hemostasis at the ureteroneocystostomy site minimizes the incidence of post-operative ureteral obstruction secondary to hema-

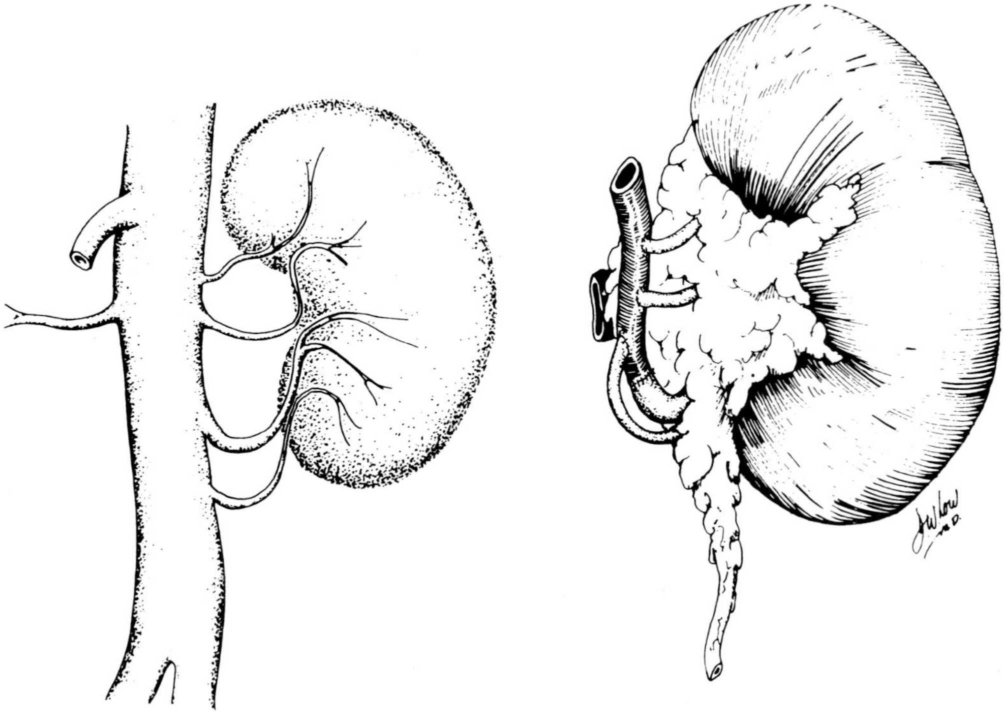

Figure 17–4. Ex vivo reconstruction of arterial vasculature from a living donor kidney with multiple renal arteries. The reconstruction of a single arterial conduit involved both end-to-side and end-to-end anastomoses of renal arteries to a segment of saphenous vein autograft. Revascularization of a lower pole renal artery best assured arterial supply to the transplanted ureter.

toma in the tunnel. The wound is closed along anatomic planes in routine fashion. Drains are not necessary and avoided because of the risk for wound and retroperitoneal infection. A Foley catheter is left in place for a minimum of forty-eight hours postoperatively.

Postoperative Follow-Up

Renal perfusion and excretion are evaluated with radionuclide scans on the first post-operative day to assess the adequacy of the revascularization and renal function. This study also provides a baseline for comparison with subsequent studies should function deteriorate or hypertension intervene. Patients are evaluated every six months with blood pressure and serum creatinine measurements. The development of sudden or uncontrolled hypertension should prompt a repeat renal scan and possibly an angiogram to visualize the renal vasculature and rule out recurrent or do novo renal artery stenosis or thrombosis.

CONCLUSION

Ex vivo renal artery reconstruction has been performed for nearly thirty years and is a valuable technique to revascularize a native or transplanted kidney with complex or pathologic vasculature. Extracorporeal repair makes it possible to avoid nephrectomy in patients with significant renal artery disease. As an adjunct to the standard renal transplantation techniques, particularly given the current shortage of donor organs, the use of donor renal allografts with multiple arteries has proven successful over the long term. As newer techniques of extracorporeal organ preservation and microvascular repair continue to develop, the indications for ex vivo surgery of the diseased renal artery or the kidney will likely expand.

REFERENCES

1. Marshall VF, Whitsell J, McGovern JH, Miscall B. The practicality of renal allotransplantation in humans. *JAMA* 1986;196:138–140.
2. Ota K, Mori S, Awane Y, Ueno A. Ex situ repair of renal artery for renovascular hypertension. *Arch Surg* 1967;94:370–373.
3. Hardy JD. High ureteral injuries. Management by autotransplantation of the kidney. *JAMA* 1963;184:97–101.
4. Belzer FO, Keaveny TV, Reed TW, Pryor JP. A new method of renal artery reconstruction. *Surgery* 1970;68:619–624.
5. Corman JL, Anderson JT, Taubman J, et al. Ex vivo perfusion, arteriography, and autotransplantation procedures for kidney salvage. *Surg Gyn Obstet* 1973;137:659–665.
6. Belzer FO, Salvatierra O, Perloff D, Grausz H. Surgical correction of advanced fibromuscular dysplasia of the renal arteries. *Surgery* 1974;75:31–37.
7. Husberg BS, Bakshandeh K, Lilly J, et al. Five cases and five unusual indications for autogenic renal transplantation. *Acta Chir Scand* 1975;141:557–563.
8. Putnam CW, Halgrimson CG, Stables DP, et al. Ex vivo renal perfusion and autotransplantation in treatment of calculous disease or abdominal aortic aneurysm. *Urology* 1975;5:337–342.
9. Belzer FO, Salvatierra O, Palubinskas A, Stoney RJ. Ex vivo renal artery reconstruction. *Ann Surg* 1975;182:456–463.

10. Bugge-Asperheim B, Sodal G, Flatmark A. Renal artery aneurysm. Ex vivo repair and autotransplantation. *Scand J Urol Nephrol* 1983; 18:63–66.
11. Dubernard JM, Martin X, Gelet A, Mongin D. Aneurysms of the renal artery: Surgical management with specific reference to extracorporeal surgery and autotransplantation. *Eur Urol* 1985;11:26–30.
12. Dean RH, Meacham PW, Weaver FA. Ex vivo renal artery reconstructions: indications and techniques. *J Vasc Surg* 1986;4:546–552.
13. Kent KC, Salvatierra O, Reilly LM, et al. Evolving strategies for the repair of complex renovascular lesions. *Ann Surg* 1987;206:272–278.
14. Sicard GA, Valentin LI, Freeman MB, et al. Renal autotransplantation: an alternative to standard renal revascularization procedures. *Surgery* 1988;104:624–630.
15. Fleshner NE, Johnston KW. Repair of an autotransplanted renal artery aneurysm: case report and literature review. *J Urol* 1992;148: 389–391.
16. Ortenberg J, Novick AC, Straffon RA, Stewart BH. Surgical treatment of renal artery aneurysms. *Br J Urol* 1983;55:341–346.
17. Novick AC, Jackson CL, Straffon RA. The role of renal autotransplantation in complex urologic reconstruction. *J Urol* 1990;143: 452–457.
18. Reilly LM, Cunningham CG, Maggisano R, et al. The role of arterial reconstruction in spontaneous renal artery dissection. *J Vasc Surg* 1991;14:468–477.
19. Barral X, Gournier JP, Frering V, et al. Dysplastic lesions of renal artery branches: late results of ex vivo repair. *Ann Vasc Surg* 1992; 6:225–231.
20. Dzsinich C, Gloviczki P, McKusick MA, et al. Surgical management of renal artery aneurysm. *Cardiovasc Surg* 1993;1:243–247.
21. Tapper SS, Meacham PW. Multi-branch renal artery lesions: surgical options and results. *Cardiovasc Surg* 1993;1:712–716.
22. Hood DB, Weaver FA. Orthotopic ex vivo renal artery reconstruction. *Am Surg* 1994;60:804–808.
23. Murray SP, Kent C, Salvatierra O, Stoney RJ. Complex branch renovascular disease: management options and late results. *J Vasc Surg* 1994;20:338–346.
24. Clume GJ, Murphy KJ, Luken L. Autotransplantation of the kidney in Treatment of Renovascular Hypertension. *Surgery* 1971;69: 326–331.
25. Jordan ML, Novick AC, Cunningham RL. The role of renal autotransplantation in pediatric and young adult patients with renal artery disease. *J Vasc Surg* 1985;2:385–392.
26. VanBockel J, van der Akker, Chang P, et al. Extracorporeal Renal Artery Reconstruction for Renalvascular Hypertension. *J Vasc Surg* 1991:13:101–111.
27. Simmons RL, Tallent MD, Kjellstrand CM, et al. Kidney Transplantation from Living Donors with Double Renal Arteries. *Surgery* 1971: 69:201.

28. Merkel FK, Straus AK, Anderson O, Bannett A. Microvascular Techniques for Polar Artery Reconstruction in Kidney Transplants. *Surgery* 1976:79:253–261.
29. Novick AC, Magnuson M, Braun WE. Multiple-artery renal transplantation: emphasis on extracorporeal methods of donor arterial reconstruction. *J Urol* 1979;122:731–735.
30. Chin JL. Microvascular reconstructive "bench" surgery for donor kidneys before transplantation: techniques and results. *J Urol* 1989; 142:23–27.
31. Chin JL. Ex vivo microvascular reconstruction before renal allograft and autograft transplantation. *Can J Surg* 1990;33:363–366.
32. Talbot-Wright R, Carretero P, Alcaraz A, et al. Bench surgery in renal transplantation. *Trans Proc* 1991;23:2327.
33. Rossi M, Alfani D, Berloco P, et al. Bench surgery for multiple renal arteries in kidney transplantation from living donor. *Trans Proc* 1991;23:2328–2329.
34. Roza AM, Perloft LJ, Naji A, et al. Living-related donors with bilateral multiple renal arteries. A twenty year experience. *Transplantation.* 1989;47:397–399.
35. Collins GM, Bravo-Sugarman M, Terasakai PI. Kidney preservation for transportation—initial perfusion and thirty hours ice storage. *Lancet* 1969;2:1219.
36. Sacks SA, Petristch PH, Kaufman JJ. Canine kidney perfusion using a new perfusate. *Lancet* 1973;1:1024.
37. Collins GM, Halasz NA. Forty-eight hour ice storage of kidneys: importance of cation content. *Surgery* 1976;79:432.
38. Belzer FO, Ashby BS, Dunphy JE. Twenty-four hour and seventy-two hour preservation of canine kidneys. *Lancet* 1967;1:536–539.

Renal Revascularization in Children

18

Henry D. Berkowitz

SURGICAL TREATMENT OF RENOVASCULAR HYPERTENSION IN CHILDREN

Renal artery occlusive disease is second in frequency only to coarctation of the thoracic aortic as the most common form of surgically correctable hypertension in the pediatric population. Corrective surgery in these children is technically challenging since vascular reconstruction must correct the current problem and yet be constructed to accommodate growth and function over a normal lifespan.

The clinical presentation of renovascular hypertension in children is markedly different than that in adults. Infants and young children frequently manifest failure to thrive, hyperkinesis and seizure disorders secondary to hypertensive encephalopathy which affect as many as 10% of these patients. In older adolescents, the hypertension is usually silent and left ventricular hypertrophy is already present by the time hypertension is discovered. This group is resistant to control with conventional drug therapy,[1] but recently angiotensin-converting enzyme (ACE) inhibitors have provided improved blood pressure control. However, these agents can precipitate renal failure and must be monitored carefully.[2]

Because the incidence of essential hypertension is negligible in infants and children, any persistent hypertension is justification to obtain detailed diagnostic studies in search of a correctable lesion unless underlying renal parenchymal disease is suspected.

Renal Artery Disease

The pediatric renovascular patient may present with a complex spectrum of lesions involving renal and visceral arteries as well as coarctation of the abdominal aorta. Bilateral renal artery involvement is reported in 14–71% of patients[1,2,3–8] and coarctation of the abdominal aorta in 14–47%.[1,2,3–9]

The renal artery lesions are different from the typical string of beads appearance of adult medial fibroplasia. The young patients present with concentrically narrowed arteries often with ostial stenosis **(Fig. 18–1)**, but lesions are located anywhere within the renal artery and may extend into segmental arterial branches or even exist as isolated segmental lesions. Histologically the lesions show atypical medial-perimedial dysplasia and secondary intimal

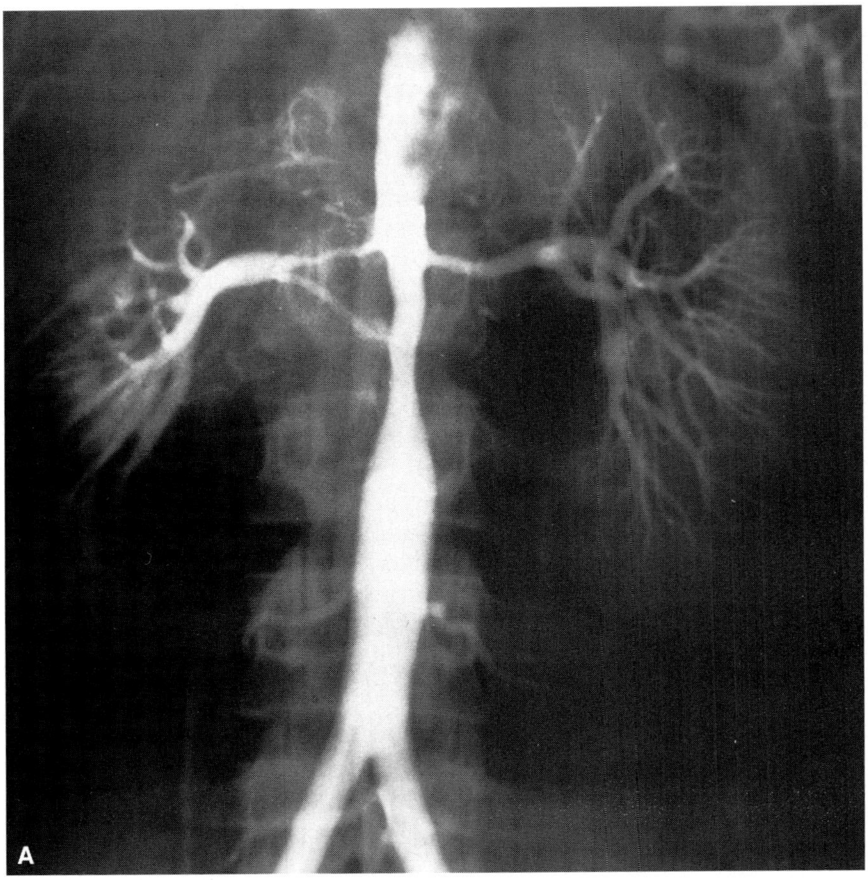

Figure 18–1. A. Preoperative arteriogram in patient with bilateral renal artery stenosis caused by concentric proximal renal artery narrowing. Arrow points to accessory lower pole renal artery. B. Same patient 4½ years after bilateral aortorenal bypass using saphenous vein which was reinforced with Dacron mesh to prevent aneurysmal dilatation. Arrow points to accessory lower pole renal artery. Triangle points to new mild aortic stenosis.

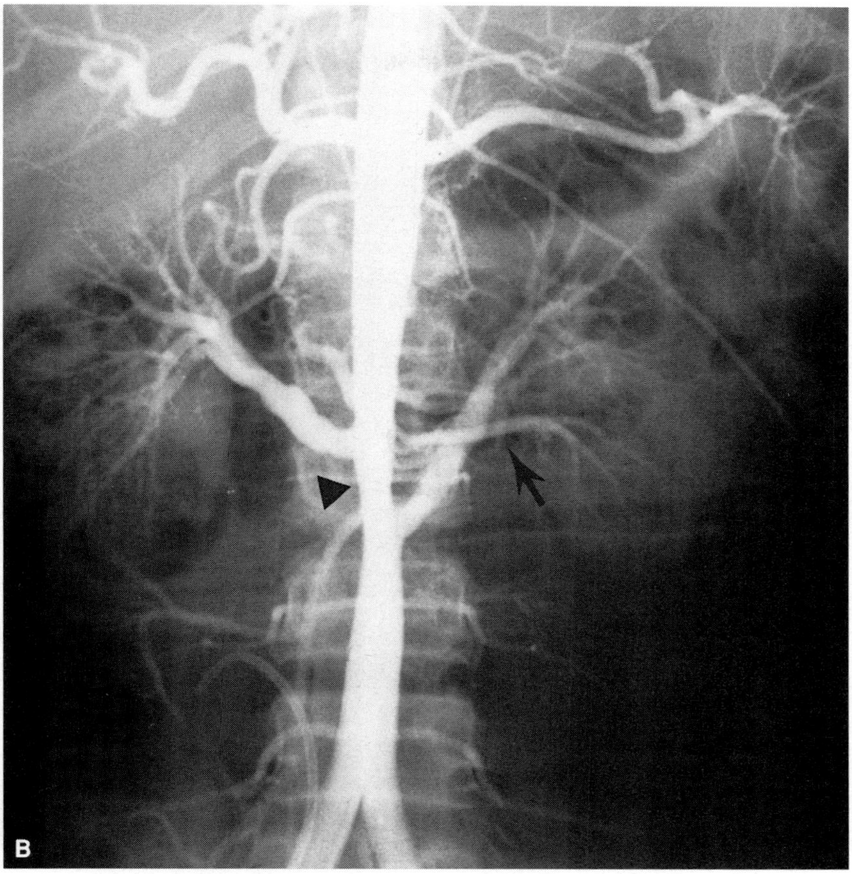

Figure 18–1. *(continued)*

fibroplasia.[8] An inflammatory arteritis is occasionally seen especially when the lesions have progressed rapidly.

Aneurysms of the renal artery may also be present in a small number of patients and usually accompany mid to distal renal artery stenosis. They are often saccular outpouchings and are frequently found at the bifurcation of a main renal artery.

Aortic Disease

Coexisting aortic lesions characteristically have a typical hourglass appearance on aortograms and produce stenoses of the infrarenal abdominal aorta **(Fig. 18–2)** but the stenosis may eventually extend proximally to obstruct orifices of the renal and visceral

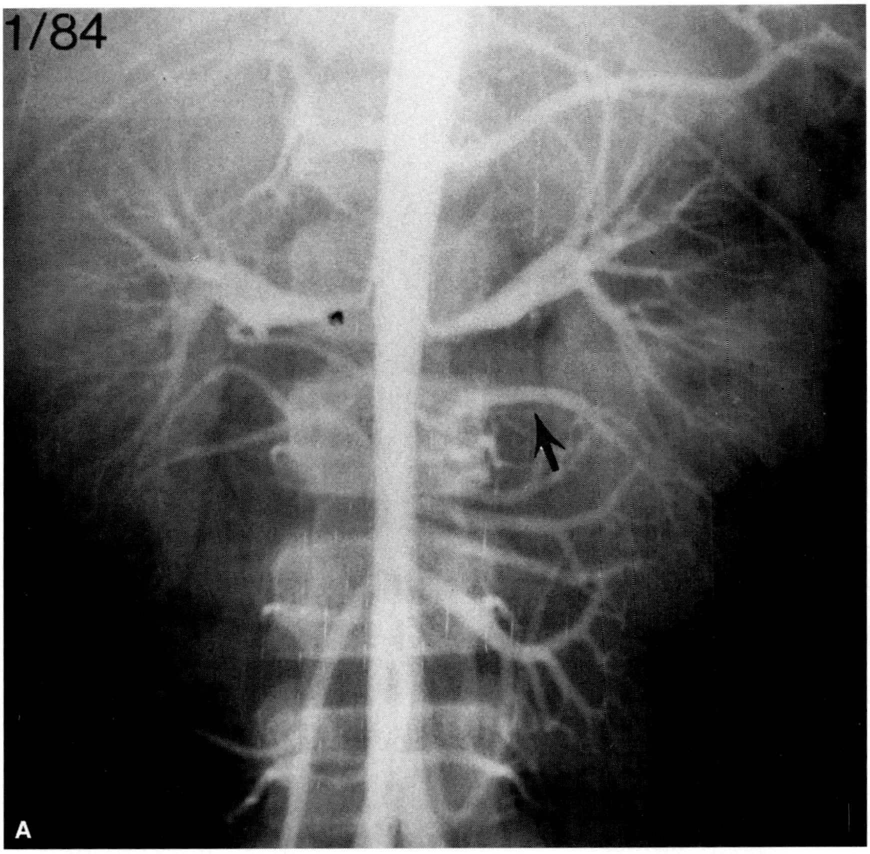

Figure 18–2. A. Preoperative angiogram showing bilateral renal artery stenosis and coarctation of abdominal aorta. B. Postoperative study at 2 months showing aortic bypass with 12 mm woven Dacron graft and bilateral aortorenal bypass with saphenous vein. Generous curve of aortic graft allows for future longitudinal growth.

arteries. This complex of lesions is referred to as the midaortic syndrome.

These lesions most likely are not present at birth, but develop and progress over a variable time course. The median age of patients with this syndrome has ranged from 12 to 17 years[2,10,11] but it has been diagnosed in patients as young as 4–5 years old. A coarctation was observed to develop in an apparently normal aorta in only 5 months, but more commonly these lesions develop over several years.[12] During this time the suprarenal aorta and, ultimately, the origin of the superior mesenteric artery (SMA) and celiac arteries may become constricted.[13] The inferior mesenteric

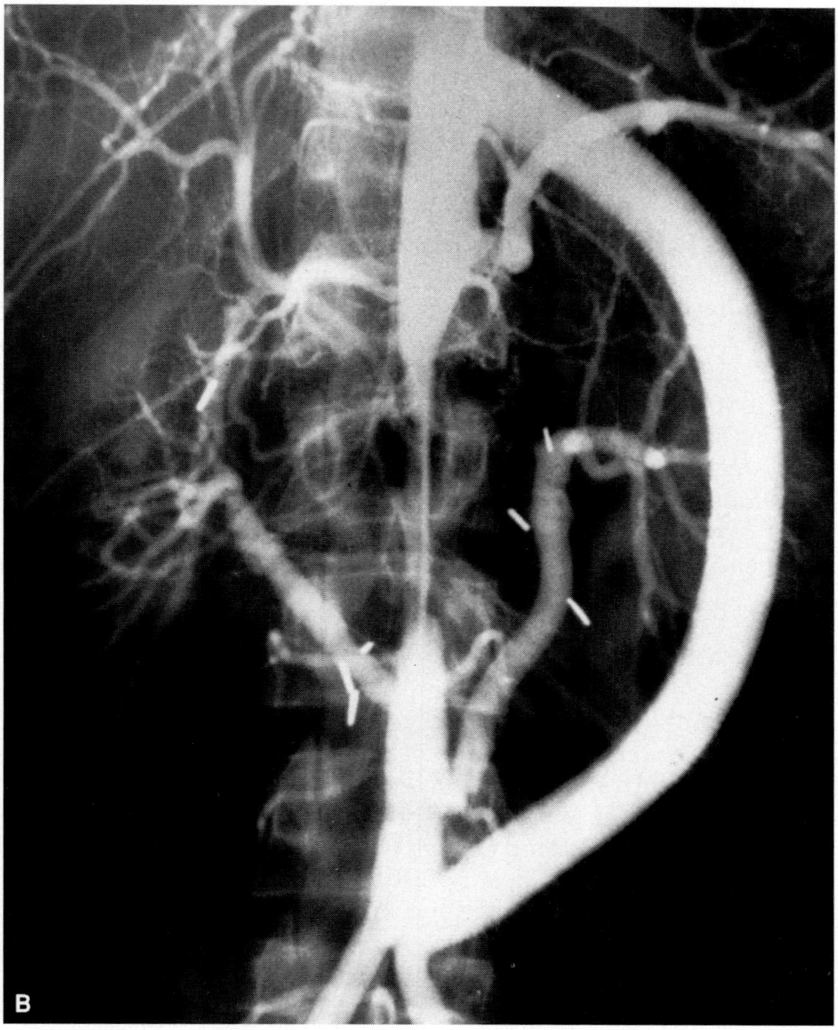

Figure 18–2. *(continued)*

artery (IMA) is characteristically spared and this allows large collaterals to develop between the SMA, celiac and the IMA which perfuse the uninvolved distal aorta and iliac arteries. The relentless progression of stenosis apparently is self-limited and may burn out after puberty.

The chief differential diagnoses are Takayasu's arteritis and neurofibromatosis. In Takayasu's arteritis, the patient is generally older and shows clinical signs of arteritis, including increased erythrocyte sedimentation rate, as well as malaise, fever, night sweats, anorexia, and weight loss. In addition, the frequent involvement of the pulmonary arteries may lead to dyspnea, which is not seen in patients with midaortic syndrome. Finally, the midaortic syndrome exclusively involves the midabdominal aorta, whereas Takayasu's arteritis most frequently shows a mixed type of involvement including the branch vessels from the aortic arch. Histologic examination of involved regions of Takayasu's arteritis will show inflammatory changes, a finding not usually seen in patients with the midaortic syndrome. Patients with neurofibromatosis do not show clinical signs of inflammatory disease but they have the peripheral lesions characteristic of neurofibromatosis, in addition to the midaortic lesion.

Typically, portions of the aorta and renal arteries obtained from patients at surgery show intimal thickening, intimal fibrosis, and atypical medial hyperplasia singly or in combination. No evidence of round cell or granulomatous infiltration typical of periaortic inflammatory disease (i.e., Takayasu's arteritis) is usually seen, nor are giant cells present.[12] The usual pathologic diagnosis is nonspecific arteriopathy.

Diagnosis

Arteriography is the key to diagnosis and in addition to demonstrating the renal artery lesions, it should visualize the origins of all abdominal visceral branches, as well as the abdominal aorta, aortic bifurcation and iliac arteries. Biplane examinations with rapid-sequence imaging followed by delayed imaging are necessary for the depiction of early filling and collateral arterial flow.

The proximal SMA and celiac arteries should be visualized in lateral projections to ensure they are disease-free, in case a visceral artery to renal artery bypass is contemplated. Examinations of the pelvic arteries is important if the internal iliac artery is to be used for a bypass graft.

Hypertensive urograms have limited diagnostic value because of their low sensitivity to segmental and bilateral main renal artery disease.[2,6] Both of these patterns of disease fail to demonstrate differences between kidney excretion of contrast dye, which is the basis of this diagnostic test. Urograms were not obtained in any of the patients from the most recently reported group of pediatric renovascular patients.[8]

The early surgical reports from the University of Michigan[1] documented elevated plasma renin activity in approximately 85% of patients with renovascular hypertension. Elevated renal vein renin ratios were used to indicate functional significance of the renal artery lesion. However, renin ratios were insensitive to bilateral renal artery lesions and to segmental disease, and subsequently it was determined that 20% of patients who benefitted from surgery did not have elevated renin ratios preoperatively. A modification of the renin measurements which included measurement of inferior vena cava (IVC) renin concentration permitted calculation of individual kidney renin excretion rates (and contralateral suppression).[14] This renin index (Renin systemic renal index) was 85% accurate in assessing functional significance of the renal pathology. However, at the present time most centers, including Michigan, only obtain renins selectively when there is uncertainty about the clinical significance of individual renal artery lesions.[8]

PTA of Renal Artery Stenosis

Percutaneous transluminal angioplasty (PTA) has not been successful in managing either the renal or aortic lesions in children. Unlike adult fibrodysplasia which affects the midportion of the renal arteries, the majority of lesions in the pediatric population are stenoses involving the proximal renal artery segments and represent true hypoplastic vessels characterized predominantly by adventitial elastic tissue.[10] These particular lesions simply stretch with balloon inflation and return to their original contour with balloon deflation without remodelling the stenotic segment. Two patients in the University of Pennsylvania series were failures of preoperative PTA[2,12] but two postoperative suture line stenoses were successfully dilated and averted surgery. Some stenotic lesions limited to the midportion of the main renal arteries represent true medial fibroplasia and benefit from PTA, but surgical therapy remains the primary treatment and provides the most durable restoration of renal blood flow and preservation of renal tissue in children.[15]

Surgical Repair

Surgery is usually performed in one stage even when bilateral renal artery lesions and a concomitant midaortic stenoses must be repaired to provided a suitable origin for the renal arteries or bypass grafts. While it is desirable to wait until a child is fully grown before undertaking this complex surgery, often this is impossible because the severity of the hypertension and the threat of losing functioning renal mass make early surgery mandatory.

Surgical exposure is obtained through a midline or chevron incision and medial rotation of the viscera gives excellent exposure of the distal right and left renal arteries, the proximal aorta up to the diaphragmatic hiatus and the visceral vessels. It is seldom necessary to extend the incision into the chest. This approach is relatively easy in children because they usually do not have abundant retroperitoneal fat.

The proximal anastomosis to the aorta is completed first by cross clamping the aorta and removing a button of aortic tissue with a punch. The graft is spatulated and sewn in place end-to-side using multiple continuous suture interrupted at three or four points to allow for future growth.

Distal graft to renal artery anastomoses is completed in an end-to-end fashion. These anastomoses are facilitated by spatulation of both the renal artery and the graft to increase the anastomotic circumference. The anastomosis is completed in most children using either discontinuous running monofilament sutures or interrupted sutures to allow for future growth.[16] Operative dilatation of stenoses in segmental renal arteries, originally advocated by the Michigan group has fallen into disfavor because of a relatively high incidence of thrombotic complications[8] and is not recommended.

The internal iliac artery is recognized as the preferred graft for pediatric revascularization, although it occasionally develops aneurysmal degeneration or stenosis.[6] Vein grafts routinely undergo aneurysmal dilatation when used for pediatric renal bypasses and this represents a major deterrent to their routine use.[17] However, the aneurysmal changes manifest themselves within the first two postoperative years and then remain remarkably stable.[2] There have been no reports of vein graft rupture and only a few late stenoses. However, continued expansion or the formation of mural thrombus in the dilated graft has prompted reoperation in a small number of cases. Plication of the dilated graft has salvaged some of these aneurysmal bypasses.[1] Vein graft dilation was prevented by surrounding grafts with a Dacron mesh tube, and resulted in long-term stabilization of the grafts according to a report from the University of Pennsylvania.[2] Despite the inadequacies of using vein grafts, there may be circumstances when use of a vein proves to be the only option available for renal revascularization in children.

Direct renal reimplantation, used sparingly in older reports was the preferred technique of treating renal artery stenosis in the most recent series reported from the University of Michigan.[8] Proximal renal artery lesions were excised and the renal artery was directly anastomosed to the aorta or an adjacent renal artery using interrupted sutures. This has now become the preferred technique of renal reconstruction at that center and it is attractive because it eliminates the inherent problems associated with the internal iliac and vein graft.

The midaortic stenosis is usually bypassed with a 12–14 mm Dacron graft inserted with enough redundancy to allow for future growth **(Fig. 18–2B)**. There have been no late complications related to inadequate graft length or diameter. The graft is anastomosed in an end-to-side fashion to the proximal supraceliac aorta and the distal end is placed just above the aortic bifurcation below

Table 18–1. Pediatric Renovascular Hypertension: Comparative Results of Surgical Treatment

Medical Center	Patients	Arterial Reconstruction Total	Arterial Reconstruction % Bilat	Nephrectomy	Cured (%)	Improved (%)	Failure (%)	Operative Mortality (%)
University of Michigan 1963–1993 (8)	57	67	23%	7	79	19	2	0
Cleveland Clinic 1955–1977 (3, 4)	27	22		11	59	18.5	18.5	4
University of California Los Angeles 1967–1977 (5)	26	19		11	84.5	7.5	4	4
Vanderbilt University 1962–1977 (6)	21	15	14%	8	68	24	8	0
University of Pennsylvania 1984–1987 (2)	17	29	71%	0	76.5	23.5	0	0
University of California San Francisco 1960–1974 (7)	14	10		4	86	7	0	7

Adapted from Stanley JC, Brothers TE. Surgical treatment of renovascular hypertension in children. In: Ernst CB, Stanley JC (eds): Current therapy in vascular surgery, 2nd ed. Philadelphia: BC Decker, 1991, 875–880.

the inferior mesenteric artery. This distal segment of aorta rarely becomes stenotic and is also an excellent site for the proximal anastomosis of the aortorenal grafts. The bypasses can also originate from the aortic graft. An alternative repair of the midaortic lesion uses a primary patch aortoplasty with PTFE graft or Dacron. The patch must be large enough to accommodate future growth of the aorta. This technique is especially appealing for the very young patient and requires less dissection than insertion of an aortic graft.

Visceral artery stenoses are repaired along with the aortic and renal lesions if preoperative visceral ischemic symptoms are present. It is unclear that all of these lesions should be repaired prophylactically in the absence of symptoms. However, one benefit of doing so would be to provide a potential for hepatorenal or splenorenal bypass in the future, if a primary renal bypass graft failed.

Results

A summary of results from the major series of pediatric renal revascularization patients is shown in **Table 18–1.** The cumulative surgical experience with pediatric renovascular hypertensive patients reveals excellent results with respect to control of hypertension and preservation of renal function. Although differences exist between institutions regarding primary arterial reconstructions versus primary nephrectomies, improved vascular surgical techniques have increased the likelihood of success for revascularization. The long-term results indicate that the repairs are durable and continue to function even after significant growth has occurred. Operative mortality for these extensive procedures was 0% in 3 series and ranged from 4% to 7% in the remaining 3 series. These excellent results support an aggressive surgical approach towards renovascular hypertension for the pediatric patient.

REFERENCES

1. Stanley JC, Fry WJ. Pediatric renal artery occlusive disease and renovascular hypertension: Etiology, diagnosis and operative treatment. *Arch Surg* 1981;116:669–676.
2. Berkowitz HD, O'Neil JA. Renovascular hypertension in children: Surgical repair with special reference to the use of reinforced vein grafts. *J Vasc Surg* 1989;9:46–55.
3. Novick AC, Straffon RA, Stewart BH, et al. Surgical treatment of renovascular hypertension in the pediatric patient. *J Urol* 1978;119: 794–805.

4. Benjamin SP, Dustan HP, Gifford RW Jr, et al. Stenosing renal artery disease in children: Clinicopathological correlation in 20 surgically treated cases. *Cleve Clin Q* 1976;43:197–206.
5. Stanley P, Gyepes MT, Olson DL, et al. Renovascular hypertension in children and adolescents. *Radiology* 1978;129:123–131.
6. Lawson JD, Boerth R, Foster JH, et al. Diagnosis and management of renovascular hypertension in children. *Arch Surg* 1977;122: 1307–1316.
7. Stoney RJ, Cooke PA, String ST. Surgical treatment of renovascular hypertension in children. *J Pediatr Surg* 1975;10:631–639.
8. Stanley JC, Zelenock G, Messina LM, et al. Pediatric renovascular hypertension: A 30 year experience of operative treatment. *J Vasc Surg* (in press).
9. Stanley JC, Fry WJ. Pediatric renal artery occlusive disease and renovascular hypertension: Etiology, diagnosis and operative treatment. *Arch Surg* 1981;116:669–676.
10. Stanley JC, Graham LM, Whitehouse WM, et al. Developmental occlusive disease of the abdominal aorta, splanchnic and renal arteries. *Am J Surg* 1981;142:190–196.
11. Messina LM, Goldstone J, Ferrell LD, et al. Middle aortic syndrome: Effectiveness and durability of complex arterial revascularization techniques. *Ann Surg* 1986;204:331–339.
12. Lewis VD, Meranze SG, McLean GK, et al. The midaortic syndrome: Diagnosis and treatment. *Radiology* 1988;167:111–113.
13. Graham LM, Zelenock GB, Erlandson EE, et al. Abdominal aortic coarctation and segmental hypoplasia. *Surgery* 1979;86:519–529.
14. Stanley JC, Gwertz BC, Fry WJ. Renal: systemic renin indices and renal vein renin ratios as prognostic indicators in remedial renovascular hypertension. *J Surg Res* 1976;20:149–155.
15. Guzzetta PC, Potter BM, Ruley EJ, Majd M, Bock GH. Renovascular hypertension in children: Current concepts in evaluation and treatment. *J Pediatr Surg* 1989;24:1236–1240.
16. Stanley JC, Brothers TE. Surgical treatment of renovascular hypertension in children. In: Ernst CB, Stanley JE eds. *Current Therapy in Vascular Surgery.* 2nd ed. DBC Philadelphia: 1991, pp 875–880.
17. Stanley JC, Ernst CB, Fry WJ. Fate of 100 aortorenal vein grafts: Characteristics of late graft expansion, aneurysmal dilatation, and stenosis. *Surgery* 1973;74:931–944.

Index